OXFORD MEDICAL PUBLICATIONS

Counselling in Primary Health Care

Counselling in Primary Health Care

Oxford General Practice Series • 30

Edited by

JANE KEITHLEY

Director of the Institute of Health Studies,
University of Durham, and Lecturer in Social
Policy, University of Durham

and

GEOFFREY MARSH

General practitioner
Stockton-on-Tees

OXFORD   NEW YORK   TOKYO
OXFORD UNIVERSITY PRESS

Oxford University Press, Great Clarendon Street, OX2 6DP
Oxford New York
Athens Auckland Bangkok Bogota Bombay Buenos Aires
Calcutta Cape Town Dar es Salaam Delhi Florence Hong Kong
Istanbul Karachi Kuala Lumpur Madras Madrid Melbourne
Mexico City Nairobi Paris Singapore Taipei Tokyo Toronto
and associated companies in
Berlin Ibadan

Oxford is a trade mark of Oxford University Press

Published in the United States
by Oxford University Press Inc., New York

First published 1995
Reprinted 1996, 1997

A catalogue record for this book is available from the British Library

Library of Congress Cataloging in Publication Data
Counselling in primary health care / edited by Jane Keithley and Geoffrey Marsh.
(Oxford general practice series : no. 30) (Oxford medical publications)
Includes bibliographical references and index.
1. Mental health counselling. 2. Health counselling. 3 Primary
care (Medicine). I. Keithley, Jane. II. Marsh, G. N. (Geoffrey Norman).
III. Series. IV. Series: Oxford medical publications.
[DNLM: 1. Counselling–methods. 2. Primary Health Care. W1 OX55
no. 30 1995 / WM 55 C85585 1995]
RC466.C68 1995   362.2'04256–dc20   94–34882 CIP
ISBN 0 19 262354 0

Printed and bound in Great Britain by
Biddles Ltd, Guildford and King's Lynn

Contents

Contributors

Viv Ball was a counsellor in primary care in Derbyshire. Her work included team development and research. In addition, she was actively involved in postgraduate medical education. She was Chair of the Counselling in General Practice Group of the British Association for Counselling. Very sadly, she died in 1994.

Tim Bond is a staff tutor in counselling in the Department of Adult and Continuing Education at the University of Durham and is Deputy Chair of the British Association for Counselling. He is an accredited counselling practitioner by the Association for Student Counselling and the British Association for Counselling. He has researched and written extensively about counselling ethics, including reports sponsored by the Department of Health and the Department of Employment. Recent publications include *HIV counselling* (BAC 1991) and *Standards and ethics for counselling in action* (Sage 1993).

Marie Campkin is a general practioner in North London, former vocational training course organizer, and council member of the Balint Society; she recently undertook training in psychotherapy. She is interested in the interface between general practitioners and people working in primary care as counsellors and psychotherapists, and the possibility of Balint groups as one means of promoting their mutual understanding and cooperation.

Simon Cocksedge is a general practitioner in Chapel-en-le-Frith, Derbyshire, a course organizer for vocational training in general practice, and a part-time lecturer in general practice at the University of Manchester. His main professional interests are counselling (he has undertaken further training in this field and currently works part-time as a counsellor) and palliative care (he is Chairman and Medical Adviser of High Peak Hospice).

Roslyn Corney is professor of psychology at the University of Greenwich. Previously she was a senior lecturer at the Institute of Psychiatry. Her research has mainly focused around mental health issues in general practice, in particular the evaluation of treatment offered by counsellors, social workers, and community psychiatric nurses.

Jane Dammers is a general practitioner in an inner-city practice in South London. She has worked closely with counsellors and therapists, and helped to promote their attachment to local practices through her work as lecturer in the Department of General Practice and Primary Care at Kings College School of Medicine and Dentistry. With Jan Wiener she has convened national conferences to explore relationships between counsellors and general practitioners, and was a member of the BAC working party which has recently published guidelines on good practice for employing counsellors in primary care settings.

Colin Forth RMN, Diploma in Community Psychiatric Nursing, is a community psychiatric nurse at North Tees General Hospital, Stockton, assigned to Norton Medical Centre. He trained at Long Grove Hospital, Epsom, and previously worked as a CPN in the Carshalton/Sutton area of Greater London. His interests include researching the standard of nursing care when administering 'depot' medication in the community. Currently he is involved with the resettlement of institutionalized patients.

Roland Freedman is a member and past chairman of the Council of the Institute of Psychosexual Medicine. He holds clinics for patients with psychosexual problems at a teaching hospital in Newcastle and at the Family Planning Association and also in the private sector. He runs training seminars in psychosexual medicine for doctors. He is an honorary clinical lecturer in primary health care at Newcastle University Medical School. He is an FRCGP and has recently retired from full-time general practice. He is a member of the British Association of Counselling and a medical advisor to the Newcastle branch of Relate.

Margaret Graham is an accredited counsellor and has worked for 16 years in a general practice in the West Country. She has a professional background in social work and was author of the paper: 'An alternative method of employing a social worker in general practice', published by the *Journal of the Royal College of General Practitioners*, January 1982. She is currently in training as a psychotherapist and also has a private counselling practice, to which many clients have been referred by GPs.

Jill Irving is a counselling psychologist. She chaired the first in a series of working parties which have helped the British Association of Counselling with the formulation of guidelines for the employment of counsellors in general practice. Her interest in this field stemmed from her work as a surgery counsellor. She has recently retired from clinical practice.

Sue Jennings is Senior Research Fellow in the Academic Unit of Obstetrics and Gynaecology at the London Hospital Medical College. She is director of the Diploma in Fertility Counselling there, as well as Principal Fertility Counsellor. Having pioneered the training and practice of dramatherapy for many years, she is currently researching the integration of artistic theory into counselling and psychotherapy. Her many publications include: *Dramatherapy with families, groups and individuals* (RKP), *Dramatherapy theory and practice 2* (Routledge), and *Counselling in reproductive medicine* (In press, Blackwell Scientific).

Jane Keithley is Director of the Institute of Health Studies at the University of Durham and the Chair of Community Health Care North Durham NHS Trust. She has a background in nursing and as a lecturer in social policy. Her

PhD thesis was a study of counselling in general practice, and her teaching and research interests include health policy and primary health care.

Geoffrey N. Marsh has been a general practitioner in Stockton-on-Tees for 35 years. During that time he has developed a comprehensive primary health care team and carried out a number of research studies into teamworking. Counsellors have been members of that team for approximately 25 years. In 1974 he was a Visiting Associate Professor at the University of Iowa, USA, and from 1978 to 1980 he was RCGP Wolfson Visiting Professor to Canada. He has a special clinical interest in general practice obstetrics.

Pip Mason is Head of Education for Aquarius, the Midlands-based alcohol and drug agency. She is also an honorary research associate of the School of Psychology at the University of Birmingham. A nurse by profession, she has worked in the addictions field since 1975, both in a counselling role and as a trainer. She has a special interest in brief interventions and is currently researching the role that specialist alcohol counsellors can play in a general practice setting.

Dorothy Poingdestre has been a member of the Diaconal Order of the Methodist Church since 1971, into which she was ordained in 1977. She gained her Certificate of Qualification in Social Work in 1985. Her work conducting funerals as a hospital chaplain, then as a social worker in a busy general hospital led her to specialize in working with the dying and bereaved. She has been a senior social worker in a Hospice since 1987.

Nancy Rowland is a counsellor and researcher. Her main area of interest is in counselling in medical settings, and she is currently researching the evaluation of counselling in primary care at the Centre for Health Economics, University of York. A book on the economic evaluation of counselling, co-authored by Keith Tolley, is to be published in 1995.

Jo Soldan is a clinical psychologist at the Institute of Medical Genetics in Cardiff where she is involved in clinical work and research with families who have a range of genetic conditions. She offers consultation and support to the Multidisciplinary Health Care Team involved in genetic counselling in Cardiff, and teaches on the psychological aspects of counselling on the Welsh National Board's Diploma Module in Genetic Counselling.

Eddy Street has qualifications in clinical and counselling psychology. He is employed within the National Health Service as a consultant clinical psychologist leading a team of psychologists who provide services to children and families. He has a particular interest in working with those families with genetic and handicapping conditions. His past research interests include investigations into family therapy skills training, and, more recently, the effects of chronic illness on family functioning. He has published widely, including *Counselling for family problems* (Sage 1994).

Sheila Thompson CQSW, is a freelance writer and teacher on groupwork and counselling. She was formerly a principal social worker at St Joseph's Hospice in Hackney, London. Her publications include Thompson and Kahn *The group process and family therapy* (Pergamon Press, 1988).

Keith Tolley is a lecturer in health economics at the University of Nottingham and was previously Research Fellow at the Centre for Health Economics, University of York. His research interests include the economic analysis of counselling, health promotion, and AIDS. He is currently completing a book with Nancy Rowland on the cost-effectiveness of counselling in health care, to be published by Routledge.

Jan Wiener is a research psychologist and Jungian analyst. She currently works in the health service in the Psychotherapy Clinic at Claybury Hospital, Essex and in private practice. She is particularly interested in working with general practitioners, and for the past eight years she has been the practice psychotherapist in an inner London group practice. She is a founder member of a staff team of GPs (from the Department of General Practice, Kings College) and analysts (from the Society of Analytical Psychology) who convene workshops with GPs and counsellors working in a general practice setting.

Preface

Jane Keithley and Geoffrey Marsh

THE RISE AND RISE OF COUNSELLING

In 1974, one of us (GNM) submitted a paper on counselling in general practice to the *British Medical Journal*. It was rejected. It appeared that the *BMJ* did not consider this subject as relevant to mainstream medicine. Fortunately, it was salvaged by the *Journal of the Royal College of General Practitioners*, albeit with some diffidence (Marsh and Barr 1975). In 1982 the co-editor of this book (JK) wrote a PhD thesis on the outcome of counselling as provided by counsellors in a primary health care team (Keithley 1982). This was one of the first major assessments of the operation and outcomes of counselling in a medical setting in the UK. Yet by 1992, when we first considered editing this book, there were 93 books in the local medical library that included the word 'counselling' in their title; counselling had taken off! Nevertheless, there was no one substantive book for all members of the primary health care team. We decided to edit one.

It has long been recognized that a substantial proportion of the problems brought by patients to general practitioners, nurses, health visitors, midwives, and other members of the primary health care team are associated with stress, relationships, and psychological or psychosomatic responses to difficulties in their lives. It is now almost the conventional wisdom that counselling can provide valuable support and help to such people. However, how far doctors are themselves adequately equipped and willing to take on a counselling role as 'priests of our secular society' has been the subject of considerable debate. The growth of the primary health care team (PHCT) with members from different professional backgrounds, including, in some cases, specialist counselling, has presented the opportunity to consider different ways in which counselling could be provided to patients.

BUT WHAT EXACTLY IS COUNSELLING?

Many GPs would frankly admit that they are unsure of what counselling actually is. They wonder what goes on in the counsellor's room, in those 50 minute or hour-long sessions. Other GPs would argue that they counsel all the time, building on an established relationship of trust with their patients. Yet others would maintain that counselling is not, and should not be, part of their professional practice, nor even part of primary health care—hiding behind the phrase that 'this is not a clinical problem'. This book attempts to sort out these different approaches and attitudes. It defines and explains counselling, and considers how far it can be differentiated from counselling skills and from other forms of help with psychological, psychosocial, and psychiatric problems.

WHAT DO COUNSELLORS DO AND SAY?

This book seeks to address counselling in primary health care from as broad a range of perspectives as possible. It thus includes contributors from a variety of disciplinary and professional backgrounds: for example, medicine, nursing, social work, psychology, sociology, social policy, and economics, as well as those whose primary professional affiliation is to counselling itself. Most of the authors are practising counsellors and some concentrate on conveying their 'hands-on' experience with clients. This variety of contributions reflects the heterogeneous nature of the contemporary provision of counselling in this setting—counsellors come from different professions, devote different proportions of their working week to counselling, and have different amounts, types, and levels of training. Nevertheless, all our contributors would assert that counselling is a distinctive activity, with a common core. The nature of this activity is most fully described in Chapter 1 by Tim Bond, but the common theme of counselling as facilitating the client's work and, through the counselling relationship, increasing the client's capacity to take control of his or her life recur in many others, especially those addressing specific problem areas in which counselling may help. The consequent degree of overlap has not, however, been edited out, as the contributors approach this common core from a diversity of backgrounds and link it to the particular theme of their chapter. In many chapters, they also describe scenarios and case histories which illustrate their work. These help to clarify the nature of counselling, not only in terms of the theoretical underpinnings and the aims of counselling, but also in terms of more pragmatic aspects of professional practice, such as the usual number and frequency of meetings, coping with waiting-lists and emergencies, and so on.

WHO SHOULD COUNSEL?

One of the major issues recurring in this book is that of who is the most appropriate person to be the counsellor. First, what are the advantages and disadvantages of providing counselling in the setting of the PHCT. Secondly, if such a service is to be provided, who should have that responsibility? Should it be the GP him or herself? Should it be another member of the PHCT who develops this role alongside their original role, for example a nurse? The distinction between practising counselling and counselling skills is important here. Alternatively, is it best to appoint an individual for whom counselling is their sole activity? Or is counselling something which *all* those concerned with the health of individuals should see as part of their responsibilities? These questions are tackled throughout the book—and do not always produce the same responses.

Another important aspect of the issue of who should counsel is that of the appropriate preparation and support for the role. What should a general practice, in seeking to appoint a counsellor as part of the PHCT, be looking for in terms of training, qualifications, and experience? How can the adequacy and appropriateness of the proliferation of courses in 'counselling' be judged? The chapter by Cocksedge and Ball addresses these vital questions. In terms of continuing support for the counsellor, several other contributors point to the distinctive emphasis in counselling on the importance of regular supervision. In some senses, therefore, the training is never at an end (is there a lesson here for GPs and other health professionals?).

WHO SHOULD BE COUNSELLED?

As already noted, there is a psychosocial element in a substantial proportion of GP consultations. In which cases should the GP, or other members of the PHCT, embark upon, recommend, or refer the individual for counselling? Those who are the most enthusiastic proponents of this form of help would probably reply that almost everyone can benefit from counselling support. However, even if this is so, the scarce resources of primary health care mean that some filtering or rationing mechanism is inevitable. Our choice of chapter headings in Part II of the book suggests the problem areas in which it is most frequently suggested that counselling has a role to play. The longest chapter in this section, by Irving, describes counselling for interpersonal relationships and psychological problems, and the case histories illustrated there will strike a familiar note to many GPs and other PHCT members. In addition, several of our contributors address the issue of what types of individuals in which sets of social circumstances may benefit from counselling.

DOES COUNSELLING OFFER VALUE FOR MONEY?

The counselling bandwagon is evidently rolling. This makes it important to ask how much it is costing, in terms of training and of providing the service, and how much it will cost if unchecked in its growth. Value for money has increasingly been accepted as an important criterion by which to judge various aspects of health care. The new GP contract and the current implementation of the NHS reforms have encouraged doctors (especially fundholders) and other team members to think carefully about the efficient management of scarce resources. This book thus contains two important chapters relating to questions of efficiency and effectiveness: one on the researcher's perspective on counselling (by Corney) and another on evaluating counselling from an economic perspective (by Rowland and Tolley). How can GPs, the primary health care team, and the counsellors themselves monitor the quality, efficiency, and effectiveness of the counselling service? What quantitative and qualitative criteria should and can be used to assess the process and outcomes of such a service? What evidence do we have about the impact and outcomes of counselling in primary health care? Are there any savings in other areas of provision of care (is it cost-effective) or does it just produce a 'feel good' factor which rapidly evaporates? Assessment from published and unpublished research of the actual and potential impact of counselling on individuals with various problems is attempted in this book. It should help practices to ascertain whether what they have established is actually helping their patients, as well as suggesting ways of monitoring and evaluating services which they plan to provide. This book examines the evidence on outcomes, tackling the substantive question of 'Does it work?' and the methodological question of 'How can we tell?'.

HOW TO GO ABOUT IT

In the majority of practices, no formal counselling is provided. So the issues surrounding establishing and managing such a service are considered, including early preparation and finance, payment systems, costs, and other resource issues. Integration into the primary health care team, referral arrangements, workload, recording, and confidentiality are all important issues that need to be addressed and are discussed in this book, as are the effects of counselling on the primary health care team itself. Because of the hands-on experience of many of the contributors, factors in the success or failure to provide counselling services are apparent. Why some services break down and others flourish becomes evident. At the end of Chapter 2 there is a list of organizations, publications, and other resources which should be of use to general practitioners and practice managers wishing to introduce, develop, and monitor counselling services.

SO WHO WILL FIND THIS BOOK VALUABLE?

This book aims to be an encouragement to practices to set up and maintain counselling services as part of their provision for the broader holistic care that their patients are increasingly expecting. It will be a valuable resource to those practices who already have made provision, in whatever form, for a counselling service. It will enable them to evaluate what they are currently providing. Any need for changes will become apparent. In addition it will be the substantive text for practices considering establishing counselling services within their own team. Its readership will, therefore, include not only general practitioners, their trainees, and their students, but also practice managers who are increasingly responsible for the cost-effectiveness and the standards of the practices that they run. Nurses, health visitors, midwives—all using counselling skills refined by years of experience—will be made aware of the concept of counselling as an entity. They will be clearer in their own minds as to whether they wish to counsel themselves or, perhaps more usually, be able to assess when specialist counselling help is appropriate. Counsellors themselves, already working in primary health care teams, will have a text that shows where they themselves 'fit' and also the potential of their team colleagues.

For those counsellors currently not working in the primary health care field at all, the book provides an overview of such work, orientated particularly around the team setting. If the varied and wide-ranging contributions encourage some of them to become involved in this field, our editorial endeavours will have been worthwhile.

Above all we hope that after reading this book all primary health care team members will feel somewhat at a loss if they currently do not work alongside a counsellor, and increasingly deprived if this state of affairs continues into the future.

Durham   J. K.
Stockton on Tees   G. N. M.
September 1994

REFERENCES

Keithley, J. (1982). Marriage counselling in general practice: an assessment of the work of marriage guidance counsellors in a general medical practice. Unpublished PhD thesis. University of Durham.

Marsh, G. N. and Barr, J. (1975). Marriage guidance counselling in a group practice. *Journal of the Royal College of General Practitioners*, **25**, 73–5.

Part 1
Counselling

1 The nature and outcomes of counselling

Tim Bond

INTRODUCTION

There is a great deal of confusion about what is meant by counselling in society in general and in medicine in particular. The widespread confusion is compounded by 'counselling' having been a fashionable term to be applied to all sorts of situations, for example double-glazing counsellor, debt counsellor, diet counsellor, etc.

Whilst the term 'counselling' in general usage can mean something quite precise, it is just as likely to be used as a label to make a familiar activity seem more trendy. Although there are numerous different meanings given to counselling in medical settings, I think most of the confusion around 'counselling' arises from three different usages, which are mutually incompatible. Because the same term is used for each of these different activities, it is very easy for two people to assume they are talking about the same thing when this is not the case. I have heard health workers talking about 'the desirability of a patient receiving counselling' and for the conversation to go on for some minutes before it becomes apparent that one person is advocating a series of sessions of psychosocial support to help with a general mood of anxiety and depression, in contrast to the other person who is thinking in terms of some practical advice about the patient's child-care problems. These misunderstandings often become apparent if the conversation continues for several minutes. However, in the hurried exchanges between people working in a busy practice, differences in meaning can go unnoticed. This can be confusing for staff. What is expected when someone is asked to counsel someone? It is even more confusing for patients. I have had some say to me that 'Dr . . . has been giving me counselling, but it was rather different from what you are doing'. The patient's perplexity could be the result of the doctor and myself having trained in different methods of counselling. More often, the confusion seems to arise from the different meanings of counselling currently in use in medical settings.

CURRENT USAGE OF 'COUNSELLING'

There are wider and narrower uses of 'counselling'. Some of the narrower uses are mutually exclusive.

Generic use

There are a variety of reasons why some people prefer to use 'counselling' in its wider meaning. Stephen Murgatroyd (1985) is antagonistic to the exclusive use of 'counselling' by a select few working in specialized roles, who are trained, certificated, and members of professional bodies. Therefore, he argues in favour of the deprofessionalizing of counselling in order to make its methods available to as many people as possible. In his view, counselling and helping are synonymous. Philip Burnard's views (1989, 1992) are of particular interest because his preference for the wider usage of 'counselling' is based on his experience of working in health care settings. As a nurse tutor, he was concerned to discover that nurses are reluctant to use facilitative skills with patients. This is not merely a matter of skills, but of an attitude and a belief that the nurse knows best, or at least better than the patient. This is contrary to the growing practice of involving patients in decisions about their own care. Therefore, Burnard is interested in extending the nurse's skills to include more facilitative interventions which involve the patients in making decisions for themselves about their treatment. He draws on John Heron's six categories of therapeutic intervention as the underpinning model. Heron (1990) divided the possible interventions into authoritative and facilitative. Authoritative interventions include: prescriptive (offering advice), informative (offering information), and confronting (challenging). Facilitative interventions include: cathartic (enabling expression of pent-up emotions), catalytic (drawing out), and supportive (confirming or encouraging). Burnard concluded that it is desirable for nurses to use the full range of interventions and, therefore, defines counselling as the effective use of verbal interventions involving 'both client-centred AND more prescriptive counselling', (his emphasis). He is, therefore, taking an all encompassing view of counselling.

In contrast to this wider definition of counselling, there are two narrower definitions in popular use which are mutually exclusive.

Counselling as advice

The first of these regards counselling as the same as giving advice. This view has had a long tradition which reaches back to at least the seventeenth century. In 1625 Francis Bacon, the essayist, wrote 'The greatest Trust, betweene Man and Man is the Trust of Giving Counsell'. It is a reasonable inference that he is thinking of advice because as he develops his argument he identifies the 'Inconveniences of Counsell'. These include 'the Danger of being unfaithfully counselled, and more for the good of them that counsell than of him that is counselled'. He also states that only people with expertise are suitable to provide 'counsell'. In modern dictionaries, both 'counsel' and 'counselling' retain the general meaning of 'advise' (Allen 1990). This usage is still commonplace in legal and medical circles. Recently, when I was working on a report about HIV counselling, a doctor was so committed to the use of 'counselling' to mean 'advising' that he wrote to me to express exasperation at all the fuss being made about counselling which he regarded as merely a 'popular term for giving advice to people' (Bond 1992). However, modern dictionaries also acknowledge the existence of a more specialized use of 'counselling' as a method used by trained professionals to help someone resolve personal, social, or psychological problems (Allen 1990). This more specialized usage has a shorter history, of at least 70 years, which I will consider next.

Counselling in psychological and social care

The use of the word 'counselling' in its narrowest meaning, first became popular in the 1920s in the USA. The term emerged in reaction against the exclusivity of psychoanalysis and psychotherapy. When Carl Rogers started working as a psychologist in America, he was not permitted to practise psychotherapy which was restricted to medical practitioners. Therefore, he called his work 'counseling' (US spelling) (Thorne 1984). It seems probable that Rogers took the term from vocational counselling that had been developed as part of a radical community action programme by Frank Parsons (1854–1908) when he established a counselling centre in the North End of Boston, a deprived city area. Rogers also had a rational agenda. The person-centred nature of his method meant that counselling itself was part of a movement to democratize talking therapies by emphasizing the importance of the client's contribution. This has remained an important tradition, even though as counselling has developed many new models for practice have developed. In all of these, there is an emphasis on counselling as the principled use of relationship, having the aim of enabling the client to achieve his own improved well-being. Two major ethical principles are closely associated with this way of counselling: respect for the client's capacity for self-determination and the importance of confidentiality. This is the use of the term 'counselling' espoused by the British Association for Counselling. The definition used within the *Code for counsellors* (BAC 1992*a*) makes specific reference to the client's capacity for self-determination.

Counselling is the skilled and principled use of relationships which develop self-knowledge, emotional acceptance and growth, and personal resources. The overall aim is to live more fully and satisfyingly. Counselling may be concerned with addressing and resolving specific problems, making decisions, coping with crises, working through feelings and inner conflict, or improving relationships with others.

The counsellor's role is to facilitate the client's work in ways that respect the client's values, personal resources, and capacity for self-determination.

Sometimes 'self-determination' is referred to as 'autonomy' or 'independence'; the choice of word often depends on personal preference, but the essential meaning remains the same. It is about a client increasing his or her capacity and inner resources to take control of his or her way of living. The concept is fundamental to counselling and acts as the cornerstone of its values from which the ethical principles are derived and ultimately standards of practice are set.

The Counselling in General Practice Working Party of the Royal College of General Practitioners adopted the use of the term 'counselling' to refer to a trained counsellor undertaking counselling as defined by the British Association for Counselling with its distinctive ethic and philosophy (Sheldon 1992).

COUNSELLING AND ADVICE

The *Code for counsellors* states:

Counsellors do not normally give advice (BAC 1992*b*).

Advice is generally thought of as an opinion given or offered as to future action. It usually entails giving someone information about the choices open to them and, then from a position of greater expertise or authority, a recommendation as to the best course of action. Rosalind Brooke (1972), writing about Citizens' Advice Bureaux, describes the advisory process as having two aspects. The advisor may interpret information in order to present it in a way which is adapted to the needs of the enquirer. The advisor may also offer an opinion about the wisdom of obtaining a solution in a particular way.

This description highlights the difficulty 'advice' poses for the counsellor. The aim of counselling is to enable the client to discover his/her own wisdom rather than have wisdom imparted to them from the counsellor. The counselling process is intended to increase the client's ability to take control personally rather than depend on another. This difference between counselling and advice does not mean that advice is an inappropriate way of offering help. It is a different method and perhaps more suitable for practical problems than making decisions about relationships, or coping with transitions, or other psychosocial issues.

In more recent times the emphasis on the impartiality of advice-giving means that skills developed in counselling are being increasingly applied to advice-giving. There has been a shift away from authoritative advice-giving to emphasizing the importance of helping the patient or client to form his/her own opinion. The increased emphasis on informed consent in all medical procedures is one facet of this trend. The guidance given to workers in Citizens' Advice Bureaux is equally applicable to the new style of advice-giving in medicine.

The adviser should structure the interview to enable clients to explore the problem fully and choose their own course of action. Advisers should not, for the sake of speed or their own satisfaction, encourage clients to become dependent . . . (NACAB 1990).

When advice is delivered in this way, supported by the use of counselling skills, it is much closer to the methods and process of counselling than when it is given authoritatively.

COUNSELLING AND PSYCHOTHERAPY

There is no universally accepted distinction between the terms 'counselling' and 'psychotherapy'. There are well-established traditions which use the term interchangeably. On the other hand, the terms are sometimes used in ways which distinguish them from each other. The criteria for the distinction varies according to the speaker's point of view. The potential distinguishing characteristics identified by Brammer and Shostrum from a search of American literature are identified in Table 1.1.

There is a need for a similar systematic study of the differentiation between counselling and psychotherapy in Britain. It seems likely that some of the findings of Brammer and Shostrum about the differences will also be applicable on this side of the Atlantic. They trace a history of counselling as dealing with problems which are primarily pressures

Table 1.1 *Characteristics of counselling and psychotherapy (Adapted from Brammer and Shostrum 1982)*

Characteristics	
Counselling	Psychotherapy
Educational	Reconstructive
Situational	Issues arising from personality
Problem-solving	Analytic
Conscious awareness	Preconscious and unconscious
Emphasis on working with people who do not have severe or persistent emotional problems	Emphasis on 'neurotics' or working with persistent and/or severe emotional problems
Focus on present	Focus on past
Shorter length of contract	Longer length of contract

from the outside environment rather than deeply embedded difficulties resulting in rigid neurotic patterns. In this sense, counselling is about helping people who have the capacity to cope in most circumstances, but who are experiencing temporary difficulties, or making transitions or adjustments in their life. Issues arising from difficult relationships at home, making decisions, coping with serious illness, bereavement, addiction, etc., may all be within the scope of counselling. If issues are merely symptomatic of something deeper, or the client is experiencing more entrenched problems such as persistent phobias, anxiety states, low self-esteem, or difficulty in establishing relationships, then psychotherapy may be more appropriate. This would imply that there is a difference in training and expertise between counsellors and psychotherapists. But neither counselling or psychotherapy are regulated in the UK and this means that they do not have established national standards. Anyone can set themselves up as either a counsellor or psychotherapist with little or no training or following extensive training. Therefore, it is not possible to assume that the psychotherapist always has a different area of experience or is better trained than the counsellor. This situation seems certain to persist for many years to come. However, even if this situation were resolved so that counsellors and psychotherapists are required to have a minimum standard of training before becoming authorized practitioners, it seems increasingly probable that the boundaries between counselling and psychotherapy would overlap. Counsellors are divided in their views about this. Psychodynamically trained counsellors are most inclined towards accepting that the two roles ought to be distinguished in the ways suggested in Table 2.1. Counsellors from a humanistic tradition tend to argue that the terms are interchangeable and that both roles require the same minimum standards of training. Nancy Rowland (1992), writing about counselling in general practice, takes the view that the similarities and differences depend on the training and orientation of individual practitioners rather than being inherent in the activities themselves.

COUNSELLING AND COUNSELLING SKILLS

One of the most important distinctions to emerge in recent years is that between counselling and counselling skills. It is also a distinction with considerable implications for medical practice. Unfortunately, it is also one which has been subject to considerable misunderstandings.

The most obvious misunderstanding is based on the idea that 'counselling skills' is a label for a set of activities unique to counselling. Although the term 'counselling skills' is sometimes used on this basis, it is quickly discredited because any attempt to list specific 'counselling skills', for example active listening, paraphrasing, using open questions, reflective responses, etc., quickly looks indistinguishable from lists labelled social skills, communication skills, interpersonal skills, etc.

In order to understand what is meant by 'counselling skills', it is useful to examine the two words separately. Here the use of the word 'counselling' is an indication of the historical source of the concept. It serves to indicate that whilst these skills are not unique to counselling, it is the way they have been articulated in counselling that has been useful to other roles which employ counselling skills. For example advice-giving has a much longer history than counselling skills, but the tendency has been to concentrate on the content of the advice rather than the way it is delivered. However, the methods which advisers use to communicate with clients can be adapted to improve the way advice is given and hence maximize the client's involvement in the decision-making. 'Counselling' in this context is acknowledging the source of the concept and method of communication. Similarly, nurses, tutors, personnel managers, social workers, and many others have all recognized that there are advantages in adopting the methods of communication used in counselling to aspects of their own role. One way in which an outside observer might detect that counselling skills are being used is in the pattern of communication. This is illustrated in Table 1.2.

Imparting expertise involves the expert in communicating his/her knowledge and expertise to the recipient which takes up most of the consultation time available. This contrasts with conversation where both participants tend to contribute for equal lengths of time and in a pattern which flows backwards and forwards. The use of counselling skills will usually change the pattern of communication in favour of the recipient, who speaks for most of the available time. Part of the expertise in using counselling skills is learning how to communicate briefly in ways which do not interrupt the flow of the speaker, but at the same time help the speaker to address more effectively the issues which concern them. When counselling skills are being used, an outside observer might notice that the recipient is encouraged to take greater control of the agenda of the dialogue than in the other styles of communication. In other words, the values implicit in the use of counselling skills are similar to those of counselling, placing an emphasis on the client's

Table 1.2 *Detection of counselling skills in the pattern of communication*

Differences in communication		
Style	Pattern of flow	Time ratio
Imparting expertise	Interactor $\Rightarrow$ Recipient	80:20
Conversation	Interactor $\Leftrightarrow$ Recipient	50:50
Counselling Skills	Interactor $\Leftarrow$ Recipient	20:80

capacity for self-determination in how help is sought as well as for any decisions or actions that may result (Bond 1989).

Other things which might be apparent to an outside observer include the way the recipient is encouraged or enabled to participate in deciding the agenda for the total transaction. In other words, the values implicit in the interactions are similar to those of counselling, with an emphasis on the client's capacity for self-determination.

The term 'skills' in 'counselling skills' is sometimes taken in a very literal sense to mean 'discrete behaviours' but this is not the way 'skills' is understood in the social sciences. Skills which are used to enhance relationships can be distinguished from 'physical skills' as in sport or work, and 'mental' and 'intellectual' skills not merely on the basis of observable behaviours. They are inextricably linked to the goal of the person using them. For instance, Michael Argyle (1981) defines 'socially skilled behaviour' as 'behaviour effective in realising the goals of the interactor'. In the context of counselling skills, those goals are to implement the values of counselling by assisting the self-expression and autonomy of the recipient.

One of the ways in which an independent observer might be able to distinguish between 'counselling skills' and counselling is whether the contracting is explicit between the two people. This is highlighted in one of the alternative definitions for counselling which is still in popular use.

People become engaged in counselling when a person, occupying regularly or temporarily the role of counsellor, offers or agrees explicitly to offer time, attention or respect to another person or persons temporarily in the role of client (BAC, 1984).

This definition was originally devised to distinguish between spontaneous or *ad hoc* counselling and formal counselling. The overt nature of the latter involving 'offers' and explicit agreements was seen as 'the dividing line between the counselling task and the *ad hoc* counselling, and is the major safe-guard of the rights of the consumer' (BAC 1985). The definition also provides a useful basis for distinguishing when someone is using counselling skills in a role other than that of counsellor or when they are counselling.

The *Code of ethics and practice for counselling skills* contains a useful test for the distinction.

1.2 Ask yourself the following questions:

a) Are you using counselling skills to enhance your communications with someone but without taking on the role of their counsellor?

b) Does the recipient perceive you as acting within your professional caring role (which is NOT that of being their counsellor)?

i. If the answer is YES to both these questions, you are using counselling skills in your functional role and should use this document.

ii. If the answer is NO to both, you are counselling and should look to the *Code of Ethics and Practice for Counsellors* for guidance.

iii. If the answer is YES to one and NO to the other, you have a conflict of expectations and should resolve it.

Only when both the user and the recipient explicitly contract to enter into a counselling relationship does it cease to be 'using counselling skills' and become 'counselling' (BAC 1989).

There are three frequent misconceptions that I encounter in discussions about counselling skills. These are:

1. *Using counselling skills is always a lower-order activity than counselling*

This need not be the case. Perhaps it is just as well, because arguably the user of counselling skills may be working under more demanding circumstances than the counsellor who usually has the benefit of more extended periods of time which have already been agreed in advance. In comparison, the user of counselling skills may be working more opportunistically with much less certainty about the duration of the encounter. Users of counselling skills can be more or less skilled just like counsellors. However, using counselling skills is not a role in itself but something important to enhance the performance of another role. This means that the capacity to use counselling skills effectively will depend not only on being skilled in their use but also on someone's competence in their primary role, for example nurse, tutor, etc. For all these reasons, using counselling skills can be more skilled than counselling. It certainly cannot be assumed that using counselling skills is a lower-order activity.

2. *People in occupational roles, other than counsellor, cannot counsel*

This would mean that doctors, nurses, youth workers, etc. cannot counsel but can only use counselling skills. This is not the case. With appropriate training, counselling supervision, and clear contracting with the client in ways consistent with counselling, it seems to me anyone can change roles to that of 'counsellor'. There are important issues about keeping the boundaries between different roles clear and managing overlapping roles or dual relationships, but these are separate issues (Herlihy and Corey 1992).

It seems reasonable to me that not every doctor wants to become a counsellor. It is a specialized activity which appeals to relatively small numbers of health workers and, realistically, probably only a few of these have the time to devote to it. On the other hand, my experience is that most doctors who have been trained in the use of counselling skills have found them useful in consultations with patients (See Chapter 15)

3. *Anyone with the occupational title 'Counsellor' is always counselling*

This is not the case. As the concept of counselling has narrowed down into a specifically contracted role, there is a need for counsellors to distinguish between when they are counselling and when they are performing other roles, including training, supervision, managing, etc. In each of these other roles a counsellor is likely to be using counselling skills. The BAC has produced codes of ethics and practice for other roles closely associated with counselling including:

- *Code of ethics and practice for counselling skills* which applies to members who would not regard themselves as counsellors, but who use counselling skills to support other roles.
- *Code of ethics and practice for the supervision of counsellors* which exists to guide members offering supervision to counsellors and to help counsellors seeking supervision.
- *Code of ethics and practice for trainers* which exists to guide members offering training to counsellors and to help members of the public seeking counselling training.

Copies of guidelines and information sheets relevant to maintaining ethical standards of practice can be obtained from the BAC office, 1 Regent Place, Rugby CV21 2PJ.

Telephone helplines: guidelines for good practice is intended to establish standards for people working on telephone helplines (sponsored by British Telecom). A new edition was produced in late 1992, single copies of which are available from BSS, PO Box 7, London W3 6XJ.

BACKGROUND OF COUNSELLORS WORKING IN PRIMARY HEALTH CARE

The background of counsellors working in primary health care settings is quite varied. Many have been trained either by Relate, formerly known as the National Marriage Guidance Council. This training consists of over 150 hours of formal training and between 170 and 220 hours of closely supervised counselling practice. The use of Relate-trained counsellors in primary health care has a long and successful history (Corney 1986; Marsh and Barr 1975). Alternatively, others have been accredited by the British Association for Counselling, which requires 450 hours of training and 450 hours of supervised practice. As there are only about 500 accredited counsellors nationally, it is not realistic to expect that all counsellors in primary health care will be accredited. Currently, it is probably more realistic to expect counsellors to be eligible for BAC accreditation, in terms of length of training and experience, or to be working towards accreditation.

The Counselling in Primary Health Care Trust distinguishes what it regards as essential and desirable in a counsellor. Their criteria are summarized in Table 1.3.

The training and background of counsellors is considered in detail in Chapter 4.

Table 1.3 *What is essential and desirable in a counsellor* (adapted from *Work specification for counsellors working in GP practices*. Counselling in Primary Care Trust, 1992).

Criteria	Essential	Desirable
Education and professional qualifications	450 hours training	BAC accreditation
Knowledge	One theoretical approach to counselling.	Variety of counselling theories and methods
	Psychosomatic disease and psychology of chronic or terminal illness.	Psychotropic drugs and their side effects
	BAC code of ethics— particularly about confidentiality	Psychopathology by visiting admission unit of psychiatric hospital
Experience	250 hours *supervised* counselling over 2 years	At least 300 hours gained over at least 3 years
Personality	Dependable	Aware of boundaries around punctuality
	Considered approachable by a wide range of patients*	Friendly*
Physical attributes	Good enough health and sufficient sight and hearing not to make special demands on clients	Able to work under pressure and to monitor and manage own stress level
Special circumstances	A constructive member of a multidisciplinary team	Understanding of culture of medical settings and willingness to develop appropriate counselling skills among team members

* Added by author

ETHICS AND STANDARDS OF PRACTICE
FOR COUNSELLORS

Counsellors have developed reasonably comprehensive ethics and standards of practice. Inevitably, because counselling is such a new role, the standards are still evolving. However, it is useful to be aware of a number of key issues.

Confidentiality

For medical staff and counsellors alike, confidentiality is both an ethical and legal requirement. However, the implementation of confidentiality is different. Medical services are provided on the basis that the treatment needs to continue even if the person providing it changes due to rotas or other reasons. Information about patients is, therefore, not usually confidential to a single person but is shared across a team on a confidential basis in order to ensure continuity of treatment. In contrast, the counselling relationship depends on the client's trust in a particular individual and there is no assumption that the counsellor is interchangeable. Similarly, confidentiality is regarded as personal to the counsellor and client unless the client gives consent for information to be shared. This also has implications for record keeping. The Code of Practice which accompanied the Human Fertilisation and Embryology Act, 1990 provides a useful example of how counsellors and team members can manage confidentiality about personal information relating to patients.

The code states:

6.24 A record should be kept of all counselling offered and whether or not the offer is accepted.

6.25 All information obtained in the course of counselling should be kept confidential subject to 3.24.

3.24 If a member of the team has a cause for concern as a result of information given to him or her in confidence, he or she should obtain the consent of the person concerned before discussing it with the rest of the team. If a member of the team receives information which is of such gravity that confidentiality **cannot** be maintained, he or she should use his or her own discretion, based on good professional practice, in deciding in what circumstances it should be discussed with the rest of the team.

This code of practice assumes a slightly more rigorous separation of records and practice over confidentiality than the procedures advocated by Dr June McLeod (1992) in her contribution to the Counselling in General Practice Working Party. The HFEA code would simply require that an entry of whether a patient was offered counselling and whether the offer was accepted or rejected was entered on the medical records. In contrast, McLeod recommends that counsellors complete a card with a brief record of dates, progress, and outcome of counselling to be kept with the medical records. The counsellor's working notes would be kept separately and would be confidential to the counsellor. Whatever method is adopted, it is important that the patient is informed about the limits of confidentiality. It is an accepted principle that discussions of confidential information, whether obtained in medical or counselling consultations, should be discussed with colleagues only after the patient's consent has been obtained, unless exceptional circumstances override the need for consent.

After misunderstandings about what constitutes counselling, tensions arising from differences about the practice of confidentiality are the second major source of difficulty which can frustrate the most effective use of counsellors in primary care. The counsellor's view of this is explored more fully in Chapter 14.

Counselling-supervision

In most professions, supervision is mandatory for trainees and for those in a probationary period after training. In contrast, counsellors are required to have regular and continuing counselling-supervision. The code for counsellors states:

B.3.1 It is a breach of the ethical requirement for counsellors to practise without regular counselling supervision/consultative support (BAC 1992*a*).

Counselling-supervision is not in any way a managerial relationship. Managerial issues should be dealt with between the counsellor and the medical practice. The counselling-supervisor is someone who is experienced as a counsellor and independent of the situation in which the counselling is provided. The supervisor's role is directed towards helping the counsellor to develop his/her own standards of practice and foster an 'internalised supervisor'. The tasks of supervision can be categorized thus:

- Formative—learning new methods and insights;
- Restorative—getting personal support and relief from the consequences of being exposed to others' emotional pain as well as that of the counsellor's;
- Normative—ensuring adequate standards of ethics and practice are maintained.

These three tasks were first described by Francesca Inskipp and Brigid Proctor (1989). As a result of my study of good practice in HIV counselling, I have added a fourth:

- Perspective—stepping back to take an overview of the total pattern of work with clients and to review the interface between counselling and other methods of helping or treating clients, including interprofessional relationships.

These tasks have to be held in balance with each other so that one does not predominate over the others. For example, if the restorative were to dominate over the others, counselling-supervision would become indistinguishable from personal counselling. The counsellor's 'internalised supervisor' needs to be an all rounder.

Discussions in supervision are anonymous. The identity of individual clients is protected in the interests of preserving confidentiality.

A minimum frequency of supervision recommended by the British Association for Counselling is one and a half-hours per month, but some counsellors have more frequent supervision because of the difficulty of their cases or because they find it increases their efficacy.

Prohibition of sex with clients

Unfortunately, a small number of counsellors abuse their position of trust by entering into sexual relationships with clients. This phenomenon is shared with all the caring professions. So far as I am aware, no such accusations have been made against counsellors in primary care. However, the belief that counsellors have sex with clients is sufficiently commonplace to be worthy of consideration.

There is no doubt that any sexual activity between a counsellor and a current client is regarded as unethical by the British Association for Counselling. Sex with former clients is considered unethical in many circumstances, particularly if the subject matter of the counselling concerns relationship or sexual difficulties. The British Association for Counselling is currently conducting a consultation with members in order to decide how to regulate changes in relationship with former clients.

Counsellors who are members of the British Association for Counselling view sexual intimacy with clients in ways which parallel health care workers' relationships with patients. Counselling inevitably involves psychological intimacy rather than physical exposure and, therefore, requires trust. Clients also sometimes imbue counsellors with power, or experience a sense of dependency. For all these reasons, counsellors need to be scrupulous about maintaining personal boundaries between themselves and clients. When a complaint of sexual misconduct has been upheld, counsellors have been expelled not only from BAC, but also from the British Psychological Society and the Association of Humanistic Practitioners. This does not stop someone continuing to practise as a counsellor, for it is an unregulated occupation, and anyone can set up as a counsellor. However, it illustrates the importance of ensuring that a counsellor adheres to an appropriate code of ethics and practice for the protection of clients and the primary health care team in which the counsellor is working.

COUNSELLING IN PRACTICE

What does counselling look like in actual practice? Many counsellors are restricted in the number of sessions that can be offered to individual patients in the first instance. Six to ten sessions of 50 minutes appears to be usual (Rowland 1992). Clients with exceptional needs who are showing significant progress could be offered up to the same number of sessions again.

The counselling relationship is probably most widely thought of in terms of stages. In the initial stage, the emphasis is on trust-building and enabling the client to describe the situation which is causing the difficulty. With some clients this may remain the major activity, because the client regains a sense of control and order in the process of exploring the issue which causes them concern. With most clients, however, it is necessary to move on to a second stage which is primarily directed at creating a change which will give the client additional resources to assist with the problem. This may involve gaining new insight, learning new skills, redefining personal goals, or reassessing important relationships. A third stage involves considering alternative ways of applying the new resources and then putting them into action.

All counsellors probably use rather similar approaches in the initial stage. The aim is to provide an enabling relationship characterized by warmth, genuineness, and empathy. These are qualities which are widely considered essential to the effectiveness of counselling (Truax and Carkhuff 1967) and certainly to the stage of trust building. The counsellor may also attempt to negotiate a contract with the client about the practical arrangements, confidentiality, and the therapeutic goal of the client. These negotiations help to increase the client's sense of control and also identify the focus of the counselling. In this way the client is encouraged to focus on what he/she is really concerned about. Many other strategies and techniques may be used to this end. The counsellor's task is to notice what a client experiences as significant, and to build up a picture of what is said, what is implied, and what is left unsaid. Gradually a picture of the client's perception emerges and this forms the foundation upon which the counsellor builds.

The next stage in the counselling relationship will vary according to the theoretical model of the counsellor. There are probably over 200 different published models of counselling. I will describe three of the most widely used. Psychodynamic counselling is within the traditions originally founded by Sigmund Freud but often considerably modified. The counsellor's concern is the client's internal relationships within that person. These feelings may have their origins in early childhood and may no longer rely on the promptings of an external person to evoke them. The aim of successful counselling in this model is to enable a person to balance the potentially conflicting demands of basic psychological needs, the demands of conscience, and the external realities of the situation (Jacobs 1988). Person-centred counselling was developed by Carl Rogers and is superficially quite different from a psychodynamic approach. In contrast with psychodynamic counselling, which emphasizes the counsellor's ability to understand the effect of past influences on the client's present experience, a person-centred counsellor seeks to use the current relationship between client and counsellor as the source of new personal development and emphasizes the role of the client as the expert in selecting what is important and healing to him or her. The quality of the relationship is extremely important and is sometimes described as '*trying to put the loving into helping*' (Mearns and Thorne 1988). In contrast again, cognitive behavioural counselling is primarily directed towards changing the way someone 'self-talks' in order to achieve beneficial changes (Trower *et al.*, 1988). Some counsellors are purists and work exclusively with one model. Others are committed to drawing on a range of models in order to find the method best suited to a particular client. It is generally considered better to be systematically rather than randomly eclectic as this reduces the risk of presenting the client with mixed messages and potentially confusing the client's problem further (Culley 1991).

WHO WILL BENEFIT FROM COUNSELLING?

A wide range of people appear to benefit from counselling. Anyone who is capable of expressing themselves verbally and who has usually been quite resourceful in the way they have coped with life until they become troubled by a particular issue will almost certainly benefit. Sometimes counselling can be useful to people who have a long history of not coping, but this is much less certain.

There are certain issues which are generally considered as being suitable for counselling:

- bereavement;
- recovery from trauma due to accident, major disaster, major medical treatment, diagnosis of serious illness, or physical/sexual abuse (post-traumatic stress syndrome);
- terminal illness;
- coping with anxiety associated with major transitions in life, for example adolescence to young adulthood, changes in occupation, moving out of work due to redundancy, retirement, or changes in relationships;
- stress management;
- problems associated with the use of alcohol or drugs;
- interpersonal and relationship problems;
- sexual problems;

- family planning;
- infertility;
- HIV/AIDS;
- psychological and the less severe psychiatric problems;
- decision making about the best course of treatment when the patient has alternatives to choose between.

Many of these issues are discussed in more detail elsewhere in this book. It is not unusual for several issues to be closely related. For example, the diagnosis of a major illness will not only be the start of a process of personal adjustment but may also involve the patient in planning what to tell a partner, and perhaps reassessing personal relationships. There may also be a need to learn how to manage personal anxiety better. When someone presents with multiple issues, the counsellor's role is to help them prioritize the issues to be addressed. Typically the choice is made on the basis of what is most urgent, or causing greatest discomfort, or most likely to create the possibility of other successes if it improved. Depressed patients are an exception to this general rule for prioritizing the issues. Often it is better to start with the most manageable issue and work progressively towards the most demanding so that a sense of confidence and of regaining control can emerge. This approach counters the sense of helplessness and dispiritment associated with depression.

An important factor to take into consideration in deciding who could benefit from counselling is the aptitude of the counsellor. His or her training and experience may be decisive in who will be the most helped by counselling. However, counselling is possible only when the client becomes actively committed to the process. Therefore, the most important factor is the client's attitude to the offer of counselling. A positive attitude considerably increases the likelihood that the client will take advantage of the opportunities offered in counselling.

WHO IS UNSUITABLE FOR COUNSELLING?

Not everyone is suitable for counselling. However, there appears to be no agreed classification of the situations unlikely to be helped by counselling. Probably the aptitude of individual counsellors is a more important factor than any general list. Nonetheless, experience suggests that some situations may be less suitable for counselling. These include:

1. The person who does not want counselling. Counselling requires the active involvement of clients and, therefore, is essentially a voluntary activity.
2. The person who consistently externalizes problems on to other people or attributes his/her problems to his/her state of physical health. For

example, a client who attributes her emotional fluctuations exclusively to premenstrual tension and is unwilling to take any role in managing her situation other than to demand tablets from a doctor is unlikely to be suitable for counselling. In contrast, someone who wants to do what she can to improve her situation or is willing to explore whether there could be other factors contributing to her changes in mood is much more suitable for counselling. The counselling is most likely to complement any medical treatment.

3. Someone who has no insight into his/her condition due to a personality disorder, or severe psychiatric disorder is unlikely to benefit from short-term counselling.

4. People with undiagnosed clinical conditions which would account for their problems. For example, counselling cannot help a tired, weepy patient who has untreated thyroid deficiency or pernicious anaemia because the appropriate tests have not been conducted. This situation is quite different from the patient who has done the rounds of all the possible medical specialities without any physiological explanation for the problems being discovered. In these circumstances, counselling may help a client to explore whether the problems could have psychological or social origins.

Some clients may be suitable for counselling but can be made unsuitable by being given unrealistic expectations of the counselling. It is important that the referrer conveys a realistic hope that counselling will be beneficial. Counselling can sometimes help people to solve problems. However, in many situations there is no immediate solution. Counselling cannot bring a loved relative back to life or remove the inevitable tensions of looking after an adolescent dependent, but it can help people to manage their bereavement or difficult relationships better.

THE EFFECTIVENESS OF COUNSELLING VERSUS ACCEPTABLE OUTCOMES

It is important to consider the effectiveness of counselling and what are the outcomes. There are problems in answering these questions. Some of the problems relate to the nature of counselling itself. It is difficult to quantify the input of the counsellor in comparison to a medicine or to a surgical procedure. Psychosocial factors are by nature often elusive and difficult to quantify. Many workers in primary care recognize the difficulty in assessing the contribution which verbal communications and the emotional climate of the relationship make to the well-being of the patient. There are also potential difficulties in identifying what changes can be ascribed to particular aspects of the counselling.

For example, I remember seeing someone after an attempted suicide who was experiencing social isolation, difficulties with her mother, and problems arising from an inability to say 'no' to people in need of her help.

The counselling, at her direction, focused on these last two problems, but when I asked her what had been most useful, her response surprised me:

It is the experience of being listened to. You remember when I started I talked about my loneliness and feeling I am the only one with these problems. I have taken you as a model and have started listening to other people and I have discovered many other people have similar problems.

The other topics addressed in counselling had been useful but for her this was the most useful.

It is also possible that beneficial changes are due not to the counselling but to events occurring in other aspects of the client's life.

The final methodological hurdle to be overcome is in deciding what constitutes a beneficial outcome in order for counselling to be considered effective. Is it sufficient that the client reports feeling better? Or is some more observable physiological or behavioural change required? In Chapter 17 of this book, Roslyn Corney examines these issues from a researcher's perspective and outlines ways in which qualitative and quantitative methodologies have been applied to assess the effectiveness of counselling. Studies about the effectiveness of counselling are important for the medium-and long-term development of counselling.

Primary health care teams require more readily available indicators of the results achieved by investing resources in counselling. In some cases these gains may be demonstrated better by secondary indicators. In the opinion of Dr Graham Curtis Jenkins, the Director of the Counselling in Primary Care Trust, acceptable outcomes might include:

• reduction in GP consultations;
• patients in receipt of counselling making more appropriate use of consultations with health care staff;
• reduction in prescribed medicines;
• reduced referrals to psychiatric out- and psychiatric patient clinics admissions;
• reduced costs in managing some patients.

Eventually the monitoring of these secondary gains may accumulate to be used as benchmarks for the effectiveness of a particular counselling provision. Changes in the secondary gains may reflect changes in the quality of counselling being provided, if the kind of issues referred and method of referral are constant.

MONITORING COUNSELLING

Regular and systematic monitoring of the counselling is important. The current advice is to keep the monitoring of the counselling simple. The British Association for Counselling (1992*b*) suggests restricting routine monitoring and auditing:

How many patients seen, how often, from which partner, appointment failures and reasons for referral. This can be done at 6 monthly intervals, and part can appear in the annual report.

Even such basic auditing will expose important issues, such as whether referrals are evenly spaced across the practice or mainly from a few sources. Changes in the pattern of appointment failures may be indicative of the underlying problem. It is reasonable to start with the rebuttable assumption that failure to attend first appointments may indicate problems with referral or reception. On the other hand increases in failure to attend second or subsequent appointments may indicate dissatisfaction with the counselling facilities, with the counsellor, or the patient's deteriorating mental or physical health.

During my study of good practice in HIV counselling (Bond 1992) counsellors and their managers were invited to identify the criteria for monitoring the quality of counselling being provided. I have adapted their suggestions to primary care as possible ways of augmenting the simple audit already mentioned.

1. *Service delivery*:

(a) **Precounselling information**: is a leaflet or other means of explaining to patients what counselling entails readily available?
(b) **Approachability**: are the counselling services attractive to intending clients? Are they provided by people who are acceptable to the clients in terms of gender, ethnic, cultural, and social background? Can clients choose a counsellor who is likely to satisfy their requirements?
(c) **Accessibility**: has the location of the counselling sessions been considered in terms of its nearness to likely users of the service and its accessibility by public and private transport? Is access to the premises possible for people with difficulties with mobility or in wheelchairs? Are there arrangements for counsellors to visit clients in hospital, at home, or at other venues if these are more appropriate?
(d) **Availability**: does the availability of the service correspond to clients' needs, for instance during weekdays, evenings, or at weekends?
(e) **Continuity**: are the services provided with sufficient continuity to gain the confidence of potential client groups? Is counselling staff turnover taking place at an acceptable rate?
(f) **Confidentiality**: are the established practice and procedures about confidentiality understood and implemented by staff? Are any limitations on confidentiality communicated to clients?
(g) **Statement of standards and ethics**: is there a readily available statement or code of practice which sets out the standards and ethics of the counselling? Is the code available to clients?

2. *Client participation in monitoring*:

(a) **Client feedback**: is client feedback sought regularly about the services provided to them?

(b) **Complaints procedure**: is there a procedure to deal with complaints from clients? How does the agency respond to the complainant? How does the agency learn from complaints and revise its practice?

3. *Staffing*:

(a) **Selection**: what are the selection criteria for counsellors? What are the selection procedures?
(b) **Training**: what provision has been made to ensure counsellors receive appropriate basic training for their role? What provision has been made for the continuing training of counsellors?
(c) **Supervision and support**: what are the arrangements for supervising counsellors by management, and for independent supervisors for counselling supervision/consultative support?

4.*Co-operation with others*:

(a) **Liaison with other staff and agencies**: how effectively do counsellors and their managers liaise with other service providers within the same agency and between agencies?
(b) **Reputation of the counselling service**: what is the reputation of the counselling service amongst other agencies? How are these views collected and responded to?

5. *Counsellors can contribute to the monitoring by the following methods*:

(a) **Client's manner**: changes in the client's manner towards becoming more competent and assertive in counselling sessions were generally thought to be positive indicators.
(b) **Changes attributed to counselling by clients**: constructive changes that are attributed to the counselling by the client are considered to be positive indications of the usefulness of the counselling. However, the counsellor also needs to consider the possibility that the changes were exclusively due to other factors or a combination of counselling and other factors.
(c) **Clients keeping pre-arranged appointments**: attendance at pre-arranged second and subsequent counselling sessions may be an indication that the client is getting something of value from the sessions.
(d) **Returning for further sessions**: clients who return for further sessions after an interval without counselling may be demonstrating with their feet a belief that counselling has helped them previously.
(e) **New clients recommended to seek counselling by former clients**: the recommendation of counselling by former clients is generally considered to be a very positive indicator.
(f) **Informal feedback from clients**: some counsellors ask for informal feedback at the end of sessions about what has/has not been useful to the client. This can be extremely informative.

6. *Other members of the primary care team or the practice manager may wish to participate in the use of any of the following*:

(a) **Monitoring attendance for appointments**: significant changes in the frequency of non-attendance for appointments usually indicates changes in the client-group's perception of the counselling service. Generally a reduction in missed appointments is considered to be a positive indication unless there is evidence of excessive dependence on the counsellors.

(b) **Distributing questionnaires to current and former clients**: questionnaires can be a useful means of obtaining information from clients who are able to read and write and who are confident enough to express their views in writing. An alternative approach is to use structured/semi-structured interviews by a skilled interviewer, although problems over confidentiality often make this approach impossible.

(c) **Using an independent consultant**: the independence of the consultant adds to the credibility of the monitoring.

(d) **Monitoring complaints and unsolicited positive feedback**: reviewing complaints and unsolicited feedback can be very informative.

This list is the accumulation of methods adopted by a variety of agencies. It is not envisaged that any single practice would attempt to undertake all the activities suggested in any single review. The list is intended to stimulate consideration of alternative methods and issues to be taken into account during monitoring. One way of using the list would be to select one topic from the list for specific attention during the routine monitoring and to change the topic periodically so that over an extended period there has been a wide-ranging consideration of the quality of the counselling available.

Formal monitoring is no substitute for regular meetings between the counsellor and other members of the primary health care team. If a new counsellor has been appointed, these meetings are necessary in order to establish how the counsellor works and to provide opportunities for team members to express their hopes and misgivings and to plan the detailed integration of the service into the work of the practice (McLeod 1992). Extra meetings are a burden on professionals who have many other demands on their time. However, it has been shown that regular meetings are beneficial both to the primary health care staff and to counsellors (Marsh and Barr 1975). They are the best means of ensuring that referrals are appropriate and that expectations are realistic. Of benefit to the counsellor is the breaking down of isolation. These meetings do not need to be all of the same kind. June McLeod (1992) suggests different ways of meeting members of the primary health care team:

(1) discussing particular patients with particular doctors or other staff;

(2) reporting back in general terms, particularly discussion of practical problems;
(3) opportunities for more detailed discussions of referrals and outcomes and opinions about the counsellor's role;
(4) using the counsellor to offer support and training in basic counselling skills for other team members.

A variety in the kinds of meetings between the counsellor and other staff reduces the burden on any individual member of staff and helps to disseminate knowledge about the service throughout the practice.

CONCLUSIONS

Counselling is a relatively new activity in primary health care and nationally. The need to establish sound professional standards is paramount. A great deal of progress has been made within the Counselling in Medical Settings division of the British Association for Counselling and the Counselling in General Practice Working Party of the Royal College of General Practitioners. Work about clarifying the nature of counselling, the implications of its particular values, and methodology will be continued within national bodies such as these. However, the justification for the provision of counselling must be the outcomes for individual patients in the first instance and the secondary benefits this additional service brings to the work of other members of the primary health care team.

REFERENCES

Allen, R. E. (1990). *The concise Oxford dictionary of current english*, Oxford University Press, Oxford.
Argyle, Michael (ed.) (1981). *Social skills and health*. Methuen, London.
BAC (1984). *Code of ethics and practice for counsellors*. British Association for Counselling, Rugby.
BAC (1985). *Counselling: definition of terms in use with expansion and rationale*. British Association for Counselling, Rugby.
BAC (1989). *Code of ethics and practice for counselling skills*. British Association for Counselling, Rugby.
BAC (1992a). *Code of ethics and practice for counsellors* (revised version of earlier editions in 1984 and 1990). British Association for Counselling, Rugby.
BAC (1992b). *So you want to start a counselling service: advice to doctors*. British Association for Counselling, Rugby.
Bond, T. (1989). Towards defining the role of counselling skills. *Counselling, Journal of the British Association for Counselling*, **69**, 3–9.
Bond, T. (1992). *HIV counselling*. British Association for Counselling, Rugby; Daniels Publishing, Cambridge.

Brammer, L. M. and Shostrum, E. L. (1982). *Therapeutic psychology*. Prentice Hall, Englewood Cliffs, New Jersey.

Brooke, R. (1972). *Information and advice guidance*. The Social Administration Research Trust, G. Bell and Sons, London.

Burnard, P. (1989). *Counselling skills for health professionals*. Chapman and Hall, London.

Burnard, P. (1992). *Perceptions of AIDS counselling*. Avebury, Aldershot.

Corney, R. N. (1986). Marriage guidance counselling in general practice. *Journal of the Royal College of General Practitioners*, **36**, 424–6.

Counselling in Primary Care Trust (1992). *Work specification for counsellors working in GP practices*. Counselling in Primary Care Trust, Staines.

Culley, S. (1991). *Integrative counselling skills in action*. Sage Publications, London.

Herlihy, B. and Corey, G. (1992). *Dual relationships*. American Association for Counselling and Development, Alexandria, USA.

Heron, J. (1990). *Helping the client—a creative practical guide* (revised version of *Six category intervention analysis*, 1975, 1986, 1989 previously published by University of Surrey). Sage Publications, London.

HFEA (1990). *Code of practice*. Human Fertilisation and Embryology Authority, London.

Inskipp, F. and Proctor, B. (1989). *Skills for supervising and being supervised*. Alexia Publications, St. Leonards on Sea, East Sussex.

Jacobs, M. (1988). *Psychodynamic counselling in action*. Sage Publications, London.

Marsh, G. N. and Barr, J. (1975). Marriage guidance counselling in a group practice. *Journal of the Royal College of General Practitioners*, **25**, 73–5.

McLeod, J. (1992). The general practitioner's role. In *Counselling in general practice*, (ed. M. Sheldon), pp. 8–14. Royal College of General Practitioners, London.

Mearns, D. and Thorne, B. (1988). *Person-centred counselling in action*. Sage Publications, London.

Murgatroyd, S. (1985). *Counselling and helping*. British Psychological Association, Leicester and Methuen, London.

NACAB (1990). Quality of advice: NACAB membership scheme requirements, 3(1). In *National homelessness advice service—guidance on CAB minimum housing advice standards*. National Citizens Advice Bureaux, London.

Rowland, N. (1992). Counselling and counselling skills. In *Counselling in general practice*, (ed. M. Sheldon), pp. 1–70. Royal College of General Practitioners, London.

Sheldon, M. (1992). Preface. In *Counselling in general practice* (ed. M. Sheldon). Royal College of General Practitioners, London.

Thorne, B. (1984). Person-centred therapy. In *Individual therapy in Britain* (ed. W. Dryden), p. 105. Harper and Row, London.

Trower, P., Casey, A., and Dryden, W. (1988). *Cognitive-behavioural counselling in action*. Sage Publications, London.

Truax, C. B. and Carkhuff, R. R. (1967). *Towards effective counselling and psychotherapy training and practice*. Aldine, Chicago.

2 The theory and practice of counselling in the primary health care team

Jane Dammers and Jan Wiener

INTRODUCTION

Most doctors, nurses, and other primary health care workers see themselves as involved in 'counselling' in the broadest sense of the word, be that talking with a patient about the effects of smoking, or listening to somebody recently bereaved and offering some words of comfort and support. A wide range of activities which commonly go on in primary care may be referred to as 'counselling', from talking with patients in an unstructured way to giving information, advising about a range of investigations and treatments, giving guidance on the best course of action, and engaging in truly non-directive, patient-led counselling—the last is a major theme in this book. In this chapter we outline how ideas derived from the disciplines of counselling and psychotherapy have been incorporated into primary care over the past 40 years, and describe how counselling is practised within the primary care team. We are particularly interested in the work and extended role of practice counsellors and suggest the value of a psychodynamic approach to looking at the relationships between counsellors, doctors, and their patients. We have found this useful as a way of understanding why particular patients are referred and how practice counsellor attachments can best be fostered. We also look at the professionals' needs for support when dealing with difficult emotional problems in the uncertain environment of general practice.

As a general practitioner and psychotherapist/counsellor we have worked together over a number of years. We struggled together with patients in general practice, learning most about ourselves and our work by talking about the patients we found most difficult. We have led, and taken part in, groups for general practitioners and counsellors working together and we are interested in how the two disciplines can effectively develop a common language and work well together. JW also provides supervision for counsellors working in general practice. In 1989 the Society of Analytical Psychology (SAP), a London-based society which trains Jungian analysts and hosts a wide range of public events in the field of analytical psychology and related topics, invited the Department of General Practice and Primary Care, King's College School of Medicine and Dentistry, London to run a joint workshop for general practitioners and counsellors. The aim was to look at emotional problems in general practice. This was the beginning of a mutually rewarding liaison leading to yearly events attended by general practitioners and counsellors from all over the country. As well as providing opportunities for participants to explore, in small groups, some of the stresses and strains of working in general practice, the collaboration of the SAP and Kings helped the staff group to learn more about unconscious processes, group facilitation, and the particular environment of general practice.

THE DEVELOPMENT OF A PSYCHOTHERAPEUTIC APPROACH IN GENERAL PRACTICE

There has been a growing interest in how psychotherapy and counselling can help to deal with the many and varied emotional and psychological problems which patients bring to their doctors every day. Developments in a psychotherapeutic approach have mostly been in response to the needs of patients, in an attempt to provide more skilled resources at the primary care level. Doctors, nurses, and others have developed their own counselling skills, and attachments of specialist counsellors have grown rapidly in the last ten years. Ideas and practices derived from counselling models have also been used to develop ways of supporting professionals working in primary care. A psychodynamic approach to thinking about what goes on in a practice can be very helpful, as a way of exploring difficulties with patients or problems in partnerships, in order to find creative solutions.

These ideas are not new. Forty years ago Michael Balint, a psychiatrist and psychoanalyst, and Enid Balint, a psychoanalyst, pioneered research work with general practitioners in an effort to explore the doctor–patient relationship and the potential for psychotherapy in general practice (Balint 1964). Balint saw the doctor as the most powerful 'drug' available to treat emotional problems, but pointed out that very little, if any, research had been done into how this 'drug' was most effectively used, when it might be harmful, and what its side effects might be. He outlined a model of listening to the patient, understanding, and making as complete a diagnosis as possible, and then using this understanding to make interventions to therapeutic effect. He worked with 14 general practitioners who brought cases for discussion and elucidation in the group. Together, they tried to discover what was really troubling the patient and what was going on between the doctor and patient. The doctors made a number of interventions, and by following the cases over several years, the accuracy of the diagnoses and the success of the interventions could be tested. Attention was given to the thoughts, feelings, flashes of insight, and fantasies which encounters with patients generated as these were very useful in developing an understanding of the patient.

Balint (1964) also wrote about the difficulties of developing a common language between psychiatrists and general practitioners. Medical terminology for physical diseases is highly developed and precise, so that a general practitioner can refer a patient with, say, a duodenal ulcer and be confident that his hospital colleague will understand him. Terms used to describe emotional problems, particularly the very wide range of problems found in general practice are much less helpful—for example, a diagnosis of 'neurosis' does not tell us very much. Balint considered 'the man in the street' would be able to make this sort of diagnosis just as well as a doctor. He predicted that the development of a dialogue would be a hard task and take a long time to achieve.

Carl Rogers' exposition of a client-centred approach to counselling (Rogers 1951) also had a major influence on general practice. He emphasized the importance of empathy, warmth, and genuineness on the part of the listener who could help the client to explore, understand, and reframe his or her experiences. He believed that patients/clients would find their own solutions to problems and that they were the best, probably the only people who could find appropriate solutions. Offers of gratuitous advice were likely to be unhelpful. Many doctors have tried to develop this style in their consultations, spending more time listening and allowing patients to explore their own ideas, and less time talking themselves (Pendleton *et al.* 1984). This is not always easy to do if the doctor has been trained in a more directive style. There is also a genuine conflict because doctors are quite properly called upon to advise their patients and to tell them, for instance, how to take a course of treatment. What seems important is that the doctor should be conscious of what he/she is trying to do and be in a position to choose different styles as appropriate.

The ideas put forward by Michael Balint and Carl Rogers have been extensively used in vocational training for general practice, which itself has had a major impact on the development of general practice over the past 20 years. Many vocational training half-day release schemes use a 'Balint Group' style to encourage trainees to discuss cases and reflect on their own reactions to patients and the problems which they bring. The experience of discussing difficult issues and feelings in a group can serve as a useful foundation upon which to foster the confidence that it is possible and helpful to discuss work with colleagues. Trainees and trainers are also encouraged to tape or video some of their consultations as a way of assessing themselves privately or, usually more beneficially, in a group. Tools have been developed to 'score' consultations on agreed criteria (Cox and Mulholland 1993). How good is the doctor at listening? Is the doctor patient-led or proscriptive? What happens when a patient raises a difficult issue or becomes distressed? By sharing this material with others, doctors can learn much about themselves and make observable changes in their approach to patients.

A climate has, therefore, been created in which many doctors and nurses working in primary care think critically about their relationships with patients, their style of consultation, and the balance between a directive or a patient-led approach. Many have also developed a wider interest in counselling and psychotherapy, and, at the same time, there has been a rapid increase in the training of counsellors. It is not surprising then that the two disciplines of counselling and primary care have been drawn closer, to see what each can offer the other, and to explore ways in which, together, they can provide something useful to patients.

WHO UNDERTAKES COUNSELLING IN PRIMARY CARE?

Counselling as part of day-to-day work in the practice

All members of the primary care team may draw on counselling skills to help them in their work. Practice receptionists, who are in the front line of patients' requests for help, require great skill in dealing sensitively with those who are distressed, frightened, and ill. The way they respond to patients has knock-on effects throughout the practice. The Department of General Practice at King's College, London, has been running courses for receptionists since 1984, drawing on communication and counselling skills to develop effective ways of dealing with upset, and sometimes difficult patients. Some receptionists have become sufficiently interested to go on to do short courses in counselling in adult education centres. Counselling skills can also be useful for practice managers in some of the personnel and teamwork aspects of their job, and are commonly taught on practice managers' courses.

Talking with patients has always been an important part of the work of nurses and health visitors. Their basic training emphasizes a counselling role and there are many short courses on counselling in particular specialty areas, for instance lifestyle counselling to reduce the risk of coronary artery disease, bereavement counselling, contraceptive and psychosexual counselling, HIV counselling, counselling carers, and so on. Practice nurses often develop particular interests and expertise in some of these areas. Community midwives are similarly trained in many areas of counselling— preconceptual counselling, genetic counselling, counselling and miscarriage, counselling parents of premature babies, counselling and stillbirth . . . the list goes on. Most courses for professionals working in primary care do at least pay lip service to addressing the 'counselling' aspect of whatever topic is on the agenda. However, there is often more emphasis on the giving of information, advice and guidance, and less on the adoption of a client-centred approach.

General practitioners vary in how much counselling they do. Some set aside long sessions, usually at the end of a surgery or outside surgery hours, to give more time to a few patients. This may be in response to a crisis or because the doctor has an interest in doing some in-depth work. Attending a short course in counselling or family therapy can foster confidence to spend more time with patients in this way. Ideas can be tried out and incorporated into the doctor's normal work pattern. However, a proper training in counselling takes several years and the necessary skills cannot be learned over a couple of days. It would be unwise for a doctor to embark on more formal counselling work with patients without considering further training, appropriate supervision, and the possibility of some personal counselling or therapy for himself.

Counselling as part of a specialist attachment

Hospital- and community-based mental health teams, social services, and some voluntary organizations have sought to extend their services more effectively into the community by attaching their workers to general practice. Attachments have provided opportunities for closer liaison and understanding between different disciplines, and for the development of professional skills and experience while working with a wide variety of clients as part of a medical team. These attachments have usually been welcomed by general practitioners as they provide more resources and facilitate referrals for specialist help.

In the 1970s there was a rapid growth in the building of local authority health centres and incentives to develop and expand existing premises, and a trend to establish larger group practices. The provision of good premises, with enough space for health visitors, district nurses, and community midwives to work alongside a group of general practitioners, also made attachments of community psychiatric nurses, clinical psychologists, and counsellors possible. Social worker attachments also flourished; much of their time in general practice was taken up with counselling patients, as well as dealing with very practical needs and giving advice. Some were excluded from statutory work as it was felt it could conflict and interfere with their counselling role in the general practice setting. However, from the late 1980s onwards, social service departments experienced difficulty in recruiting staff in inner city areas, financial constraints, and increasing amounts of the statutory work associated with child abuse. As a result social workers now have far less time for counselling work and many practice attachments have been withdrawn.

The National Marriage Guidance Council, now Relate, started to place some of their counsellors in group practices and health centres in the 1970s. By the mid 1980s about half the local councils were involved in such schemes (National Marriage Guidance Council 1985). There were a variety of funding arrangements; the counsellors were not usually employed directly by the practice, and may or may not have made a contribution towards the cost of the premises, but they were often able to make a small charge to the patient on a sliding scale, just as they would have done on their own premises. More recently, local councils have been able to negotiate funding directly through the FHSA or with fund-holding practices, and there are now an estimated 170 Relate counsellors currently working in general practice (Relate, personal communication). Some social workers and Relate counsellors who have become very interested in counselling in general practice, have negotiated individual contracts and funding directly through the practices, continuing their work and expanding their hours in the process. Mental health teams have developed numbers of different attachments for clinical psychologists, psychotherapists, community psychiatric nurses, and, in a few instances, psychiatrists. Their work is usually a combination of assessment and treatment and they are often helpful in providing direct access to hospital-based services, if appropriate. These attachments are usually funded by the health authority, but there are also examples of imaginative schemes of joint funding between a health authority, an FHSA, and a practice. A worker may be attached to three or four practices and also retain a base in the community mental health unit where he or she has supervision and is in contact with other mental health team workers.

Many of these attachments have flourished; some have only been a limited success. In their guidelines for counsellors working as part of a medical team in primary care, the National Marriage Guidance Council (1985) warns that only experienced counsellors should be deployed. This acknowledges the complexity of the work in general practice, the diverse nature of the problems the patients bring, and the complexity of relationships within the primary health care team. They recognize the problems for professionals working within different conceptual frameworks and are concerned about potential professional isolation and dilution of a counselling approach if dominated by a medical model. Unfortunately, the health centre building programme was curtailed in the 1980s and the development of premises became almost entirely the responsibility of individual general practitioners. Lack of adequate accommodation, particularly in inner city areas, is now a significant obstacle to the expansion of a wide variety of services, including counselling, in general practice.

THE EMPLOYMENT OF PRACTICE COUNSELLORS

Counselling as a profession has expanded rapidly in the last ten years and the British Association of Counselling (BAC) enrolled its 10000th member in May 1993. The first reference to a practice counsellor was made by

Marsh and Barr (1975)—by practice counsellor we mean someone who has had training in counselling or psychotherapy and is working in a practice primarily, and usually solely, as a counsellor. In the late 1980s, a few FHSAs started to recognize counsellors and were prepared to reimburse 70 per cent of their pay. This provided a major impetus to employment and was widely publicized in the weekly magazines for general practitioners. Other interested practices were encouraged to pressurize their own FHSAs to follow suit. In 1988 the Royal College of General Practitioners published an occasional paper on counselling in general practice (McLeod 1988) and later devoted one of its clinical series to the same subject (RCGP 1992), thereby acknowledging important developments in this area. The counselling in Medical Settings (CMS) division of the BAC helpfully published guidelines for counsellors working in practices (Rowland and Hurd 1985) and for general practitioners employing a counsellor (Irving and Health 1985) which have just been revised (CMS 1993). These raise issues of competency and accreditation, supervision, access to records and record keeping, confidentiality, communication, and terms and conditions of employment including professional insurance and ultimate clinical responsibility.

It is difficult to trace accurately the growth in the number of practice counsellors over the years. In the past, most FHSAs did not recognize counsellors for the staff reimbursement scheme and so they were employed in a number of ways which has made them hard to identify. Quite a few worked on an entirely voluntary basis with no external record of their existence. Others were employed by practices as 'receptionists', their pay made up by claiming more hours than they actually worked. A few were paid directly by the patients. It is likely that the number of practice counsellors overall runs parallel to the membership of the Counselling in Medical Settings (CMS) division of the BAC. CMS had 319 members in 1985, 408 in 1989, with a big increase to 704 members in 1992 (BAC/CMS personal communication 1993). The total number of practice counsellors will have been perhaps two or three times more than this, as not all are members of CMS, but the figures do give some idea of the trend in the last eight years.

Sibbald *et al.* (1993) surveyed about one in 20 general practices in England and Wales to ascertain accurately, for the first time, the number and distribution of practice counsellors. Of these 134 (9 per cent) of 1542 practices had a practice counsellor—giving an estimate of 2600 practice counsellors altogether in England and Wales. Overall 484 (31 per cent) of practices had one or more people undertaking counselling as a distinct activity; 95 (6 per cent) had a clinical psychologist, 181 (12 per cent) a community psychiatric nurse, and 74 (5 per cent) a variety of other people, including practice nurses and health visitors. Large practices and training practices were more likely to offer a counselling service. Health regions showed considerable variation in the provision of practice counsellors and clinical psychologists, with high levels in Mersey, North-Western, Northern, and South-Western regions. This is probably related to patterns of funding, with increased probability where FHSAs reimbursed the counsellors' costs. The main barriers to providing counselling reported in this study were financial constraints and lack of space.

Choosing a counsellor

If a practice wants to set up a counselling service, how do they go about it? Different trainings, expertise, and interest among counsellors and therapists can be quite confusing. The quality of the relationships the counsellor establishes with the patients is most important, critically influencing the success of therapy. The counsellor's personality and capacity to learn and adapt to the demands of general practice, and the ability to work as a member of a team, are as important as professional qualifications.

Many attachments are opportunistic. The practice may be approached by a qualified counsellor who works privately in the area and is interested in extending his/her experience in primary care (a problem if the counsellor is also a patient of the practice). Alternatively, local health authorities and voluntary agencies seeking attachments may approach practices to find out who is interested and has the necessary resources to accommodate a counsellor. Training institutions are increasingly keen to find a variety of work placements for trainee counsellors under supervision, and may contact local practices.

A practice which is actively seeking to employ a counsellor would do well to contact their FHSA and find out if they, or anybody else locally, has an interest in practice counselling. We suspect that most appointments are made through local connections and personal recommendation, rather than through formal advertising. The Department of General Practice at King's, has run a successful scheme where interested practices were put in touch with local counsellors, providing guidelines for their employment, and running a group to support the work. Several FHSAs have established schemes to promote counselling in general practice. JW has worked with Kensington and Chelsea FHSA to foster counsellor attachments and promote discussion of their work. Derbyshire, Oxfordshire, and Cambridgeshire FHSAs have all drawn up guidelines for the employment of counsellors, helped with appointments, provided access to supervision, and organized groups and workshops for general practitioners and counsellors working together. The BAC standards of accreditation are helpful as a baseline for competency, and the local branch of the BAC can provide useful contacts (see also Chapter 4).

HOW DO COUNSELLORS WORK IN
GENERAL PRACTICE?

Developing relationships and learning a common language

There has been little work to date which explores the progress of attachments and what makes them flourish or founder. When professionals from two different disciplines come to work together, they need to understand, value, and trust each other if they are to provide effective patient care. We would like to draw on our experience to discuss some areas which may be problematic, in the belief that if they are acknowledged and thought about, a closer and more productive relationship can evolve.

There may be real interprofessional problems of rivalry—who does the patient love most? In addition, there may be envy of the amount of protected time a counsellor has with a patient, misunderstanding confounded by the use of jargon, and fear of seeming ignorant about the others' field of expertise. Both doctor and counsellor can feel de-skilled, imagining the other to be better at meeting the patients' needs. Each may fantasize that the other can deal with difficult problems more easily, and with less stress. There may be mutual anxieties about professional competence, professional responsibility for the patient, and confidentiality.

Doctors have relationships with their patients extending over many years. They can feel reluctant to share their patients with others for fear of spoiling the relationship they have built. They may feel that they should be able to deal with the patients' distress themselves and that they are letting the patient down if they refer them to somebody else. They may be sceptical about counselling, or know little about it and when it might be appropriate for a patient.

Counsellors and therapists come from a variety of backgrounds and differ widely in the amount and type of training they have had. Einzig *et al.* (1992), in a survey of 24 organizations running BAC registered, or equivalent, counselling courses, found that only one had specifically incorporated issues pertinent to counselling in primary care into their course. Another ran a postgraduate supervision training programme for counsellors working in general practice. The counsellors' previous experience may have been quite narrow and it may be difficult, initially, to assess and work with the very wide range of patients who present in general practice. The medical model can be quite overwhelming and the counsellor may feel isolated in the work, particularly if he/she is not in touch with other practice counsellors, or does not have adequate supervision. The experience of working alone in private practice is very different to working in a team, and entrenchment in a specific theoretical orientation may result in blinkering.

If doctor and counsellor are to find a way to work together and 'learn a common language', they need to be flexible, have a willingness to learn from each other, and be open to new ideas. It is essential to make time to meet to reflect on how the attachment is going, discuss the patients who have been referred, and look at the outcome of the counsellor's assessments, for instance decisions about treatment, and work. One of the main reasons for an attachment failing to reach its full potential, is when there is inadequate protected time to discuss these issues properly. The busy general practitioner is usually the culprit. We suggest that the fleeting communications in the corridor, which are so common in general practice, are of limited use and are an effective way of avoiding real discussion of some of the difficult and painful issues which arise when dealing with emotional problems. It often takes a year or two for a counsellor to settle into a practice and develop an effective way of working. This is a real difficulty with short-term student placements.

Models of working

We have identified two main models of working, characterized by variation in the boundaries of confidentiality. Whatever the boundaries of confidentiality are, they should be made explicit, and the patient's consent sought before information is shared on any level. In the first model, the counsellor–patient dyad is the prime relationship and strict confidentiality is maintained within it. Information about patients at the time of referral is minimal; their names may simply be entered into the counsellor's appointment book. The counsellor does not discuss the case with the referring doctor except possibly to say when the counselling is starting and finishing. The model is very common in counselling outside general practice and may be used at the beginning of an attachment as all parties feel their way. If it continues, it is likely to severely restrict the potential of an attachment and there is a danger that the counsellor becomes a dumping ground for patients whom the doctors find most difficult. The counsellor can become isolated, struggling in vain with these patients, as there is no structure for talking about what is going on. Professionals may use confidentiality as a screen to hide behind and avoid confronting some of the difficult issues and feelings we have discussed, which a closer working relationship entails.

In our second model, the counsellor is truly part of an interdisciplinary team of general practitioners, practice nurses, health visitors, and others who are involved in the joint management of patients. Confidentiality is maintained within the boundaries of the practice as a whole. The counsellor is interested in the information and feelings the referring doctor has about a patient, is prepared to share his/her own assessment and give reports on progress as appropriate. As the counselling comes to an end, a conscious effort is made to hand the patient back to the doctor. The counsellor may attend practice meetings to understand more about the life and concerns of the whole practice, and may also be called upon to help the whole practice, including receptionists, to deal with a difficult patient—the so-called 'heartsink patient' who is not going to be 'cured' but is best held and tolerated in the practice. Similarly, when the practice is distressed, say over the death of a child, or a complaint by a patient, the counsellor may help to facilitate discussion. Some counsellors might extend their role further, acting as a consultant to the practice to help with internal problems such as disagreements among partners, or informally 'lending an ear' to let a problem be aired without offering any specific advice or intervention. However, as an employee, it may be inappropriate to enter into this kind of relationship with an employer, and the counsellor may have to resist strong attempts to be drawn in. With time, good humour, and good communication, many attachments will move from the first model towards the second, with full integration of the counsellor into the primary care team.

Assessment and treatment

It is helpful to keep in mind the distinction between assessment and treatment. All too often they can become merged and counselling begins before a proper assessment of the patient's difficulties, defences, and likely ability to use counselling productively has been made. Assessment is a very important part of a counsellor's work in a practice. It can be difficult and relatively little previous experience in this area may have been gained. One of the functions of assessment is to decide which patients *not* to treat. Edwards (1983) talks of five categories of patient for whom individual counselling or psychotherapy seems to be contraindicated. They are:

1. In many cases of psychosis, borderline and latent psychosis, where dangers exist of the development of persisting psychotic transferences and the release of primitive aggression.
2. People with dependent personalities of long standing, who form attachments that cannot be resolved and for whom separation, or the threat of separation leads to disintegration.
3. People with personality disorders or psychoneuroses with rigid defences of an obsessional, paranoid, or schizoid type. There may already have been previous attempts at therapy with little change or improvement.
4. People with histrionic personalities who have shown intense acting out, self-destructive, attention-seeking, or manipulative behaviour.
5. People with severe addiction to alcohol, cannabis, or heroin.

In addition, it may not be appropriate to refer severely depressed patients who are at risk of suicide. In the process of self-exploration, patients often feel worse for a while before they begin to feel better, and the risk of self-harm may be exacerbated. Those who are severely depressed may initially be too incapacitated to be able to use therapy, and a course of antidepressant medication and/or referral to a psychiatrist may be appropriate in the beginning.

Patients in all these categories are familiar in every practice; the general practitioner cannot tell them to go away! Indeed, it is the doctor's job to provide continuing 'primary care'. An experienced counsellor can have a useful role in supporting the doctors in their management and prevent unproductive referrals to numerous outside agencies. Joint assessments can often clarify what help *can* be usefully offered, and when it is fruitless to battle against persistent defences, how dependency can be managed, and contracts made to maintain containing boundaries with manipulative patients.

Approaches to treatment will vary according to the patient's problem and the counsellor's training and skills. Cognitive techniques, anxiety management, behaviour therapy, and social skills training can all be useful. Humanistic approaches including encounter groups, co-counselling, and meditation might also be drawn on. We have noticed that as counsellors become more experienced in general practice they tend to draw on a wider range of skills and therapies, and may embark on further training to broaden their areas of expertise.

There has been much debate as to whether there is any place for long-term counselling in general practice. The fear is that the counsellor's waiting list will become too long and some general practitioners initially specify that the counsellor should only see patients for short-term work, say six sessions. Again we have found that with experience, many counsellors develop a flexible approach, quite different to that in private practice. Sometimes an assessment is enough; the patient's problem has been defined and they are happy to be returned to the general practitioner to continue to work with them. A few sessions of brief focused treatment is helpful to many, some of whom will later decide to go on to long-term therapy. After a short course of weekly treatment, some patients may continue to see the counsellor on an irregular or infrequent basis, say once a month. For others, the counsellor may leave the door open, offering to see them again in the future if they are getting into difficulty. The counsellor's work usually takes on some of the characteristics of general practice—a flexible approach to a very wide range of problems, deployment of a diversity of skills, and an open-minded attitude to the timing and frequency of sessions.

REFERRALS

Good counselling depends on good referrals. It is worth questioning why a general practitioner refers a particular patient at a particular time. Among all the patients a doctor sees with emotional problems, why does he/she choose to work with some personally, refer some to the counsellor or other agency, and ignore or do very little work with others? Some referrals are quite straightforward, but others are more problematic. We have examined our own work to determine how the power of the patient, some of the unconscious processes in the doctor, and also the environment of the practice, can all affect referrals. We would like to present our findings in some detail, as a useful way of illustrating some aspects of a counsellor's attachment to a practice.

The power of the patient

Certain groups of patients are difficult to help and are likely to arouse feelings in the doctor which are hard to manage. We all know that 'heartsink patients', whom we prefer to call 'difficult practice patients', are a problem to manage and contain in the practice. They have often been referred to a wide range of potential helpers but always appear back in the practice to persecute the doctor, and often the receptionists too! Psychosomatic patients produce symptoms as a substitute for expressing feelings and are difficult to help; counselling may exacerbate their illness. Patients with compulsive problems, for example an eating disorder, may metaphorically 'throw up' any offers of help as they are more comfortable using 'substances' to control their inner processes. Teenagers with problems may not want to attend the practice, seeing doctors and therapists as parent or authority figures against whom they must rebel. Disturbed families can be slippery as there is usually evidence of splitting within the family in terms of who really has the problem. This can make treatment and management decisions difficult. Elderly people may be neglected, as there is a common belief that older people are too set in their ways to be able to accept help and change. Ethnic minority groups are often inaccessible to 'talking help' across languages and cultures—there is much work to be done to provide more appropriate help to these groups at a primary care level. Finally, borderline/psychotic patients are bound to be difficult because their disturbance and anxiety will inevitably affect us in what can be a very confusing and disorientating way.

Tom Main (1957) explains why some kinds of patients can be difficult. They convey great suffering, but at the same time an insatiability so that 'every attention is ultimately unsatisfying'. Behind this suffering he believes that there is an inbuilt attack which demands that the helper takes what can be a masochistic responsibility—you must go on helping me as so far nothing you have done is making me better.

In psychodynamic language, we are in the area of transference and counter-transference. Jung (1966) talked about the 'old idea of the demon of sickness'. According to this, a sufferer can transmit his/her disease to a healthy person whose powers then subdue the demon. He also used the analogy of a chemical reaction, between doctor and patient which implies not only possible change in the patient, but a necessary preparedness for change in the helper if the patient is to get well. The doctor needs to try and find a way of handling the emotions aroused in him/her by the patient, to tolerate misrepresentation and even attack, and may need to sacrifice his/her own wishes for speedy, definitive returns.

Freud and Jung recognized the importance of the transference, that is the patient's unconscious tendency to project parts of the self and inner world into the helper, but it is only since the 1940s that countertransference, that is the helper's response to the patient's transference, has been the subject of serious scrutiny. Jung (1966) felt it futile for the helper to erect defences of a professional kind against the influence of the patient: 'by doing so he only denies himself the use of a highly important organ of information'.

Patients are bound to affect the doctor. If the doctor can reflect on this and think about what belongs to the patient and what is part of the doctor's own inner world, it can help in the assessment of the patient. Hopefully, the doctor can take on board the painful, inner problem of the patient, understand and assimilate it, and then give it back to the patient in a repaired form whereby the patient can then understand and integrate it in a creative way. At times, the power of the patient may be such that the doctor's capacity to think and reflect is impaired. This can lead to the substitution of action for thought and the possibility of a hasty referral.

An example of a powerful patient

We would like to present a case example where unconscious factors inhibited appropriate courses of action which would have been in the patient's best interests. It took place when we were working together as general practitioner and counsellor in an inner London group practice.

Case history 1

The patient, whom we shall call Michael, was 28-years-old and is homosexual. He was diagnosed as having insulin-dependent diabetes in his late teens. When he registered with the practice he was initially seen by the trainee, who was anxious about him and asked one of the partners to see him. His diabetes was badly out of control, he was eating compulsively, running dangerously high blood-sugar levels, and failing to monitor his diabetes most of the time. He was depressed, almost suicidal, and felt that he could not manage to sustain a sexual relationship. He felt that nobody loved him and he was clearly in a vulnerable state. He generated considerable anxiety in the doctor who sought out the counsellor with a degree of urgency asking her to see Michael as soon as possible. He had activated in the doctor a strong wish to help and she felt that he might be a suicide risk. He was chaotic, out of control, and appeared to be unmanageable.

He introduced himself to the counsellor as 'diabetic, half-blind, and queer'. Michael was a very striking, rather feminine-looking man who always wore black clothes and dyed his hair blonde. He talked about his eating problems and his frequent wish to binge. He worked irregular hours in a restaurant, was always surrounded by food and drink, and had no proper meals. He felt that he could not make relationships, and had only had one relationship of any significance in the previous five years. Significantly he did not stress his diabetes at all to the counsellor. She thought about the possibility of long-term psychotherapy for him and decided to see him herself in the practice for a few sessions to explore his problems in making relationships.

It was only when the doctor and counsellor presented Michael at a consultation seminar that they realized that Michael was slowly committing suicide by failing to take responsibility for his diabetes. He was splitting off his illness, failing to own it. This self-destructive activity had led to some collusion from both the doctor and counsellor who were paying more attention to his relationship problems than to his physical illness. The main and immediate problem of his diabetes had been by-passed. Having understood this, the doctor and counsellor decided to try to actively manage him jointly in the practice. They saw Michael together and set up a contract whereby he would see the doctor and counsellor alternately once a fortnight. The doctor would focus on establishing a programme to help him to control his diabetes; the counsellor would focus on why he was abusing himself in such a way.

He attended his therapy sessions, but failed to come to most of his appointments with the doctor, perpetuating the split which we had observed. The joint management was, therefore, not really successful and he remained out of control. However, he was held in the practice, and may have gained something from the relationship with the practice. Eventually he moved away, but did ask the counsellor to help him to find a general practitioner in his new area.

This example shows how an unconscious split in the patient between physical and emotional problems can lead the doctor and counsellor to become split in similar ways. This might be called a neurotic countertransference reaction in the professionals. Michael is the kind of patient who is likely to arouse conflicting feelings. The doctor felt a great deal of urgency, the counsellor took a longer-term view. The doctor was dealing with blood sugars and the practicalities of self-monitoring and giving insulin injections in the restaurant environment, while the counsellor focused on the patient's sexuality and relationships, knowing little about the ins and outs of diabetes. The professionals might have become seriously split if they had not worked together or if they had erected defences under the guise of confidentiality. However, Michael actually helped them to become more conscious of what they were doing, which led to attempts to work more closely together in a mutually supportive way, and offer him better care. It is often these patients who present a 'muddle' and generate intense feelings, from whom most can be learned.

We might expect that practice counsellors would see quite a number of patients with serious physical illness, for example patients dealing with the stress and anxiety of a newly diagnosed condition may well benefit from counselling, as may those living with the difficulties of long-term illness or disability, and this is explored further in Chapter 11. However, talking with many counsellors, we have the impression that very few patients with physical illness are in fact referred. Perhaps doctors are consciously or unconsciously anxious about the potential split of mind and body, counsellor and doctor. The doctor may feel unhappy about being left to deal with the physical concerns of the patient while somebody else supposedly deals with the emotional aspects of their illness. Very few counsellors have any specific training in working with people with physical illness and they may not feel very confident to do so. The doctor may be reluctant to refer the patient, seeing the counsellor as inexperienced in this area. Training programmes need to address this issue and it is worth thinking about this area when styles of referral are being reviewed.

Unconscious factors in the doctor and counsellor which affect referrals

One of the strongest pressures on general practitioners is to 'do something', to take some action which will make the patient better. To achieve a cure is one of the main objectives of a medical approach. As Tom Main says, 'cured patients do great service to their attendants' (Main 1957). The treatment of psychological problems is not so much about cure, but rather about trying to help people to understand themselves better so that they can manage their lives more effectively. A psychodynamic approach places great value on subjective rather than objective knowing, so that the doctor's personal responses to the patient may be used as a valuable tool for diagnosis and treatment. For instance if the doctor feels depressed by a patient, it is likely that the patient is depressed too; similarly if the doctor feels very angry, the patient may well be feeling, but not expressing, anger. However, using our own antennae can be tricky because, as we have outlined, some patients overwhelm us with their feelings whereas others are inaccessible.

Patients can stir up the feelings of the doctor or counsellor in a number of different ways. Crudely, there are two different responses which may be made:

1. *The omnipotent approach*: rushing around trying to do everything. This may foster over-dependent relationships and encourage patients to project too much power into the doctor and not take responsibility for their own difficulties.
2. *The defensive approach*: switching off from the patient's distress. Reaching for the prescription pad is one way of avoiding the Pandora's box

of emotional problems; concentrating on physical symptoms, investigations, and referrals is another. We could view the six-minute consultation as a device to avoid really getting to know our patients.

We have found that the following groups of patients can have a powerful effect, sometimes making the doctor or counsellor behave uncharacteristically:

1. Psychosomatic patients can generate anxiety about the possibility of missing real physical disease
2. Patients who present problems of such enormity and great urgency can be overwhelming and create intense pressure to do something immediately (Michael is a good example).
3. Seriously depressed patients can project their depression, paralysing the professionals, and engendering feelings of hopelessness.
4. Self-destructive patients, including patients with addictions, can be very disturbing and feel intolerable.
5. Professionals may enjoy a certain amount of dependency from patients because it makes them feel needed, but they may well feel anxious and uneasy when dealing with very highly dependent and vulnerable patients.
6. Sometimes the patient's problem is too close to home—for instance, a recent bereavement of their own may make it very difficult for the professional to work with bereaved patients for a while.
7. Patients who are out of touch with their feelings can leave the professionals feeling helpless and out of touch too.
8. Professionals may 'act out' in response to a very likeable patient, in an attempt to make it all better; this is not actually in the patient's best interest.
9. Finally, there are those patients who, for one reason or another, the doctor or counsellor simply does not like or want to help.

When the doctor can share some of the thoughts and feelings about a patient, it can help the counsellor to understand why that particular patient is being referred. Together they can then think about the potential doctor/patient/counsellor relationship. It may become clear that the referral is more to do with how the doctor feels than what the patient wants or needs. Sometimes the counsellor can help the doctor to deal with the feelings the patient is projecting into him/her, enabling useful work to continue with the patient without making a referral. At other times the counsellor may agree to see the patient for a while, until the doctor is able to tolerate and work with the patient again. It is important to remember that patients have chosen to bring their emotional problems to the doctor and an immediate referral to somebody else may leave them feeling rejected and pushed on, before they have taken the important step of putting what is troubling them into words, in the presence of someone else.

Sometimes referrals to the counsellor seem to be 'inappropriate', or the patient does not turn up. In our own work, we found a number of these patients who seemed to have been pushed by the doctor to see the counsellor because the doctor was finding difficulty in working with the patient often for one of the reasons listed above. Unless this is understood, the counsellor may well have the feeling of being 'dumped' with impossible patients, and the doctor/counsellor relationship may be harmed. On the other hand, if feelings about very difficult patients can be acknowledged, they can be used constructively to make diagnoses and appropriate management plans. The doctor/counsellor relationship may be enhanced and more patients managed effectively on a long-term basis within the practice.

An example of unconscious factors in the doctor affecting referrals

The following illustrates what can happen when a doctor is unable to separate his/her own difficulties from the patients', leading to a series of 'inappropriate' referrals.

Case history 2

A woman doctor referred a series of women to a counsellor, with what the doctor called 'eating problems'; many of these women were mildly overweight. Most of them were not motivated to seek help, in fact they did not see themselves as having a problem with eating or their weight. They felt that they had been told by the doctor that they ought to see the counsellor. It took some time to realize that the doctor was herself getting thinner and thinner, verging on anorexia! In this case the issue was not addressed directly between the counsellor and doctor as it seemed too much of an intrusion on the doctor. However, having understood what was happening, the counsellor was able to let the patients leave without worrying too much about them.

Practice dynamics and their effect on referrals

When we looked at our own referrals, we realized that in some cases the patients and their particular problems mirrored some of the problems the doctors were experiencing in the practice as a whole. The following examples illustrate how a patient may become a symptom of the practice dynamics.

Case history 3

One of the female partners, who had been in the practice for about six months, began to refer a number of middle-aged, depressed women who were struggling to make a life for themselves after their children had left home. In many cases their husbands were emotionally unavailable. The counsellor began to realize that some of these women did not really want to see her, but had been 'sent' by the doctor. The counsellor had a good relationship with this doctor and it was possible to talk about what was going on. What emerged was that the doctor had been left with a large number of older, middle-class women when another woman partner left the practice. When asked why she was making all these referrals, the new doctor came to see that she was experiencing difficulty with these women because they reminded her of her own mother, who had recently been widowed. The referrals reflected some of the difficulties experienced by the practice in adjusting to changes in the partnership, as well as something of the doctor's personal struggles with her internal world.

Case history 4

A second incident arose at a time when there was a period of intense conflict in the practice, making it extremely difficult for the doctors to work together, and leading eventually to the practice splitting up. Some of the conflict centred on major financial problems. Within a 2-month-period, two patients were referred for assessment: one was in danger of being declared bankrupt; the other was involved with shady, possibly fraudulent dealings!

Isabel Menzies Lyth's work on containing anxiety in institutions is helpful here (Menzies Lyth 1988). She believes that primitive anxieties are always present in any organization or social structure. Influenced by the writings of Melanie Klein and Wilfred Bion, she explores how the very structure of an institution can be seen as a form of defence, designed to avoid or minimize personal experiences of doubt, guilt, anxiety, and uncertainty. However, at times, the structure is actually anti-supportive to staff: 'the need of the members of the organization to use it in the struggle against anxiety leads to the development of socially structured defence mechanisms, which appear as elements in the organization's structure, culture and mode of functioning'. 'Busyness' in general practice is surely a good example of a defence against uncertainty and anxiety.

In each of the above examples, where events in the practice and the particular difficulties faced by each doctor are affecting referrals, time can be wasted in the pursuit of a course of action which leads into a cul-de-sac. The doctor may not consciously make the link between what is going on and the way patients are being dealt with; the patients do not understand why they are being referred; the counsellor may wonder about patterns in referral. Clearly it is helpful if the counsellor is sufficiently immersed in the practice to know something about what is going on. Reviewing referrals, and finding time to reflect and talk about them is a most effective way of minimizing the often unconscious actions which are actually unhelpful to patients.

Outside influences on referrals

Although our main focus is on unconscious and internal forces, both within the doctor and within the practice, we would like to make some reference to the changes taking place in general practice and the NHS, and how these can affect referrals for counselling and therapy. Since the new contract, general practitioners have had to devote considerable time and energy to developing new financial and management strategies to implement the ever-changing government requirements. This may have left some doctors with diminished personal resources to devote to patients who are asking for extra time and attention to help with emotional problems. Our own experience is that, sadly, more time is now spent talking about administrative problems and much less about patients and their care. At the same time we know that the recession with its attendant increase in unemployment and poverty adversely affects the physical and emotional health of our patients, whose needs are becoming greater.

Menzies Lyth (1988) makes the point that public and government pressures can place incompatible demands on what she calls 'the humane institutions', that is those who deal with human beings as their throughput. A general practice may be said to have custodial, therapeutic, and financial objectives. Trying to meet one set of objectives may seriously inhibit success in achieving others. This can lead to confusion and doubt.

Recent media coverage suggests that stress is an increasing problem for doctors. Personal pressure, lack of resources in health and social services, and seemingly overwhelming need among patients can lead the stressed doctor into an ever more narrow, tunnel-vision view of the range of possible avenues available to help the patient. Lethargy and repetitive behaviour which result from stress tend to restrict the doctor's capacity to think imaginatively and discuss possible options with the patient. The doctor may unconsciously avoid discussion of emotional issues and fail to diagnose depression and anxiety in his patients. Or, he may make rather hasty referrals, be it to a counsellor or a hospital out-patient clinic, to try to relieve himself of some of the patients and their problems. Working closely with a counsellor, sharing some of the stress, discussing patient assessments and possible management options, can be a creative way of getting out of the tunnel and into the light.

CHANGES IN A COUNSELLOR'S WORK OVER A PERIOD OF TIME

After two years of working together in the practice, we decided to look in detail at our referrals as we were interested in what sorts of patients had been referred and why, and what had happened to them when they came to see the counsellor. Over the two years the three doctors had made 101

Table 2.1 *Referrals from general practitioners to a counsellor in one practice; comparison of two 2-year intervals*

	Number of patients	
	1988/9	1990/1
1. Assessment and referral for long-term work—taken up	28	14
2. Assessment and referral for long-term work—NOT taken up	14	3
3. Assessment followed by short-term work in the practice	12	25
4. Assessment followed by joint management with a doctor in the practice	14	20
5. Assessment only—patient expressed no wish for further help	14	16
6. Patient left in the middle of the initial assessment	11	11
7. Patient failed to attend the initial assessment	8	12
Total number of patients seen in each 2-year-period	101	101

referrals to the counsellor, who was employed for four hours a week in a practice with approximately 6000 patients. Two years later we repeated the same exercise to see if the patterns of work had changed over the course of time. The outcome of referrals in the first two years, and again two years later, are presented for comparison in Table 2.1.

The limited number of hours that JW, the counsellor, was employed restricted her almost entirely to assessment and short-term work although, there were a few patients whom she saw intermittently, and one patient she took on privately. This last case was unusual as there was a policy to refer patients elsewhere for private treatment, but it was felt that this particular patient would benefit from continuing care in the practice.

The most significant change over the four-year-period was that as time went on, fewer patients were referred outside the practice for long-term work. Also, the counsellor took longer to make her initial assessment and took on a greater proportion of patients for short-term work. She became more flexible in her approach to treatment, and more difficult patients were taken on for active joint management with the general practitioner. The doctors also became more confident in their ability to assess and manage patients themselves and more open to talking about some of their patients with the counsellor, without actually referring them. The number of patients for whom assessment, or incomplete assessment, was either enough or perhaps too much, remained constant. Interestingly, the number of patients who failed to turn up remained about the same too, although we had expected it might decrease.

Over time, the doctors and counsellor began to learn a common language. The doctors developed a more realistic understanding of what the counsellor could, and could not, do. The counsellor came to understand the milieu of general practice and appreciate the doctors' work, particularly with patients who had long-term difficulties. Time was made to review the work, discuss problems, learn from mistakes, and understand each other's strengths and weaknesses. The relationship with the counsellor as part of the practice team was valued more and more, not only by the doctors but by the paramedical staff and receptionists as well. Her role broadened into a wider ranging consultancy to the practice as a whole.

SUPPORT FOR GENERAL PRACTITIONERS AND COUNSELLORS WORKING TOGETHER

Support for doctors

Those who work with patients and support them in trying to untangle, understand, and make progress with difficult psychological and emotional problems, owe it to themselves and to their patients to find the best avenues of support for themselves. We believe that general practice has much to learn from counselling and psychotherapy, where it is the norm to seek consultation for day-to-day work issues arising with clients and colleagues. Counsellors and therapists expect to discuss their cases in detail, either with an individual supervisor and/or in group seminars, in order to disentangle what belongs to the client and what belongs to them. They hope to be helped to think imaginatively about the client, and creatively about possible interventions and options for treatment. Many will have been in therapy themselves and had the opportunity to explore and hopefully come to terms with past painful experiences, and are thus less likely to unconsciously project their feelings into others. All this can of course stir up envy amongst doctors, most of whom are aware of the stress they are under and their own unmet needs, and which might alienate them from counsellors and therapists. Alternatively, doctors can learn from the therapy model and work to develop more supportive structures for themselves.

Within the medical profession, general practitioners have done more in this respect than any other specialty, but many still feel quite isolated and lonely in their work. What avenues are open for general practitioners to express their own needs? Some confide in spouses or partners at home, but endless stories of patients and intrigues in the practice can place stress on personal relationships. Colleagues can be helpful, particularly if there is enough time to talk and the doctors are prepared to reveal something of their own feelings. This can be difficult in competitive partnerships when discussing problems might feel tantamount to admitting failure, ignorance, or incompetence. 'Young practitioner groups' which often arise from vocational training schemes, and 'trainer groups', can provide a forum for discussion, but they are often limited by focusing on topics or administrative problems—anything in fact to avoid actually discussing the doctor himself. An external facilitator who is experienced in group dynamics can help these groups to move on. Balint groups have provided many doctors over the years with opportunities to discuss cases; however their existence is patchy. They have thrived in North London, for example, but there has never been a group in South London. A few general practitioners seek supervision to pursue a specialist area such as family therapy or dealing with drug addiction, and an unknown number are in therapy themselves. We know of some practices which have employed external facilitators to help to sort out problems within the practice and partnership, with various degrees of success.

General practitioner/counsellor case discussion groups

Both authors have personal experience of groups for general practitioners and counsellors working together. One was established as part of a project in the Department of General Practice, King's College, London, to facilitate counselling in general practice, and was co-led by JD and a practice counsellor. The other, in which the authors participated together, was set up in Parkside Clinic, a National Health Service psychotherapy clinic in Paddington, London. The clinic organized placements for trainee therapists in local practices and invited the general practitioners to attend a fortnightly seminar together with the therapists and two facilitators. In some areas, FHSAs have made it a condition of funding that the doctors and counsellors should attend meetings at the FHSA to discuss how the attachments are working.

There can be difficulties when trying to convene such a group which brings people from two professions together. We have found that levels of experience and sophistication in a group environment vary. Counsellors are much more used to this sort of activity and more open to revealing information about themselves and patients. The first group found it very difficult to discuss cases. When a doctor and counsellor were invited to talk about a joint patient, the doctor often said little, underestimating his/her own assessment of the patient and deferring to the counsellor. Clearly many doctors and counsellors found little time to communicate in the practice, and were embarrassed to say things which ideally would have been talked about beforehand. Anxieties about confidentiality, and reluctance to comment on a case referred by another doctor in the practice who was not there, also surfaced. The group often got side-tracked into focusing on topics and generalities, exchanging information on local resources, and discussing terms and conditions of employment. This had its uses—very low rates of pay were upgraded, and doctors were persuaded that time for discussion and supervision should be included in the counsellor's schedule. After about 18 months the doctors stopped coming to the group, saying they were too busy. The counsellors continued to meet and started to talk about cases. However, when the the GP co-leader went on maternity leave, rivalries surfaced among the counsellors about different levels of training and approaches to their work, and the group finally broke up.

The Parkside group has continued to meet and does manage to discuss cases. This may be because the counsellors/therapists are themselves a cohesive group. They also meet independently, and have a forum outside the joint group where they can discuss some of the difficulties of working in general practice. The Parkside group has similar difficulties in sustaining the interest and attendance of general practitioners.

Groups are potentially useful to facilitate the learning of a common language, but the difficulties of getting two professions to really talk and share their work should not be underestimated. These are not supervision groups; there is a fine line to tread to facilitate discussion at a useful level, without members risking too much or having expectations of the group which cannot be fulfilled. Powerful emotions may be unleashed and distress can be evident, particularly in those who have nowhere else to share some of the difficulties in their work. Some of these feelings may need to be dealt with elsewhere. The group leaders need to be experienced and be able to manage this.

Conferences and workshops

The authors have instigated a number of workshops and conferences over recent years. The staff team has always comprised a group of thera- pists and general practitioners working together. Initially this involved a collaboration between staff at the Parkside Clinic and the Department of General Practice and Primary Care, King's College. More recently Jungian analysts who are members of the Society of Analytical Psychol- ogy have worked closely with staff from King's and some local general practitioner trainers to evolve a model of work based on psychodynamic thinking.

We have held several national conferences for general practitioners and counsellors working together, to explore the potential for work in general practice and the relationship between doctors and counsellors. Participants have come from all over the country, many feeling quite isolated in their own areas. There is clearly scope for more local work- shops and for the establishment of a network of support among interested practices.

Organizations interested in counselling in primary care

A number of organizations interested in facilitating the development of counselling in primary care are listed in Appendix 3.2.

SUMMARY

Employing a practice counsellor can facilitate the work of general practice in a number of ways. The counsellor is a direct resource for patients, providing assessment, short-term work, and sometimes a longer-term relationship. The counsellor can support the doctors and others in the practice in managing patients, particularly those we refer to as 'difficult practice patients' who are best looked after in general practice. We have shown how, as a member of the team, and by looking at patterns of referral the counsellor can develop insight into the practice dynamics. The counsellor may be able to help the practice to deal constructively with difficult situations, particularly when they affect patient care—as they usually do. We consider the most useful input can be in terms of ways of thinking about problems, using a psychodynamic approach, and being imaginative about what sorts of help might be available.

Time needs to be devoted to fostering the relationship between counsellors and primary care. The full potential of a counsellor may not be realized in a practice for a couple of years as it takes a while to learn a common language. In time, members of the practice may become more orientated towards a counselling model, take more time to reflect on what is going on and think more about their own and others' feelings.

APPENDIX 2.1

PRACTICALITIES OF EMPLOYING A COUNSELLOR

The BAC guidelines (BAC 1993) are an excellent basis for good practice. We would like to refer briefly to a few issues which we have found can cause some difficulties and are worth considering and discussing, particularly at the beginning of an attachment.

Terms of employment

All employees need a proper contract, stating hours of work, rates of pay, sick pay entitlement, notice, grievance procedures, and so on. Sometimes those employed on a very part-time basis seem to miss out on this, but the doctor does have a legal responsibility. More difficult questions such as exactly how the counsellor is to work, and what the balance between assessment, short-term and long-term work is to be, are harder to write down and may change. There may be an initial struggle between the counsellor and the doctors about the style of work, which will usually settle down in time. The counsellor's hours need to include not only time to see patients but also time to talk to doctors and attend meetings, time to write up notes and do other administrative tasks, and time for supervision.

Confidentiality and record keeping

Most practices include the counsellor within the boundary of confidentiality of the whole practice and allow him/her to see the patients' medical record. We have found it helpful if the counsellor makes an entry in the notes when the counselling starts, when the patient is seen, and when the counselling finishes. It is also extremely useful to know if the patient does not attend, as they often come to see the doctor instead, who can then discuss with them why they have not taken up the offer of counselling. A few patients may not want any record of their visits to a counsellor to be in the medical notes.

All counsellors should keep proper records of their work. It would be extremely unusual for these to be kept in the patient's notes, and a locked filing cabinet needs to be provided in the practice for the counsellor's private use. Under the Data Protection act patients have a right to see their medical records. It is unclear as to whether this would include the notes of a counsellor employed by the practice, but it is probably safest to assume that it might. The amount of written information passing between doctor and counsellor seems to vary enormously. The initial referral may be a detailed typed letter, or just a name in an appointment book. Some counsellors copy their initial assessment to the doctor, and/or write a summary when the counselling is finished; others communicate nothing at all in writing.

The boundaries of confidentiality vary considerably among practices; whatever they are, they need to be explained to the patient at the beginning of any counselling. Broadly, confidentiality can be approached in two ways. Either the counsellor does not discuss or pass on anything without specifically asking for the patient's consent in each instance; or the confidentiality is shared with the doctor, or the practice. In the latter case the patient can expect the counsellor to discuss whatever is appropriate; the patient can stipulate if there are specific things which are to remain entirely confidential to the counsellor. Should the counsellor also tell the patient about their own supervision, and perhaps about case discussions outside the practice if they attend groups or seminars? When would confidentiality be broken because of worries about risks to the patient, or to a third party? These issues need to be discussed.

The counsellor may experience conflicting loyalties. He/she is responsible not only to the patient, but also to the doctors and other members of the primary health care team as colleagues, and to the doctors and the FHSA as employers and funders. The counsellor is professionally account-able to the appropriate training/validating organization, to their supervisor and to society as a whole. The interests of all these different bodies may conflict and vary from the belief systems of the counsellor. At times conflict between the interests of the practice as a whole, and of the individual patient, may be experienced.

Space and privacy

Some practices find it extraordinarily difficult to provide the counsellor with a room which is sound-proofed and free from interruptions. Is it the hurly-burly culture of general practice which leads people to constantly burst in with, 'Oh I'm sorry I didn't realize you were here', or an unconscious desire to find out what is really going on between counsellor and patient? Peace and quiet are essential. A counsellor usually prefers to work in one room, and clinical equipment such as sphygmomanometers, needles and syringes, and bare couches are best removed or covered up. There need to be a couple of armchairs and enough distance between them to feel comfortable—whatever the pressure on space, counselling cannot really be done in a cupboard! Like other staff, the counsellor needs to be able to summon aid quickly should the patient become very disturbed; many practices now have panic buttons in all their rooms.

Referral

Patients may make an appointment with the counsellor in a number of ways. In some practices the doctor refers to the counsellor, who then gets in touch with the patients by letter or phone. In others, after talking to the doctor, the patients are asked to fill in a short form giving their personal details and a brief outline of why they would like to see a counsellor. Asking patients to take this initiative may eliminate those who do not really want counselling. Some practices have an appointment book at reception, and patients can refer themselves. Whichever method is adopted, the need for confidentiality and privacy must be thought through. One patient described the process in his practice—'I would have had to stick my head through the hatch, a small hole about three foot square with a guillotine like shutter which comes down to close it, and shout to one of the receptionists that I wanted to see the counsellor, so that everybody in the office would know.' Not surprisingly he decided not to. We found one practice was planning, unwittingly, for an HIV counsellor to be in the surgery at the same time as the antenatal clinic. It became clear that a man waiting to see the counsellor among so many pregnant women would be very conspicuous, so a different time for the counsellor's session had to be found.

Clinical responsibility and insurance

The vexed question of 'who is ultimately responsible for the patient' inevitably arises. Perhaps the answer is that the patients are ultimately responsible for themselves! However, this would not be very helpful in a court of law, so clinical responsibility needs to be discussed and agreement reached as to whether confidentiality can be broken, if say the patient was thought to be at risk of suicide, or revealed some kind of abuse of a third party. Every professional is responsible for his or her own work. As a professional, a counsellor should be covered by personal insurance. Who pays for this has to be negotiated with the practice. By making a referral, the doctor may be seen to be *delegating* part of his/her work to the practice counsellor, thereby remaining ultimately responsible for the care of that patient.

Funding

Funding practice counsellors has always been a problem. We have mentioned that some were employed as 'receptionists', and others worked on an entirely voluntary basis. With the development and professionalization of counselling, voluntary work in general practice is now rather discouraged, being seen to undermine the role of the counsellor, when all the other primary care staff are properly paid. Working on a voluntary basis may also mean that the counsellor has no funds to pay for personal therapy or supervision, which might be neglected. The exception are students on placements, who would be expected to have supervision from their training organization.

Half the practice counsellors identified in Sibbald's study of counsellors in England and Wales (Sibbald *et al.* 1993) were employed by the practice with reimbursement from the FHSA. In some areas practices are able to claim a direct reimbursement of a percentage of the counsellor's costs; in others, practices are allocated an overall staff budget by the FHSA to spend as they see fit. Budget-holding practices decide their own priorities for allocating money in different clinical areas. Some practices made the counsellor's sessions into 'health promotion' clinics, thereby claiming monies which more or less covered the counsellor's costs. However, from June 1993, payments for health promotion clinics have been so modified that the ability of these practices to fund counsellors in the future must remain uncertain. Other sources of funding come from voluntary organizations, such as Relate and the Mental Health Foundation, and joint schemes between health authorities or trusts, FHSAs and practices. In some practices the counsellor is funded, at least in part, by contributions from the patients.

It has to be said that the future funding of counselling in general practice is unclear, and it is likely that funding will continue to come from diverse sources. Interested practices in one area should get together and approach their FHSA to draw up a strategy to try to secure funding. Those who have already employed counsellors and are convinced of their value are likely to strive to continue to find ways and means of keeping them on.

APPENDIX 2.2

ORGANIZATIONS INTERESTED IN COUNSELLING IN PRIMARY CARE

The Society of Analytical Psychology: 1 Daleham Gardens, London NW3 5BY, Tel. 071–435–7696 and the Department of General Practice and Primary Care, Kings College School of Medicine and Dentistry, Bessemer Road, London SE5 9PJ, Tel: 071–326–3016 have developed a unique collaboration to explore and develop the relationship between psychotherapy and general practice. The staff group puts on conferences and workshops and members are available as consultants to individuals or practices.

The Counselling in Medical Settings division of the British Association for Counselling: 37a Sheep Street, Warwickshire CV21 3BX, Tel. 0788–78328/9, has been very active in fostering the growth of counselling in primary care. Branches of the BAC hold regular local meetings all over the country; some of these have looked at the particular experience of working in general practice.

The Counselling in Primary Care Trust: Suite 3a, Majestic House, High Street, Staines TW18 4DG, Tel. 0784–442601 is a charitable organization, funded by the Artemis trust, set up to promote, support, and develop counselling in primary care. It aims to set up a database of counsellors working in primary care, sponsor conferences, encourage research, and establish a specific training programme.

Relate Marriage Guidance: Herbert Gray College, Little Church Street, Rugby CV21 3AP, Tel. 0788–573241 has experience over many years of working in primary care settings.

The Mental Health Foundation: 37 Mortimer Street, London W1N 8PX, Tel: 071–580–0145 has funded several initiatives promoting counselling in primary care.

The Royal College of General Practitioners: Princes Gate, Hyde Park, London SW7 1PU, Tel: 071–581–3232 has published *counselling in general practice* in its clinical series, and has a library with a section on counselling.

Community Health Councils: Some have surveyed local practices and liaised with FHSAs to promote counselling in primary care.

REFERENCES

Balint M. (1964). *The Doctor, his patient and the illness*, (2nd edn). Pitman, London.

Cox, J. and Mulholland, H. (1993). An instrument for assessment of videotapes of general practitioners' performance. *British Medical Journal*, **306**, 1043–6.

CMS (Counselling in Medical Settings). (1993). *Guidelines for the employment of counsellors in general practice*. CMS, Rugby.

Edwards A. (1983). Research studies in the problems of assessment. *Journal of Analytical Psychology*, **28**, 299–311.

Einzig, H., Basharan, H., and Curtis Jenkins, G. (1992). The training needs of counsellors working in primary medical care: the role of the training organisations. *Counselling in Medical Settings News*, November, 9–13.

Irving, J. and Heath, V. (1985). *Counselling in general practice: a guide for general practitioners*. British Association for Counselling, London.

Jung, C. G. (1966). *Collected works*. Vol. 16 *The practice of psychotherapy*, para 364/5. Routledge Kegan Paul, London and Henley.

Main, T. (1957). The ailment. *British Journal of Medical Psychology*, **30**, 129–145.

Marsh, G. N. and Barr, J. (1975). Marriage guidance counselling in a group practice. *Journal of the Royal College of General Practitioners*, **25**, 73–5.

McLeod, J. (1988). *The work of counsellors in general practice*. Occasional paper no 37. Royal College of General Practitioners, London.

Menzies Lyth, I. (1988). *Containing anxiety in institutions: selected essays*, Chapter 7. Free Association Books, London.

National Marriage Guidance Council. (1985). Surgery counselling: guidelines for Marriage Guidance work in health centres or medical group practice. *Practice Outlook*, **1**, 7–13.

Pendleton, D., Schofield, T., Tate, P., and Havelock, P., (1984). *The consultation: an approach to learning and teaching*. Oxford University Press, Oxford.

RCGP (Royal College of General Practitioners). (1992). *Counselling in general practice*,

RCGP Clinical Series. Royal College of General Practitioners, London.

Rogers, C. R. (1951). *Client centred therapy*. Constable, London.

Rowland, N. and Hurd, J. (1985). *Counselling in general practice: a guide for counsellors* (Revised 1991). British Association for Counselling, London.

Sibbald, B., Addington-Hall, J., Brenneman, D., and Freeling, P. (1993). Counsellors in English and Welsh general practices: their nature and distribution. *British Medical Journal*, **306**, 29–33.

3 Economic evaluation

Nancy Rowland and Keith Tolley

INTRODUCTION

Everybody knows that, in health care, there are just not enough resources to go round. This is, in part, a political problem; some would argue that the National Health Service (NHS) is underfunded (Light 1990). It is also partly a technological problem; medical technology is so expensive that protecting the health of all patients to the maximum degree is just not possible (Doyal 1987). Economic factors in health care are becoming more important as demands on health care systems increase beyond the ability of these systems to satisfy them (Goodwin *et al.* 1990). Demographic trends, the continuing stream of new medical and surgical advances and increasing public expectations are placing ever greater demands on the NHS. When demands for resources exceed supply, decisions must be made regarding the allocation of resources. This raises questions about treatment effectiveness and treatment cost. Clinicians with limited funds thus need information on which to base decisions about treatment programmes. This has relevance to counselling in primary care; when resources are scarce, the wide-scale adoption of counselling is unwise without first establishing its effectiveness (Martin 1988). Thus determining the effectiveness of counselling is increasingly preoccupying counsellors who may have no choice but to evaluate their programmes if they hope to receive public funds (Daniels *et al.* 1981).

This chapter stresses the importance of the evaluation of counselling, of which economic evaluation is a part. Counsellors have an ethical obligation to evaluate their work. Their regulatory body, the British Association for Counselling (BAC), considers supervision of counselling work to be essential. Supervision is a form of process monitoring and peer review and is the main method by which counsellors evaluate their work. The British Association for Counselling's Research Committee (1989) notes that evaluation of counselling is important both at the micro level (investigating whether counselling is effective in helping people with their life problems) and at the macro level (the extent to which employers and funding bodies can be persuaded that counselling is cost-effective). As is discussed in Chapter 18, there is no systematic and coherent body of research about the evaluation of counselling in general practice and many questions remain unresolved. Who does it work for? What effects does it have? How much does it cost? Is it cost-effective? General practitioners are turning increasingly to nurses, social workers, clinical psychologists, and counsellors rather than to psychiatrists for help with their patients' mental health problems. Is this an effective response? (Wilkinson 1986).

Our review of papers evaluating counselling in primary care shows that scant attention has been paid to the role of economic analysis, either in terms of assessing the cost of providing a counselling service or in attempting to quantify the costs and benefits of counselling. Few practitioners or service providers appear to be familiar with the different types of economic analysis, or understand how economic analysis can be of value as part of a wider evaluation. We surmise that practitioners and researchers overlook the role of economic evaluation for a variety of reasons. First, lack of knowledge and understanding of economics dissuades attempts to cost services. Second, economic measures are suspected of being 'crude' measures and are viewed as only partially useful (for example, Corney 1990), and third, advocates of counselling in general practice may predict that counselling will not be shown to be cost-effective or cost-beneficial, so that economic analysis is felt to be better left unexplored. Finally, some practitioners are concerned about the misuse of the 'economic argument'; that if one 'treatment' is shown to be cheaper than another, the cheaper option will be pursued regardless of other factors, which they may perceive as more important than cost. Thus, for example, if psychotropic medication were shown to be cheaper than counselling, it might be the preferred option regardless of qualitative issues such as the possible side effects of long-term medication, including dependency. Some practitioners doubt the ethics of economic analysis as a tool in decision making with regard to potentially life-saving or life-enhancing treatments. We shall come back to the ethical issues of economic analysis at the end of the chapter, but first, we shall outline the approaches to economic analysis.

TECHNIQUES OF ECONOMIC EVALUATION

There are a number of different techniques of economic evaluation, all of which can be applied to the evaluation of counselling in primary care. The choice of technique depends on the objectives of the evaluation and the time and money available for collecting data on effectiveness. All the techniques outlined below can be applied to the provision of counselling services in primary care.

Cost-minimization analysis

This is the simplest form of economic evaluation as it involves only the measurement of the costs of alternative options. The technique can be used when it is already known that there is no difference between the effectiveness of the options under consideration. Given that there is no apparent difference in their effectiveness, the analysis is designed to choose the option which produces the lowest costs. For example, the Government's limited list of prescriptions was a cost-minimization exercise. The Government argued that various drugs were commonly prescribed by GPs, some of which were more expensive than others, although they produced the same results. Assuming this to be the case, the cheapest drug was listed. The reason some doctors challenged the decision, apart from restriction of clinical freedom, was that they felt some drugs were more effective than others and thus should not be excluded (Rowland and Tolley 1991). To give another example, it would appear that some patients may enjoy as good rates of recovery from simple surgical procedures as day-patients as they would have done had they been admitted to hospital as in-patients. Decisions may then be made on the basis of cost-minimization.

Cost-effectiveness analysis

A cost-effectiveness analysis is used when both the costs and outcomes of alternate programmes differ, but the effectiveness can be compared using a single common measure. It is not necessarily about choosing the cheapest option, but assessing costs in the light of which is the most effective option. Thus in a cost-effectiveness analysis there is a single objective which is usually measured in a single common unit, for example, the number of cases of breast cancer detected. Cost-effectiveness analysis compares the cost of achieving a goal by different means (Glass and Goldberg 1977). For example, a group practice might agree that a worthwhile health objective would be to help the smokers on their list stop smoking. Alternative options to achieve this aim might include doctors' advice to stop smoking, or referral of smokers to the practice nurse for a 'stop smoking' support group. The costs of these interventions can be compared as can their relative effectiveness. The cheapest option may well be a single session of advice from the general practitioner and the most expensive may be the ongoing patient support group. If the results of this small project show that the majority of patients give up smoking after receiving advice from a high-status professional, like a doctor, then it is clear that doctors' advice to quit smoking is the most cost-effective option. If, however, the practice nurse's support group helps patients to stop smoking for longer, then while such a group may be the most costly it is also the most effective. The decision to be made here is not clear-cut and the effect of the economic analysis will have been to provide information about the differences in costs and effects in order to facilitate decision making. Relevant criteria for choosing any particular programme may be in terms of greatest outcomes, greatest outcomes for a fixed cost (or budget), or achieving a target outcome at least cost.

Cost-benefit analysis

A cost-benefit analysis involves placing a numerical value (usually money) on all the relevant costs and benefits of alternative schemes and assessing which produces the greatest net benefit. For example, a health authority might try to decide between several different schemes to provide help for people with HIV infection or AIDS and their families. They might compare the costs and benefits of employing a specialist AIDS worker, placing AIDS counsellors in hospitals, or building a hospice for AIDS patients. For a single programme to be deemed worthwhile, requires only that the benefits exceed the costs. (Care must be taken to ensure that all relevant costs and benefits are included.) However, if the health authority faces a fixed budget and a choice needs to be made between competing options, then the programme which produces the greatest net benefits should be given priority.

A comprehensive cost-benefit analysis can be used to make value-for-money comparisons between widely diverging programmes. Hence, as monetary values are being used as a common measure of outcome, the technique allows, in principle, for comparison between counselling programmes in different settings and expenditures on other public and welfare services such as health education, defence, and social services. The main difficulty in carrying out a full cost-benefit analysis is the difficulty of putting monetary values on many of the inputs and outcomes. It is in response to many of the difficult-to-evaluate intangible inputs and benefits in health care, such as how to assess the costs and benefits of enabling a patient with end-stage cancer to die at home as opposed to in hospital, that economists have designed a technique more appropriate for the health care setting—known as cost-utility analysis.

Cost-utility analysis

In general, counselling interventions are unlikely to have a large impact on life expectancy in the same way as, say, surgical treatment for coronary artery disease. The main benefit of counselling might be expected to be in terms of improvements in well-being and in social and psychological functioning. For example, the benefits of a counsellor attachment in general practice might be measured in terms of quality of life gains for the patient and his or her family. Many instruments for measuring quality of life exist which are not based on a measure of utility but which can be used to compare the output of alternative counselling options, although these vary in terms of their appropriateness and ease of use within an economic evaluation (Bowling 1990). However, health economists have attempted to devise measures specifically for evaluating the cost-effectiveness of programmes for which health is the important outcome. This is the technique of cost-utility analysis. It attempts to place a numerical value (ranging from 0 to 1) on qualitative outcomes such as quality of life or satisfaction with life.

Several such indices, known as utility scales, have been devised by health economists (Torrence 1986). As in cost-benefit analysis however, putting a single numerical value on quality of life is problematic and controversial among health researchers. Cost-utility analysis involves combining expected health state with life expectancy data, producing quality adjusted life years (QALYS) or well-years. These reflect the utility or satisfaction gained from changes in the level of a person's combined disability and distress (Williams 1985). The development and use of QALYs is of particular relevance to the discussion of ethics and economics later in the chapter.

What do economists mean by economic evaluation?

Efficiency and equity

The terms efficiency and equity have particular meaning for economists, which differ slightly from common parlance. As a society, we want to ensure that the resources allocated to the health service in general, and primary care in particular, are used to achieve the greatest possible improvement in the health of the population. To a health economist, efficiency means that health benefits are maximized for a given level of resources. In addition, as a society we have equity objectives, so we may want to ensure that health benefits are distributed fairly among the old and young, rich and poor. Thus the general practitioner's aim may be to provide health care for all patients (equity) and the question may be how to allocate resources efficiently to achieve this aim.

Money

It is often assumed that when economists talk about costs and benefits, they are talking about money; cost equals expenditure and benefit equals savings. This is not the case. When economists talk about costs, they are not talking about financial costs, although money may be a common measure against which to compare options. In the context of economic analysis, a cost is not so much a monetary effect as an 'opportunity cost'; that is the value, or worth, of resources in their next best possible use. For example, if a particular policy makes use of equipment which would otherwise only be scrapped, then the appropriate measure of the cost of this equipment is its scrap value and not, for example, what it may have cost when new, less some arbitrary depreciation (Glass and Goldberg, 1977).

Costs

In undertaking an economic evaluation of alternative counselling pro-grammes, the inputs of each scheme need to be identified and valued.

This is known as a costs-analysis and is an essential component of each type of economic evaluation. At first sight it may seem that some of the costs of individual inputs are easily measured and valued, such as the time of a newly appointed counsellor in a general practice (for example, valued using the gross salary paid). However, even if the new practice counsellor was previously employed in the health centre as a practice nurse and there is no change in salary and no extra items of cost in financial terms on the practice balance sheet, the time of this staff member could have been used in some alternative way. Moreover, there may be hidden costs, such as the existing use of staff and volunteers; or over-valued resources such as an unused office which has little or no alternative use value. In undertaking a costs-analysis, it is important to identify as many of the relevant inputs of each alternative scheme as possible. If a comprehensive list of possible costs and effects of a scheme is made, the analyst has some idea of the type of economic evaluation that is appropriate.

The relevant costs and effects to be considered depends on the perspective of the study, that is, what are the costs to whom? Economic evaluations may be conducted from a variety of perspectives. One of the most common is the society-wide perspective, which includes costs incurred by agencies other than the one initiating the scheme and clients using the service. For example, if a counsellor in general practice refers all patients with alcohol problems, previously dealt with by the GP, to an agency specializing in alcohol problems, subsequent costs are incurred by the outside agency. Individuals referred to the agency may incur costs in terms of travel and attendance time and expenses. Intangible costs such as anxiety about the referral may also be incurred. Knock on costs may involve the referred patients returning to their GP with a request for medication to help them abstain from alcohol. If these costs are underestimated or inadequate resources exist to meet such knock-on needs, the impact of the counsellor employed in the practice may be severely limited.

An economic evaluation of counselling may involve several different costing techniques. The choice of method, however, and consequently the costs and benefits that need to be measured, will vary acording to the nature of the evaluation exercise and the objectives of the programme being considered. The range of costs and effects analysed depends on the time and effort available to conduct a cost appraisal and the perspective of the evaluator. If only a little time or money is available to undertake an economic evaluation then a more limited perspective may be appropriate (for example restricting analysis of costs to the initiating agency, for example the practice).

The relevance of economic evaluation to counselling

We started this chapter by arguing for the importance of economic analysis of counselling in general practice. Economic evaluation is important so that we can build up a body of knowledge about the costs and effects of counselling and compare the costs and effects of alternative counselling interventions and programmes. It might also be argued that economic evaluation is important in the current-climate of change in the NHS. The present Government's commitment to cost-analysis and value for money cannot be doubted. The introduction to *Promoting better health* (Department of Health and Social Security 1987) states that the primary care services are the front line of the NHS. On an average working day over 1.2 million people use them. They cost over £5000 million per year. The Government's plans for primary care and its aim to improve value for money must be seen against this backdrop. The White Paper signalled the need for general practice to accept a wide range of professions working within it, and there are clear indications that the Government might be prepared to make more available to remunerate them. This means that counselling is likely to become more common in British general practice. However, given budgetary constraints, hard competitive choices have to be made between the different health professionals in the primary care team and awkward conflicts inevitably arise (Pereira Gray 1988).

The new GP contract and the implementation of the NHS reforms have encouraged doctors to think carefully about the effective and efficient management of resources. Economic analysis does not provide answers to questions but helps to clarify aims and objectives, inputs and outputs, information which assists decisions. We will now look at several studies of the economic evaluation of counselling in general practice, to consider the practicalities of undertaking such evaluation and some of the problems which arise.

THE ECONOMIC EVALUATION OF COUNSELLING IN PRIMARY CARE

There are very few economic analyses of counselling in general practice, and we have cast our net wide to include counselling as practised by clinical psychologists, nurse therapists, social workers, and others who use psychological treatments.

As Waydenfeld and Waydenfeld acknowledge (1980), counselling is notoriously difficult to assess. Most studies address the issue of validity by using multiple-outcome measures. Thus, the impact of counselling services in primary care is measured using a variety of qualitative outcome data (for example patient satisfaction, patient well-being) and quantitative data (for example consultation and prescription rates) before and after counselling. As Ives points out (1979), subjective assessments of global improvement are notoriously subject to bias and other sources of error. However, it might be assumed that an improvement in the patient's condition would be expected to be reflected by his or her interaction with the general practitioner so that the number of doctor/patient contacts and the number of prescriptions for psychotropic drugs for each patient in the months immediately preceding referral and after discharge might provide more objective measures. Given that time and medication are probably the most costly elements of primary care, they deserve attention. Attendance rates and prescriptions provide quantifiable 'hard' data, for which costs can be easily calculated. However, of the studies which utilize such quantitative measures, few attempt to assess costs.

In order to provide a brief overview of the research that has been undertaken to evaluate counselling in primary care, we will review several studies using different methodologies. Starting with studies utilizing multiple-outcome measures, but which do not include cost analysis, we will then focus on those that include cost analysis, before analysing in some detail those that attempt more complex economic evaluation.

Studies involving multiple-outcome measures

In a multicentre two-year-study Waydenfeld and Waydenfeld (1980) used 'as many criteria as they could' in assessing the outcome of counselling for 88 clients, involving 35 general practitioners and 9 counsellors. Measures included surgery attendance figures, prescriptions, and assessments by the doctors, patients, and counsellors involved. Before and after counselling comparisons, taken over six months on either side, showed that attendance at surgery fell by 31 per cent, with a similar reduction in the number of prescriptions issued. Patients, doctors, and counsellors registered high levels of satisfaction with the provision of on-site counselling. However, of the doctors interviewed, five thought their workload was unchanged, two admitted some relief, and two felt their workload had actually increased through their greater personal involvement and through discussions with the counsellor. The authors conclude that surgery counselling fills a definite need and could be considered for extension nationally.

Earll and Kincey (1982) carried out a controlled trial in which 50 consecutive potential referrals for psychological treatment from one general practice were randomly allocated either to behavioural treatment or routine general practitioner care. The patients' use of NHS resources was assessed during the treatment period and at a follow-up comparison point, when the patients' subjective ratings of their progress were also obtained. The treated group received significantly less psychotropic medication than the control group, though this difference was not maintained at the longer-term follow-up. There were no differences in general practice consultation rates, or in subjective ratings of patient improvement, though the level of patient satisfaction was high. The authors conclude that further studies should be set up to discover what GPs and clinical psychologists should do to maintain short-term effects of behavioural techniques in primary care.

In Ashurst and Ward's study (Ashurst 1979) of the Leverhulme counselling project, the hypotheses tested were:

(1) that counselling will reduce the prescription of psychotropic drugs;
(2) that counselling will reduce the number of consultations with general practitioners;
(3) that a counselling service based in the primary medical care setting will be found acceptable by patients and their general practitioners.

In a detailed report (Ashurst and Ward 1983), there were no outcome differences on the reported data from 406 patients presenting with minor neurotic disorders who were randomly assigned to counselling or to routine general practitioner treatment. Patients who received counselling (treatment) were no less likely to reduce their dependency on or use of antidepressant drugs than those who did not receive counselling (control). While treatment group patients were likely to reduce their use of tranquillizers while they were being counselled, counselling was associated with an increased likelihood of tranquillizers being prescribed subsequently. The control patients were slightly more likely to end their use of psychotropic drugs. Counselled patients used more general practitioner time, seeing their doctor slightly more frequently and for slightly longer than the controls. Patients who rejected counselling, however, were less likely to feel better and twice as likely to continue using psychotropic medication, than those who accepted counselling or the controls. While high proportions of clients valued the help they received, there was no striking difference in outcomes between the groups.

In a study focusing on quantitative data, Koch (1979) describes 30 general practitioner consultations with patients with psychological problems referred to a clinical psychologist for behaviour therapy. Consultations for advice and psychotropic drugs were compared during one year both before and after treatment and were found to be reduced by over 50 per cent following treatment. Contact with clinical psychology services, therefore, seemed to considerably reduce the demand made by these patients for general practitioner time. The mean number of consultations per patient in the year after completion of psychotherapy was 5.46, which represented a significant reduction when compared with pretreatment rates. Consultation rates for advice and psychotropic medication were significantly lower than before treatment, with little change in consultation rates for the prescription of other drugs. At follow-up it was noted that all three types of consultation rate increased slightly compared with rates during treatment. Repeat prescription rates were reduced significantly as a whole and specifically for psychotropic medication. The interaction with clinical improvement was statistically significant ($p = 0.001$). In both consultation rates and repeat prescription variables, the percentage of physical drug therapy rates was increased. Koch, therefore, advocates close liaison between clinical psychologists and general practitioners. He notes that referral criteria should be more rigorously defined and a control group monitored, so as to enable clarification of which reductions were more than part of the natural history of change. It should also show a reduction in general practitioner referrals to expensive, hospital-based psychiatric services. No attempt was made to assess costs.

However, it may be that rates of consultations and prescriptions are unrepresentative of longer-term rates or may be atypical for the particular time under study. Freeman and Button (1984) showed that three-quarters of the patients in a group practice referred to a clinical psychologist during a three-year-period, showed marked reductions in the consulting and psychotropic drug prescription rates in the six months after treatment compared with the six months leading up to treatment. However, the rates for the whole practice revealed a general decline over the period of study. Furthermore, examination of the records of all patients with at least one psychosocial problem over a six-year-period showed that encounters for psychosocial problems tended to be concentrated in a relatively short period, 'the worst year', rather than being evenly distributed over the whole six years. It is concluded that the natural history of most psychological disorders is one of crisis and remission and also that it may be difficult to interpret reductions in consulting and prescribing rates after referral to a psychologist (or counsellor) unless contemporary trends for the whole practice are known.

In the light of this, Blakey (1986) attempted to assess rates of consultation and prescription for patients referred to clinical psychologists and these patients' immediate families for three-year-periods both before and after referral. Patients and their children consulted more and had more medication prescribed before referral than control groups, this tendency being particularly prevalent in the year before referral. After the contact with the psychologist, there was a decrease in all these indices in the short term, and there were long-term decreases in psychotropic drug prescriptions for patients and in both consultations and prescriptions for their children. The results show, therefore, that the effect of the intervention was more than a short-term one.

Studies with basic cost data

Ives (1979) describes the service provided by a part-time clinical psychologist attachment to two group practices. A total of 238 patients were seen over a period of 28 months. Of those completing therapy, 72 per cent made satisfactory progress. In the three months after stopping treatment patients made significantly fewer (36 per cent) visits to the surgeries and received significantly fewer (50 per cent) prescriptions for psychotropic drugs than in the three months before referral. These changes were maintained one year later, in the three-month-period 12–15 months after discharge. On this evidence, Ives argued that the provision of such largely successful therapy for a population of patients for whom adequate treatment was previously unavailable should be expanded. He noted that the rate of referral to psychiatrists did not alter, at least at the smaller practice for which figures were available. The study includes brief mention of financial data, noting that a reduction in medication has cost-reduction benefits, although these were not quantified. Instead, in a random sample of 30 prescriptions issued by the larger practice to patients in this study, Ives estimated a mean potential cost to the NHS of £1.19 per item.

In a study which made an effort to undertake a simple cost analysis, Anderson and Hasler (1979) undertook a survey of the subjective and objective effects of counselling on the first 80 patients who used a newly established, part-time counselling service in a health centre. There was an improvement, as measured by the feelings of the patients and doctors and through some reduction in the use of psychotropic drugs and medical consultations. The cost analysis focused on the change in use of psychotropic drugs. The total cost of drugs issued to all 80 patients for a three-month-period before counselling was compared with a similar period after their counselling sessions had been completed. It was estimated that the reduction in drug costs for the total group was £76.92. This figure was based on the unit cost of 100 tablets of the prescribed strength calculated from the December 1977 issue of MIMS. The actual saving would have been much greater owing to the additional costs of dispensing fees, container allowances, and cost allowances. The cost of consultations was not calculated, although the authors note that most patients reduced their use of medical time after counselling. The authors conclude that in the short term, counselling offered an alternative to the use of psychotropic drugs and enabled some people to reduce or discontinue medication. It may also be linked with a reduction in the demand for medical time, although it is not possible to say whether this would have happened in the practice without the counselling service. However, the results of this study should be treated with caution. No attempt was made to cost the counselling service or to compare outcomes (there was no control group). Sophisticated statistical techniques were not used and the study took place over a short period of time.

Studies utilizing more detailed cost data

We will look at three studies, analysing the methods and results to give an idea of how to conduct an economic analysis. Robson, France, and Bland (1984) carried out a controlled study of a behaviourally orientated clinical psychology service based in a health centre where two randomized groups were compared. Patients in the control groups received usual primary care management; subject patients received the same, but, in addition, were able to consult a clinical psychologist in the health centre. Outcome was assessed by psychosocial and economic measures. These showed changes in favour of the subject condition, many of which were statistically significant.

What economic measures were used? In terms of outcomes, the number of visits that the patient made to the GP was calculated for 34 weeks before the patient entered the study, 10 weeks after entry (the intervention period), and 24 weeks after the intervention period. The cost of prescribed drugs was calculated from prescriptions returned by the Prescription Pricing Authority and were divided into three categories: (A) those drugs acting on the central nervous system including all psychotropic drugs; (B) drugs for gastrointestinal, nutritional and skin conditions; (c) all other drugs, that were used to control for overall changes in prescribing patterns during the study. The total net cost of ingredients was calculated for each patient monthly for one year after entering the study. The number and cost of hospital visits for patients in both subject and control groups were recorded using information on the unit cost of out-patient visits provided by the finance department of the local health district.

With regard to visits to the GP, results showed that in the 34 weeks before entering the study there were no significant differences between groups. As might be expected there was a highly significant difference between the two groups during the 10 weeks when many of the subjects were seeing the psychologist. But more interesting is the finding that 24 weeks after the end of the intervention period the subjects were still making significantly fewer visits to their doctor. Hospital referrals were too few to analyse, but there was a wealth of data about prescription costs. At both 34 and 52 weeks follow-up, the cost of drugs in category A (central nervous system) was significantly less for the subject group than for the control group. There were no significant differences in categories B and C. Psychotropic drugs were the largest and most expensive item in category A. The overall saving in the cost of drugs that are active on the central nervous system was substantial and highly statistically significant up to one year. In monetary terms, an average of £4.05 less a year was spent per subject patient on category A drugs. A mean of 114 subject patients entered the study each year, producing an estimated saving of £462. In 1981, during the clinical period of the study, a senior clinical psychologist earned £17.71 a session, which is equivalent to £1629 for two sessions a week for a 46-week-year. The authors conclude that it seems that 28 per cent of the salary of a senior clinical psychologist working in this way could be found from drug economies alone.

Similarly, Marks (1985) notes that placing nurse therapists in primary care may save more health resources than it consumes. Two cost-benefit analyses, one controlled (Ginsberg *et al.* 1984) and one uncontrolled (Ginsberg and Marks 1977) suggested that even disregarding intangible benefits, such as lessened fear and anxiety, the cost of employing a nurse was more than offset by tangible economic gains after treatment, arising from the patients having less time off work, fewer personal expenses, and a lower use of health care resources. Because most resources used in psychotherapy, or indeed in any health or social service framework, relate to the cost of staffing, exploration of the costs and impact of different therapist variables deserves high priority. The pilot, uncontrolled analysis of outcome of treatment by behavioural nurse therapists found that the overall benefits to society exceeded the costs of the programme (Ginsberg and Marks 1977). The outcome for neurotic patients treated by nurse therapists compares well with that obtained by psychiatrists and clinical psychologists (Marks *et al.* 1975, 1978) and their major selection and management decisions match those of psychiatrists (Marks *et al.* 1977). Thus with their lower training costs, nurse therapists are a cost-effective alternative to psychiatrists and psychologists for administering behavioural psychotherapies. In the long term it may cost the community less to provide nurse therapists for such patients. In an aside, Marks (1985) also notes that most of the GPs in the study of a nurse therapist in primary care wanted the nurse therapist to continue in their practice after the study was over. The funding of such placements, however, is a problem.

Let us look in more detail at the controlled clinical trial referred to above. In this randomized trial (Ginsberg *et al.* 1984) neurotic patients (mainly phobics and obsessive compulsives) in primary care were assigned either to behavioural psychotherapy from a nurse therapist or to routine care from their GP. The economic analysis in this study came from two sources, first from patients' records, yielding data about the number of visits to the general practitioner and drug usage and second, from an economic questionnaire (EQ) completed by all patients at entry into the trial and at one-and two-year follow-up. The EQ covered four main areas:

(1) family situation; marital status, household members, etc.;
(2) education—educational level attained and qualifications;
(3) work situation and employment history and income—effect of problem on work, job mobility., absenteeism;
(4) difficulty experienced in visiting therapist—time taken for visits, time from work, costs incurred, etc.

An extra section covered utilization of other care facilities, for example, visits to general practitioners, social worker, or counsellor, or domiciliary visits from any of these agencies. Visits to voluntary agencies and costs incurred were also recorded.

At the end of one year clinical outcome was significantly better in patients cared for by the nurse therapist. Economic outcome to one year, compared with the year before entering the trial, showed a slight decrease in the use of resources by the nurse therapist group ($n = 22$) and an increase in resource usage in the GP treated group ($n = 28$), mainly due to the latter's increased absence from work and more hospital treatment and drugs. Assuming that nurse therapists treat an average of 46 patients a year and that such patients treated behaviourally maintain their gains for two years, the economic benefits to society from nurse therapists treating such patients may outweigh costs. This excludes any monetary value on the substantial clinical gains from a reduction in fear and anxiety.

Results from the controlled study, compared with the previous uncontrolled study which found decreased resource use of about £100 per patient per year, found a decrease of only £24, although the control group increased their resource use over the same period by £128 per patient per year. However, the numbers are small, few economic differences were significant, and many patients either did not complete the trial or waiting list periods, or they failed to return economic data. Thus the inferences from the results must be tempered with caution.

Finally, a recent study by Scott and Freeman (1992) aimed to compare the clinical efficacy, patient satisfaction, and cost of three specialist treatments for depressive illness with routine care by general practitioners. This was a prospective, randomized study with each patient allocated to one of four groups: amitriptyline prescribed by a psychiatrist, cognitive behaviour therapy from a clinical psychologist, counselling and case work by a social worker (intervention groups), or routine care by a doctor (the control group).

The authors argued that the investment of time and skill required for both the social work intervention and cognitive behaviour therapy is quite unlike the routine management of depressed patients in primary care; most patients see their doctor for less than 10 minutes on the first occasion. Such investments in psychological treatments may be justified if they prove to be more clinically effective and/or more acceptable to patients in preventing furher episodes of depression, or by helping patients cope better with problems. Therefore, they aimed to compare how much time and money each treatment cost and how they were valued by patients. In today's NHS, the clinical efficacy of a treatment may be compromised if patients do not like it, if it takes too long, or costs too much.

Results showed that psychological treatments, even though lengthy, were most positively evaluated by patients. Social work counselling was evaluated most positively in terms of meeting needs and helping with problems. A marked improvement in depressive symptoms occurred in all treatment groups over 16 weeks. The severity of depressive symptoms declined in all treatment groups, but any differences in clinical efficacy between the specialist treatments and routine general practitioner care were small and not commensurate with the differences in length and cost of treatment.

Initial analysis of cost differentials showed that the specialist treatments involved much longer patient contact and cost the health service about four times as much as routine general practitioner care. The latter took only a handful of appointments, but practice doctors referred some patients to other NHS staff and facilities, which reduced the cost differential to threefold. The cost of drugs prescribed by the general practitioners reduced the cost differential further to twofold. (The cost may have been affected by the confirmation of the diagnosis of depressive illness in all the patients, reducing the number of medical investigations and referrals made by the general practitioners.) Detailed analysis of resource use showed that all specialist treatments involved at least twice as many appointments and from four (amitriptyline/psychiatrist) to 14 (social work counselling) times more face-to-face contact than in routine medical care. Although both cognitive behaviour therapy and social work counselling involved more face-to-face contact than amitriptyline treatment from the psychiatrist, the total costs of the three specialist treatments were similar because clinical psychologists and social workers are less expensive to employ by the hour. Face-to-face contact with the specialist therapists, as noted above, cost about four times as much as the cost of the time the general practitioners spent with their patients. General practitioner care, however, made use of other NHS personnel and resources; three patients were referred to and seen at a psychiatric out-patient clinic (staff costs, £142), one patient was referred to a psychiatric out-patient clinic and attended a psychiatric day hospital (estimated cost £444) and one patient was referred to a primary care health visitor (£33). If these additional costs are included, then the average cost per patient in the general practitioner's care rose to £47, which was still less than half the cost of any of the specialist treatments.

The average cost of all psychotropic drugs over all patients was £8.31 over 16 weeks and £7.28 in patients allocated to amitriptyline treatment from the psychiatrist (no significant difference). The cost of psychotropic drugs prescribed by general practitioners increased the average cost of general practitioner contact by a third, but the cost of amitriptyline was trivial compared to the cost of the psychiatrist's time. The authors make note of possible long-term effects, in that depressed patients treated by cognitive behaviour therapy or social work counselling may be less likely to relapse than patients treated with antidepressants alone over the one or two years after the index episode. If this is the case and patients are helped to cope more effectively with the problems that led to their depression, this may prevent further episodes of depression. Until relapse rates after treatment are measured, the cost-benefit analysis is incomplete.

Thus the authors conclude that the additional costs associated with specialist treatments of new episodes of mild to moderate depressive illness presenting in primary care were not commensurate with their clinical superiority over routine general practitioner care, but that a proper cost–benefit analysis requires information about the ability of specialist treatment to prevent future episodes of depression.

Table 3.1 *Main results from studies containing economic data*[1,2]

Study	Economic/cost assessment
Robson *et al.* (1984) Patients allocated to: • on-site clinical psychologist • routine GP care	Reduction in drug costs £4.05 per patient £462 total saving per year ($n = 114$)[3]
Ginsberg *et al.* (1984) Patients allocated to: • on-site behavioural therapy • routine GP care	Change in resource use Cost per patient over study period ($n = 48$) − £24 (Intervention group) + £128 (Control group)[4] (1981 price levels)
Scott and Freeman (1992) Patients allocated to: • amitriptylline/psychiatrist • cognitive therapy/psychologist • social work counselling/social worker • routine GP care	Average cost per patient[5] £113 £115 £121 £26 ($n = 114$)

[1] Price year for study was given only by Ginsberg *et al.* (1984).
[2] In each study the control group was routine GP care.
[3] The total saving of £462 per year was estimated to be 28 per cent of the costs of employing a clinical psychologist. Savings were found for drugs acting on the central nervous system.
[4] This produced a net benefit of £152 for the nurse therapist option.
[5] Cost of therapist time.

Table 3.1 provides a summary of the findings relating to costs and cost savings in the three main studies reviewed in this Section.

Critique of studies

Some of these studies failed to have a control group and some took place over short periods of time. Most of the studies of counselling in primary care make no attempt to cost the data. None of the studies reviewed comprehensively examine costs to the system (such as referral to a psychiatrist or time spent in hospital), often because patient numbers are too small for analysis (for example Earll and Kincey 1982). Subjective accounts suggest that counsellor attachments work well, with much consumer and practitioner satisfaction. The majority of studies have shown that after the cessation of counselling, clients make fewer visits to their doctors, fewer psychotropic drugs are prescribed and fewer referrals are made to psychiatrists. For more comprehensive reviews of the effectiveness of counselling in primary care or in medical settings generally, see Corney (1990) and Brown and Abel Smith (1985).

What do we know about the economic benefits of counselling in general practice as a result of such work? While authors are rightly cautious about suggesting that a drop in consultation rates, for example, can be presented as evidence for the cost-effectiveness of counselling (Davis and Fallowfield 1991), can we draw any conclusions about economic data from these studies? While reductions in consultation and prescription rates do not indicate the cost-effectiveness of counselling, in financial terms, there may be reductions in costs. The data from these studies could form the basis for a cost-minimization evaluation.

If we were to undertake a simple economic evaluation of counselling in primary care, we would follow Ives (1979) in arguing that an effective, carefully designed research study should be able to answer unequivocally the following questions:

To what extent can the presence of a counsellor in the surgery prevent:

(1) future patient morbidity;
(2) use of the doctors' time;
(3) use of psychotropic drugs: tranquillizers and/or antidepressants;
(4) referral to psychiatrists;
(5) admissions to psychiatric hospitals?

We would want to compare the counsellor intervention with routine general practitioner care and care from other PHCT members, and would include detailed costings to the system. What sort of data would we need to collect? Our hypothesis is that the provision of counselling services in primary care results in the improved mental health of patients consulting the counsellor compared with those consulting their doctor; that they take less psychotropic drugs, visit their general practitioner less often, and make fewer visits to psychiatrists on an out-patient or in-patient basis. Simple costings would thus include the salaries of the counsellor, general practitioner, psychiatrist, and so on. The time each professional spends with patients would need to be billed accordingly. Information can be gathered about prescription costs. Referral costs to the patient (time and travelling) and to the general practitioner buying-in psychiatric services need to be considered.

If we were to do a wider cost analysis, we would wish to assess opportunity costs. For example, if the time the general practitioner saves from referring patients with neurotic disorders to the counsellor is now spent in offering alternative services, what are these services and how much do they cost? If the general practitioner likes to do minor surgery on site, what is the cost to the system? How much does this cost the practice compared with referral for minor surgery to the local hospital? And how does this compare with the original costs of the general practitioner seeing patients with neurotic disorders? The spectrum of cost analysis can be as limited (comparing general practitioner with counsellor) or as broad (comparing costs to the practice within the community) as required, depending on the questions the researcher needs and can afford to answer.

Conducting an economic evaluation

A number of gaps have been identified in the economic evaluations of counselling reviewed in this chapter, and the studies are unlikely to provide much guidance for those wanting to undertake an evaluation in their own setting. There are a number of important steps in conducting an economic evaluation, which we will mention briefly here. First, a clear definition of the objective of the evaluation is required. For example, the primary objective might be to discover the most cost-effective approach to dealing with psychosocial problems among patients presenting in general practice. Second, a clear description of the options to meet this objective is needed. For example, viable options might be to employ a specialist counsellor in the surgery, to train selected practice doctors or other practice staff to provide all the counselling requirements, or to 'do-nothing' (which in fact is 'doing something', such as continuing with the use of 'untrained' general practitioners providing 'counselling').

Third, an appropriate study design needs to be chosen for collecting data and measuring the effectiveness of each option. The fourth step is the identification of the costs and the main outcomes or benefits of each option. In a cost-effectiveness analysis, an appropriate outcome measure needs to be chosen by which to compare options, for example, the reduction in the level of psychosocial problems among patients visiting the general practitioner. In a cost-utility analysis, outcomes are usually measured using quality-adjusted-life-years (QALYs) and in a cost-benefit analysis using monetary values. Finally a clear presentation of the cost-effectiveness results relating to each option should be provided. To go into detail about each of these steps is beyond the scope of this chapter. We would refer the reader to a text for counsellors on the practical use of cost-effectiveness analysis in health care settings (Tolley and Rowland, in press).

ECONOMICS AND ETHICS

The economic evaluation of counselling in general practice involves making decisions about the costs and effects of counselling and about the allocation of resources to finance counselling services. The ethical issues associated with the economic evaluation of counselling are rarely discussed in the literature, but they are often raised by counsellors, aware of the likely conflict between the quality and cost of care. Proponents of counselling, who advocate the development of counselling in primary care, often bemoan the fact that there are scant resources for such development. Some counsellors argue that counselling services should be prioritized in the health service budget, others are concerned about financial restraints affecting the quality of care. We consider it important to broaden the discussion of the ethics of economic evaluation in the context of the provision of health care services and to look at the issues this raises for counsellors and other health professionals. Thus we conclude this chapter with a discussion of ethics and economics in health care.

There is a fundamental conflict between those counsellors and doctors who are concerned that allowing costs to influence clinical decisions is unethical and those health economists who advocate a systematic deployment of resources. A doctor writing to the *New England Journal of Medicine* put his view clearly, 'A physician who changes his or her way of practising medicine because of cost rather than purely medical considerations has indeed embarked upon the "slippery slope" of compromised ethics and waffled priorities' (quoted in Williams 1992). We shall examine such arguments as well as the arguments for the 'rational' allocation of resources based on cost-effectiveness criteria.

The issues of ethics and economics raise many questions. As we have noted, economists start with the premise that resources are always scarce. Given this scarcity, rational decisions need to be made about their fair distribution, in general practice, hospital medicine, and throughout the National Health Service. The value underpinning the NHS is that the life and health of each person matters and that each person is entitled to be treated with equal concern and respect, both in the way health care resources are distributed and in the way they are treated by health care professionals, however much their personal circumstances may differ from those of others. Accepting the value of life generates a principle of equality. When resources are scarce, they must be allocated fairly (Harris 1987).

Harris (1987) argues that while it is true that resources are limited, it is not true that resources for health care are justifiably as limited as they are made out to be. Within health care, staff are too often forced to consider the question of the best way of allocating health budgets *per se* and consequently are forced to compete with each other for resources. Harris believes that the task of health care economics is essentially immoral, in that it seeks to find more efficient ways of doing the wrong thing—sacrificing the lives of people who could be saved. He argues that the obligation to save as many lives as possible is not the same as the obligation to save as many lives as we can cheaply or economically save. Instead of attempting to measure the value of people's lives and select those which are worth saving, any rubric for resource allocation should examine the national budget afresh to see whether there are any headings of expenditure that are more important to the community than helping people whose lives are in danger. He believes that the value of life is paramount and that where patients lives are at stake, resources should be allocated accordingly. Thus we need to re-examine priorities in terms not of the health care budget alone, but of the national budget. If this is done, it will become clear that it is simply not true that that the resources necessary to save peoples' lives are not available. The argument is that to ensure fair allocation of resources, enough resources should be made available to go round.

This is certainly a case to consider and it may well be worth politicking to transfer more funds to the health service. But in the meantime, there is not enough to go round. How should resources be distributed? Who should make allocation decisions? It is essential that health service providers act ethically in relation to their patients; how are decisions to be made?

The current climate of medical ethics

The nature of health and health care means that the patient is in the hands of the doctor, because the asymmetry in information between them results in a serious impairment of the individual's autonomy as a decision maker. The doctor is empowered by the patient to make decisions on the patient's behalf. It is, therefore, essential that the doctor acts in the patient's best interests. The clinician's job is to protect the patient and to work as best as he or she can for that individual. A relationship based on trust between the doctor and the patient is thus of paramount importance (Mooney 1984).

In the present moral climate of the NHS, medical ethics dictates that individual doctors try to maximize the health of individual patients. Each doctor following individualistic ethical objectives will be concerned to maximize the benefit for his/her patients. To this end, the doctor will attempt to gain more and more scarce resources to assist in this goal. Such an attempt—which ignores the opportunity cost to other doctors' patients—is legitimized by the ethics of virtue and of duty. Medical ethics in a sense implores the doctor to assume every other doctor's patients out of existence (and also possibly, potential future patients). Thus some clinicans are bitterly opposed to the use of economics in medical decision making. They believe that the the overriding principle governing the actions of a doctor towards a patient is that the best should be done for that patient; treatment should not rest on mathematical calculations.

Williams (1992) asserts, however, that it cannot be ethical to ignore the adverse consequences upon others of the decisions you make, which is what cost represents. 'What will it cost?' means 'What will have to be sacrificed?' and this may be very different from 'How much money will we have to part with'? He argues that a caring, responsible, and ethical doctor has to take costs into account; it is unethical not to do so! Williams acknowledges, however, that there are some important ethical issues in deciding what costs and benefits to count and how to count them.

Mooney argues that unlike medical ethics, economics embraces a concept of social as well as individual ethics. He suggests that there is a relative lack of acceptance of the ethics of the common good in medical ethics. As a result, while economics in the field of health has as an objective the maximization of the health of the community, subject to resource constraints, medical ethics pushes individual doctors to try to maximize the health of their individual patients. The fact that individual doctors' values in aggregation are not conducive to the goal of maximizing the health of the community at large from the resources available to it, may prove rather disturbing for doctors. Thus economic analysis may create discomfort within the medical profession. Mooney suggests that certain institutional alterations in the NHS, for example, new budgeting structures and the acceptance of efficiency as a social goal, are required in order to promote the type of behavioural change which will make doctors act in the interests of the common good to a greater extent than is now the case.

Alternatively, Cubbon (1991) suggests that doctors in the health service should not have to make decisions about which of their patients should be given time, effort, and resources, when this will clearly be to the disadvantage of the others, as they would feel they were playing God and their capacity to relate to patients would be undermined. Rather, economic effectiveness should be a tool in directing policy decisions about resource allocation rather than in dealing with individual patients. Thus the impersonal, calculating aspect, which makes such measurement seem inappropriate as a morality of personal relations, is less objectionable in the formulation of policy. In a modern society, planning of services will always involve assessment of costs and benefits and will entail some groups of people deliberately being deprived of benefits. The informed formulation of policies affecting the distribution of scarce resources does not go against the grain of our moral intuitions. The people who would benefit from the developments under consideration will mostly be unknown to policy makers. Often they will be unknown to anyone, because they will not yet have become ill. The point is that decisions will be made as rationally as possible. In response, Harris (1991) agrees that using measures of economic effectiveness to discriminate between patients would undermine the doctor–patient relationship, but argues that a public policy based on such data might, for analagous reasons, undermine public confidence in and respect for government and health policy makers.

Outcome measures

Against a background of permanently scarce resources, it is crucial that health care resources are used efficiently. In order to distinguish between efficient and inefficient use of health care resources we need to measure standards of treatment and their effects on individual patients. The NHS is underpinned by strongly held, but vaguely articulated egalitarian principles. One of the ethical objections to the economic approach is that it is unethical to judge the value of a person's life. Williams (1992) believes that judgements about the value of another person's life (or more correctly, the value of improvements in another person's health) are inescapable in a system which is expected to behave in an egalitarian way in discriminating between the well and the ill, and between those likely to benefit from a particular treatment, and those unlikely to do so, in order that some systematic priority setting can take place in the face of inescapable resource constraints.

Williams (1987) summarizes the arguments for and against;
Either:

1. Health care priorities should not be influenced by any other consideration than keeping people alive.
2. Everyone has an equal right to be kept alive if that is what they wish, irrespective of how poor their prognosis is and no matter what sacrifices others have to bear as a consequence.
3. When allocating health care resources we must not discriminate between people, not even according to their differential capacities to benefit from treatment.

Or:

1. Health care priorities should be influenced by our capacity both to increase life expectation and to improve people's quality of life.
2. A particular improvement in health should be regarded as of equal value, no matter who gets it, and should be provided unless it prevents a greater improvement being offered to someone else.
3. It is the responsibility of everyone to discriminate wherever necessary to ensure that our limited resources go where they will do most good.

Williams notes that at the end of the day we simply have to stand up and be counted as to which set of principles we wish to have underpin the way the health care system works. If nothing else, it is good to make our values explicit and thus accountable.

There are many sides to the ethics argument. In essence, the major standpoints are something like this. Medical ethics are fundamental in the health service and in doctor–patient relationships. Health care outcomes involve basic issues relating to the quantity and quality of life. Resources are scarce and decisions need to be made about their allocation. Should doctors act for individual patients or for the community as a whole, or should they leave such decision making to health service managers (thus not compromising their relationship with patients)? If managers and politicians make decisions, how can this be done fairly and will doctors be happy to live with the consequences?

Finally, what does this mean for those who advocate the development of counselling in general practice? Proponents of counselling will need to consider the costs and benefits of counselling to general practice and to the health service as a whole, bearing in mind that the allocation of resources to counselling will necessarily entail other treatments are foregone. The issue of ethics and economics is an, as yet, unexplored area for counsellors, and one that cannot be ignored. In a paper which questions the place of psychoanalysis and psychotherapy in the health service, Wilkinson (1986) writes that various aspects of choosing priorities in health care touch on medical ethics. He believes that it is not a question of ethics *or* economics; without a wide use of economics in health care, inefficiencies will abound and decisions will be made less explicitly and hence less rationally than is desirable. Wilkinson argues that there are pressing clinical, research, economic, and ethical reasons for an urgent review of the extent and impact of psychotherapeutic practices in the NHS. Such an understanding is needed to ensure the provision of efficient and effective mental health services within the context of general health services. The price of inefficiency, inexplicitness, and irrationality in health care is paid for in death and sickness. Food for thought for counsellors.

REFERENCES

Anderson, S. and Hasler, J. C. (1979). Counselling in general practice. *Journal of the Royal College of General Practitioners*, **29**, 352–6.

Ashurst, P. M. (1979). Evaluation of counselling in a general practice setting: preliminary communication. *Journal of the Royal Society of Medicine*, **72**, 657–9.

Ashurst, P. M. and Ward, D. F. (1983). *An evaluation of counselling in general practice*. Final Report of the Leverhulme Counselling Project. Mental Health Foundation, London.

Blakey, R. (1986). Psychological treatment in general practice: its effect on patients and their families. *Journal of the Royal College of General Practitioners*, **36**, 299–311.

Bowling, A. (1990). *Measuring health: a review of quality of life measurement scales*. Open University Press, Milton Keynes.

British Association for Counselling Research Committee. (1989). Evaluating the effectiveness of counselling. *Counselling*, **69**, 27–9.

Brown, P. T. and Abel Smith, A. E. (1985). Counselling in medical settings. *British Journal of Guidance and Counselling*, **13**, 75–88.

Corney, R. H. (1990). Counselling in general practice—does it work? *Journal of the Royal Society of Medicine*, **83**, 253–7.

Cubbon, J. (1991). The Principle of QALY maximisation as the basis for altering health care resources. *Journal of Medical Ethics*, **17**, 181–4.

Daniels, M. H., Mines R., and Gressard, C. (1981). A meta-model for evaluating counselling programmes *Personnel and Guidance Journal*, May, 578–82.

Davis, H. and Fallowfield, L. (ed.) (1991). *Counselling and communication in health care*. Wiley and Sons, Chichester.

Department of Health and Social Security (1987). *Promoting better health. HMSO, London*.

Doyal, L. (1987). General practice and the ethics of resource allocation. *Practitioner*, **231**, 1398–401.

Earll, L. and Kincey, J. (1982). Clinical psychology in general practice. *Journal of the Royal College of General Practitioners*, **32**, 32–7.

Freeman, G. K. and Button, E. J. (1984). The clinical psychologist in general practice: a six year study of consulting patterns for psychosocial problems. *Journal of the Royal College of General Practitioners*, **34**, 377–80.

Ginsberg, G., and Marks, I. M., (1977). Costs and benefits of behavioural psychotherapy: a pilot study of neurotics treated by nurse therapists. *Psychological Medicine*, **7**, 685–700.

Ginsberg, G., Marks, I., and Walters, H. (1984). Cost-benefit analysis of a controlled trial of nurse therapy for neuroses in primary care. *Psychological Medicine*, **14**, 683–90.

Glass, N. J. and Goldberg, D. (1977). Cost benefit analysis and the evaluation of psychiatric services. *Psychological Medicine*, **7**, 701–7.

Goodwin P. J., Feld, R., Warde, P., and Ginsberg, J. (1990). The costs of cancer therapy. *European Journal of Cancer*, **26**, 223–25.

Harris, J. (1987). QUALYfying the value of life. *Journal of Medical Ethics*, **13**, 117–23.

Harris, J. (1991). Un-principled QALYs: a response to Cubbon. *Journal of Medical Ethics*, **17**, 185–8.

Ives, G. (1979). Psychological treatment in general practice. *Journal of the Royal College of General Practitioners*, **29**, 343–51.

Koch, H. C. H. (1979). Evaluation of behaviour therapy interventions in general practice. *Journal of the Royal College of General Practitioners*, **29**, 337–40.

Light, D. (1990). Biting hard on the research bit. *Health Service Journal*, 25 October, 1604–5.

Marks, I. (1985). Controlled trial of psychiatric nurse therapists in primary care. *British Medical Journal*, **290**, 1181–4.

Marks, I. M., Hallam, R. S., and Connelly, J. C. (1975). Nurse therapists in behavioural psychotherapy. *British Medical Journal*, **111**, 144–8.

Marks, I. M., Hallam, R. S., Connolly, J. C., and Philpott, R. (1977). *Nursing in behavioural psychotherapy*. Royal College of Nursing, London.

Marks, I. M., Bird, J., and Lindley, P. (1978). Behavioural nurse therapists— developments and implications. *Behavioural Psychotherapy*, **6**, 25–36.

Martin, E. (1988). Counsellors in general practice. *British Medical Journal*, **297**, 637.

Mooney, G. (1984). Medical ethics: an excuse for inefficiency? *Journal of Medical Ethics*, **10**, 183–5.

Pereira Gray, D. (1988). Counsellors in general practice. *Journal of the Royal College of General Practitioners*, **38**, 50–1.

Robson, M. H, France, R., and Bland, M. (1984). Clinical pyschologist in primary care: controlled clinical and economic evaluation. *British Medical Journal*, **288**, 1805–8.

Rowland, N. and Tolley, K. (1991). Evaluating the cost-effectiveness of counselling. *Counselling*, **2**, 47–9.

Scott, A. I. F. and Freeman, C. P. L. (1992). Edinburgh primary care depression study: treatment outcome, patient satisfaction, and cost after 16 weeks. *British Medical Journal*, **304**, 883–7.

Tolley, K. and Rowland, N. *Evaluating the cost-effectiveness of counselling*. Routledge, London. (In press.)

Torrence, G. W. (1986). Measurement of health state utilities for economic appraisal: a review. *Journal of Health Economics*, **5**, 1–30.

Waydenfeld, D. and Waydenfeld, S. W. (1980). Counselling in general practice. *Journal of the Royal College of General Practitioners*, **30**, 671–7.

Wilkinson, G. (1986). Psychoanalysis and analytic psychotherapy in the NHS—a problem for medical ethics. *Journal of Medical Ethics*, **12**, 87–90.

Williams, A. (1985). The value of QALYs. *Health and Social Services Journal*, **94**, 3–5

Williams, A. (1987). Response: QALYfying the value of life. *Journal of Medical Ethics*, **13**, 117–23.

Williams, A. (1992). Cost-effectiveness analysis: is it ethical? *Journal of Medical Ethics*, **18**, 7–11.

4 Quality and training

Simon Cocksedge and Viv Ball

INTRODUCTION

The arrival of counsellors in the surgeries of general practitioners through-out the United Kingdom in recent years has not been matched by the arrival (for counsellors) of the consistent standards of quality and training which are expected of other members of the primary health care team (PHCT). It is still possible to be appointed as a counsellor in a general practice on the basis of a brief introductory course of evening classes in basic counselling skills, calling oneself a 'counsellor', and meeting a general practitioner (GP) at a party (though going on the course is not essential!).

This chapter begins by looking at the needs of those involved in counselling in primary care. After this, quality issues and training for all members of the PHCT are reviewed. Particular attention is given to the quality and training of counsellors in primary care and to GPs—unless GPs, as the gatekeepers of the National Health Service, are aware of counselling issues for their patients, counsellors in primary care will be underused. Many of the points raised relate to issues which are changing and evolving at present. Even if answers are not available, questions need to be asked.

In the context of this chapter, the underlying meaning of quality in counselling in the primary care setting is taken as the attempt to provide a consistently high standard service to everyone which is both clinically effective and cost-effective.

QUALITY ISSUES

This section considers, from the perspective of both service users and service providers, what is needed in order to ensure that counselling services are of a high standard.

What do clients/patients want or need?

Where once a person in need of help with a personal problem might have turned to a family member, a respected individual in the local community, or a minister of religion, now the family may be widely dispersed, the local community may not tangibly exist, and the role of the clergy may not be understood or accepted. Instead, the local PHCT offers an easily accessible and socially acceptable alternative in the form of the family doctor.

Such a person in need is likely to expect at least two different types of service from the PHCT. The first is the obvious professional role of a trained carer (be it nurse, doctor, physiotherapist, etc.). The second, however, is a more pastoral, listening role.

There is no doubt that listening and pastoral care are seen by the public as part of the normal work of members of the PHCT. Unfortunately, it is often safer and more comfortable for team members to focus on their professional role while ignoring their pastoral and listening responsibilities, thus reducing the quality of overall care that is offered. All members of the team need to be equipped to 'hear' messages from their patients and either deal with such messages themselves or refer elsewhere appropriately.

It is important to note that the person in need mentioned above did not turn first to the local PHCT, but to his or her local GP. People, on the whole, do not understand the concept 'Primary Health Care Team' but they do see their family doctor as their first port of call for health care and they give high priority to his or her level of attention and communication (Consumer's Association 1992). Heavy demands and expectations are thus put on the GP, who acts as the gatekeeper to the National Health Service for most people. This responsibility of gatekeeper is both powerful and crucial. It can only be fulfilled by the GP within the limits of his or her own values, beliefs, training and competence, and his knowledge of locally available services. Hence, the quality of care the patient receives from the PHCT is directly related to the ability of the gatekeeper GP to fill several roles.

The general public need all members of the PHCT to offer competent listening and pastoral care when appropriate. GPs are key figures in this.

What do general practitioners want or need?

The role of the GP in the PHCT is twofold. Firstly, he or she has a professional role as a skilled carer providing general medical services. Secondly, GPs are increasingly involved in planning appropriate services for their patients and in employing and coordinating staff to provide these services.

The GP as skilled carer

After family and friends, people are more likely to consult their GP regarding a personal or emotional problem than any other individual or agency (Corney 1990). It is widely quoted that up to 30 per cent of patients presenting to GPs have emotional problems and that GPs treat 95 per cent of patients with psychosocial problems (Goldberg and Huxley 1992). Possible reasons for this include familiarity and a pre-existing relationship. GPs are unique among caring professionals in seeing people for short interviews or consultations over a long period of time (often, literally, a lifetime). A trusting relationship may be built up during the treatment of relatively minor problems allowing deeper communication when the need arises. Other factors are availability, accessibility, the stability of the GP within the community, and the lack of stigma attached to visiting the surgery.

In order to attend to the psychosocial needs, the doctor must be able to pick up cues, to listen to the 'music' behind the words, and to hear the message a person is trying to communicate. This involves the use of counselling/listening/communication skills (referred to as counselling skills for the rest of this chapter). These skills, which must be distinguished from the process or activity of counselling, need to be part of the 'tools of the trade' for all GPs (see Chapter 1 for a discussion of the distinction between counselling skills and counselling *per se*).

Once the GP has listened and 'heard' the patient, a joint decision must be made. Either a referral is offered or help is provided by the GP alone. If the former, then the referral can be to someone within the PHCT, for example counsellor or community psychiatric nurse (CPN), or elsewhere. The choice depends on the GP's knowledge of the availability of local services and the wishes of the patient. If help is to be offered by the GP, then various factors have to be considered, including the GP's own skills and interest.

A GP may be keen to fill a counselling role, but may not have the time available. GP time is expensive and it may be more cost-effective to refer such patients elsewhere. However, patients want more time with their doctor (Consumer's Association 1992). Is the current trend for practices to employ a counsellor an escape by the doctors into a doctor-centred role? Are GPs really giving their patients what they want and need by referral to a specialist counsellor, or would these patients prefer, and be equally helped by, more time with their doctor? If so, should list sizes be further reduced? Is employing a counsellor just a safe and soft option for GPs to avoid the psychosocial problems, which might be both threatening and time-consuming? Are counsellors becoming 'the benzodiazepines of the nineties', a quick 'prescription' to get the patient out of the surgery in less than six minutes? Is considering employing a counsellor a symptom of an unmet need within the doctor or the practice? Is the possibility of referring patients to a counsellor actually a cry for help or part of a self-searching process by the GPs? Are the needs of the doctors separated from the needs of their patients? As the drift towards employing counsellors continues, these questions need to be answered, as they have wide implications for the provision of a high-quality primary care service.

For patients to receive a full and effective service from the National Health Service, their GP/gatekeeper must have the ability to get to the point of decision mentioned earlier. All GPs, whether or not they are interested in the psychological aspects of their work, must be able to listen and 'hear'. Without this ability, which must be taught as part of their training (see 'Training needs for GPs' below), GPs will offer a poor quality service to their patients.

The GP as planner and employer

Increasingly GPs, especially fund holders, are involved in the planning and provision of services within the community. Monitoring the quality of such services is implicit in this and involves assessing need and looking at what is already available locally, both in the health service (including the practice itself) and the voluntary sector. From such a review of local mental health services may come the question 'should a counsellor be employed by the practice?' If the answer to this question is 'yes' or even 'maybe', then where does the GP start? How can GPs ensure that such a counselling service is of high quality?

One important source of help is the British Association for Counselling (BAC). The BAC is a professional body for counsellors and practising members must abide by the Association's Code of Ethics and Practice. The Association is involved in standard setting for counsellors by accrediting both training courses and individual counsellors. It has also produced guidelines for the employment of counsellors in general practice (British Association for Counselling 1993). These guidelines cover the role of the counsellor, the training that the counsellor should have undertaken, and a discussion of the job description (with a sample job description outlined). In addition, funding, employment status, insurance, and professional membership along with the role of the counsellor in the PHCT are considered.

Given that counsellors are relatively recent additions to the PHCT, it is important that time is spent devising a job description. Unless this is well defined, there will be uncertainty for both the GPs and the counsellor. It is also important that the role of the counsellor is understood and agreed by all members of the team. Central issues include referral and liaison. Who can refer? Which patients should be seen by the counsellor and which by other team members such as CPNs? How do the counsellor and the GP work together? Should referral involve reviewing patients together, joint consultations, or the counsellor supporting the GP who continues to see the patient? In addition, some thought must be given to deciding what is an 'appropriate' service. How many sessions should be offered to each person? How long should the sessions be? Is long-term counselling 'appropriate' in a primary care setting? Factors such as supervision, an uninterrupted quiet room, confidentiality, audit and evaluation, records and assessments must all be discussed. Again, the BAC guidelines (British Association for Counselling 1993) will prove helpful in considering these topics. Unless the practice and the counsellor are clear about these issues, a poor quality service will be offered.

One important early task is finding the funding for a counsellor. Fundholding practices, with control of their own budget, are likely to find this easier than non-fundholders, who may have difficulty getting salary reimbursement from their Family Health Services Authority (FHSA) (there is a quality issue here in the potential for a two-tier service). Recent changes in payment for health promotion clinics have affected the funding of counsellors in some FHSAs.

Deciding on an appropriate salary may also be difficult. There is at present no consensus on how much counsellors working in primary care should be paid. What should the level of the counsellor's remuneration be relative to other members of the PHCT, such as the health visitor, midwife, or district nurse who are frequently as, if not more, highly trained? There is unlikely to be agreement on this subjective and emotive issue until the position of the counsellor in the PHCT is fully established and a national salary scale is produced. To reduce resentment, it would be best if such a scale were directly related to the salaries of comparable professional groups in the PHCT (for example nurses, social workers, etc.). Due allowance must be made for the level of training (which may have been self-financed), funding of supervision, and possibly self-employed status. For the present, GPs need to make their own judgements on this contentious issue, bearing in mind, with reference to quality, the old adage that 'you get what you pay for'.

In addition, the GP needs to find a well-trained counsellor. What does 'well-trained' mean in the context of counselling in primary care? There is no consensus on this among counsellors or among GPs already employing counsellors. A recent survey (Sibbald *et al*. 1993) has shown that three types of counsellor presently predominate—CPNs, practice counsellors, and clinical psychologists. Of the 586 counsellors surveyed, GPs reported that only between one-third and one-half had training in counselling. The qualifications of 85 were unknown to the employing GP! These are astonishing statistics. Not only are GPs employing many people as practice counsellors who have no direct training for the job (though they may have relevant parallel training), but in many cases, the GPs do not know the qualifications of their counsellors.

There is an urgent need for a national registration system ensuring a guaranteed baseline level of quality and professional competence for counsellors generally and particularly in primary care (in the way that being a Registered General Nurse guarantees a basic level of competence which is easily understood by other health care professionals). This is a crucial issue for the future of counselling in primary care (see below 'Training needs for counsellors').

How does a GP go about finding a practice counsellor? This may be difficult. The first place to ask is the local FHSA who may have a list of potential counsellors and be able to offer advice (see below 'What do FHSAs want or need?'). Secondly, it is worth approaching the BAC who may be able to advise on local contacts (for example local training courses) and who publish a fortnightly jobfile in which vacant posts can be advertised. Other possibilities for advertising include local papers and the national press (the Wednesday jobs section of *The Guardian* is widely read).

What do other members of the PHCT want or need?

Like GPs, every member of the PHCT needs to be able to respond to their patients' call for listening and pastoral care, in addition to using their normal professional skills. But, also like GPs, there is considerable variability in training and ability in relation to this among the PHCT. Some may feel that listening and pastoral care should be part of their role but feel inadequately skilled, others that they are already overwhelmed and stretched to the limit. In addition, some team members may be enthusiastic and interested in this aspect of their work, but simply not have enough time to respond adequately.

Whatever the situation, all members of the PHCT must be able to use basic counselling skills when necessary and should consider it part of their role to do so. They must also be prepared to refer patients back to the GP, to a practice counsellor, or to other appropriate sources of help. Such liaison requires good links between the counsellor and all members of the PHCT.

What do counsellors want or need?

General practice is the initial point of contact with the National Health Service for most people. This gives primary care an immediacy and accessibility which is both unique and attractive to the members of the PHCT. It is, in part, this immediacy and accessibility which draws counsellors to primary care.

At a general level, specialist counsellors want to become accepted as valued and useful members of the PHCT. They want their specific role to be understood and distinguishable from CPNs (who will be more appropriate for overt psychiatric illness, psychosis, and depression, although some may adopt a broader counselling role, see Chapter 6) and from other members of the PHCT. This distinction is generally neither well defined nor understood.

Although it is estimated that about 30 per cent of general practices at present have counsellors (Sibbald *et al.* 1993), concrete evidence to prove their efficacy and cost-effectiveness is still being accumulated (see Chapters 3 and 17). Until this is available, it may be difficult to convince sceptical members of current PHCTs that they need another colleague.

Part of being accepted is being adequately trained. Counsellors want to be fully trained and competent to work in primary care, but sadly this is not always the case. There are few BAC recognized courses. Counsellors in training will have to find their own course fees and associated expenses. There is no doubt that training aimed specifically at counselling in a primary care setting is woefully lacking at present and much needed, though some progress is currently being made in this area (see below 'Training needs for counsellors').

Counsellors in primary care need to be able to be self-directed and independent practitioners. They must be able to cope with relative isolation (counselling, like general practice, can be a lonely business), but also able to link with other professionals beyond their place of employment. Within the practice, mutual respect and teamwork are essential, involving good links, feedback, and liaison. A wider role for the counsellor as a facilitator and educator within the practice team also needs consideration. This might include attendance at PHCT meetings and discussion of problems with team members (which may be patient-related or more personal). The counsellor may be able to act as an informal facilitator for communication within the practice, enabling team members to think about their work in different ways. In addition, the counsellor may be used as a resource for advice and encouragement by team members, possibly enabling them to manage patients themselves who might otherwise have needed referral elsewhere.

Counsellors need to recognize the limits of their competence. This is a key element of training and the limits will vary from counsellor to counsellor. They will be determined by the counsellor's training (for example some Relate-trained counsellors will feel happy to take on psychosexual counselling) and by the other resources that are available locally (a knowledge of which is essential for all counsellors in primary care). The ability to recognize overt psychiatric illness is obviously essential. In addition, some counsellors may not feel happy to take on longer-term counselling/ psychotherapy.

To offer a high quality service, counsellors also need an understanding of the practical day-to-day business of organizing a counselling scheme in a general practice. This includes how to ensure appropriate referrals, a system (with good liaison) for assessing patients and if necessary referring on to others or back to the GP, adequate remuneration (varying according to training, experience, and level of responsibility) with a contract, a suitable venue (a quiet, uninterrupted room), secretarial support, supervision (which should be remunerated), and an appointments system, along with agreements on a method of maintaining records and on confidentiality issues.

What do FHSAs want or need?

FHSAs, along with District Health Authorities (DHAs), have a duty on behalf of the tax-paying public to assess health needs, to ensure the provision of appropriate services, and to be accountable for both. They need to be convinced of both the health benefits and the economic benefits of counselling in the primary care setting—as mentioned earlier, the evidence is accumulating but the case is not yet proven. They need a full understanding of counselling in general and counselling in primary care in particular. They also need a policy on the role of counsellors in primary care: who should become a counsellor in general practice, what are the guidelines on standards, funding, supervision, etc? The BAC guidelines are intended to help health service managers as well as GPs and counsellors (British Association for Counselling 1993). The key to this is having a liaison officer (who ideally will be both a health care professional and an administrator) who can operate at both a practice and a policy level, relating equally to contractors/PHCTs, DHAs, and community mental health services.

FHSAs also have a duty to protect the public from inappropriate, incompetent, or negligent health care. They may need to be involved in disciplinary and complaints procedures.

At present, there are considerable difficulties for FHSAs. Priorities and organizations vary—there is a total and inequitable lack of consistency nationally about approval and funding for counsellors in primary care. Some FHSAs have adopted a very 'hands off' stance, while others (such as Derbyshire) are heavily involved, with close liaison on standard setting, appointing counsellors, in-service training, funding, and supervision.

There is an urgent need for a national policy to set standards for counselling in general and counselling in primary care in particular (see also 'Training needs for counsellors'). Such a policy could be administered locally by FHSAs and would allow local flexibility but ensure national consistency. It would first involve ensuring that GPs and all other members of the PHCT are equipped with adequate counselling skills during their training to enable them to fulfil a listening/pastoral role in addition to their clinical role. Secondly, it would involve a national system for the funding of counsellors in primary care, so that everyone in the country has access to a counsellor. Thirdly, it should ensure that counsellors are seen as full members of the PHCT liaising closely with other team members (especially CPNs), so that their role and areas of responsibility are delineated. Finally, such a policy should establish standards of training and supervision for counsellors in primary care. As a minimum, these should be that all counsellors in primary care must be BAC accredited or possess an equivalent qualification, for example hold the Diploma in Counselling Psychology of the British Psychological Society (British Psychological Society 1993), and undertake the regular supervision required in the accreditation scheme. In addition, as specific training for counselling in primary care becomes available, it should be regarded as part of the qualifications for counsellors working in this setting.

The framework for such a national structure, for counselling generally and for primary care in particular, needs to be facilitated, perhaps even laid down centrally, by the Department of Health. Until such a scheme is in place, counselling will remain in limbo. Comparability with other professions will not be achieved and development (for instance of pay scales and career possibilities) will not take place.

Conclusions

People in need presenting to the PHCT want attention to both their psychosocial and their physical needs. If members of the team cannot attend to the 'whole' person in this way, they are failing to offer a reasonable quality of care. All members of the PHCT need to be able to use basic counselling skills. If a practice counsellor is involved, quality should be ensured by adequate training and supervision (although there are no national standards at present) coupled with efficient organization in the practice, good liaison, referral, and teamwork.

FHSAs, DHAs and the Department of Health have a duty to evaluate the mental health needs of the whole population and relate this to local communities. In relation to counselling in primary care, they need to look at quality both in terms of clinical and financial effectiveness—this requires national standards.

TRAINING ISSUES

To achieve standards, training is essential. This section looks at the training needs of those working in primary care in relation to counselling.

Training needs for GPs

As discussed earlier in this chapter, simple attentive listening by the GP using basic counselling skills will often be enough to help a person start to understand their position and then to move forward. If a problem is present that requires attention, a number of possibilities may occur. The G.P. may:

(1) fail to unearth the problem initially;
(2) ignore the issue as being outside the remit of a disease-centred approach to general practice;
(3) see the patient for a series of consultations in normal surgery;
(4) see the patient for one or more longer sessions outside normal surgery hours;
(5) refer the patient elsewhere for further help.

The training needs of GPs can be considered in the light of the above options:

1. *Failing to unearth the problem initially*: it is essential that, on entering general practice, doctors have sufficient awareness of themselves and others to be able to be sensitive to the non-somatic needs of their patients. Failure to do so may lead to frustration for both the doctor and the patient. It may also have economic implications—the over-investigation of somatization, based on a disease-centred approach, may be very expensive.

2. *Ignoring the issue*: potential GPs need to be made aware, both at medical school and in vocational training, of the demands and expectations put on to them by society to attend to the whole person, not just to physical illness. Although it is generally safer and easier to focus on the purely physical, any GP who does so is inappropriately ignoring a vast area of need.

3. *Seeing the patient for a series of consultations in normal surgery*: this is the most likely option for most GPs. A combination of time, use of basic counselling skills to listen empathically, and the appropriate medication, if necessary, will often be enough to relieve distress.

4. *Seeing the patient for one or more longer sessions*: some GPs feel happy to work at a deeper level, though there may be issues of boundaries for the patient. Further training may be helpful, but is clearly only for the minority. A GP working in this way may need supervision or further support (see Chapter 15).

5. *Referring the patient elsewhere*: the GP needs to know what other health professionals can offer his patient and what resources are available locally. These may include counsellors (employed in the practice or working privately), voluntary agencies (such as Relate and Cruse), CPNs (who may be part of a community mental health team), psychologists, psychotherapists, psychiatrists, local clergy, hospice bereavement teams, pregnancy advisory services, drug abuse, and HIV services—the list will vary from place to place.

One additional training need is that of support for GPs. Medical schools are demanding and sometimes dehumanizing places which put considerable stresses on students. Students are turned into doctors, who are seen as authority figures and who, it is assumed, are there to help others, do not fail, and do not need personal support or help for themselves. Despite all the training, many doctors entering general practice are surprised by, and unprepared for, the variety of roles expected of them. Little attention is paid to the personal development of general practitioners. How can a GP 'give' for 35 years? Is the 'return' in terms of job satisfaction and patients' gratitude, not to mention a good income, sufficient reward? Is being a doctor-centred doctor just a survival mechanism? Can an authority figure, who may have little self-awareness, ask for or receive help? Counsellors take it for granted that supervision is part of their work. No such assumption exists in general practice, which can be a very lonely place.

Training opportunities for GPs

The first opportunity to influence doctors comes in selection for medical school. It is essential that personality factors, in addition to levels of academic achievement, are taken into consideration. Once at medical school, counselling/communication skills need to be a prominent part of the curriculum (as is already the case in some places) along with an attempt to raise students' awareness of themselves and others.

As was emphasized in the Toronto Consensus Statement on doctor–patient communication (Simpson *et al.* 1991), clinical communication skills do not reliably improve from mere experience. Such skills training should be given at all levels of the curriculum and qualifying authorities should require proof of competence in counselling/communication skills. Unless such teaching is an assessed part of the curriculum, many students, often struggling to cope with the sheer volume of learning at medical school, will not value it adequately and will not attend enough sessions, resulting in a lost opportunity.

The next opportunity to produce listening doctors comes in vocational training for general practice. Unfortunately, junior hospital doctors (including GP trainees during the hospital component of their training) often receive little teaching, either regarding clinical skills or counselling/communication skills. The Royal College of General Practitioners is, however, attempting to rectify this situation (Royal College of General Practitioners 1993).

Specific instruction in the use of the consultation, and counselling/communication skills within it (Pendleton *et al.* 1984), needs to be taught and assessed during the trainee year, either by trainers or on day-release courses. Again, this is already the case in some places. In addition, an awareness, first of the pivotal role of the GP in identifying and managing psychosocial problems, secondly of the need for teamwork in primary care, and thirdly of counselling itself (as distinct from counselling skills) and the role of counsellors in primary care, must develop at this stage. Self-awareness must also be raised, with personal development seen as central, normal, and non-threatening, both for trainees and established GPs.

Once doctors become general practitioners, the opportunities for training become fewer. The trainee on becoming a principal loses the support of the trainer, often moves to a new area and may feel very isolated. A Young Principals Group or a mentorship scheme may help here. Some practices are involved in team-building, practice facilitation, and development of the individual within the group. This can be very helpful, but may prove too threatening for some. Other methods of continuing support include Balint groups and short courses as part of continuing medical education.

There are many brief courses in counselling skills which may be of interest to some GPs. An introductory course might be for 6–10 evening sessions, often organized by colleges of further education as part of an adult education programme. More extended training (generally one to three years of half-day or evening attendance, weekly) will involve theoretical and practical work leading to a certificate or diploma in counselling. These longer courses are usually college or university based (the BAC has a directory of courses). Full training in counselling or psychotherapy will only be an option for a minority.

Accredited counsellors are only allowed to practice if they are receiving regular supervision from an experienced colleague who has had further training. Supervision is seen as central to the process of counselling. It is both suprising, and sad, that no such facility exists for, or is required of, the GP. Opportunities for further personal growth along with support for practising GPs are all too rare. Some sort of continuing support or supervision, possibly linked to the postgraduate education allowance, could only improve the health of the nation's GPs.

Training needs for counsellors

Patients who are referred to a practice counsellor will assume that the counsellor is a professional trained to the same standard as the other members of the PHCT. Sadly, as demonstrated above, this is not always the case. To appoint a counsellor in general practice on the basis of an evening introductory course in basic listening skills is the equivalent of sending someone on a first aid course and then offering them a post as a district nurse.

Counsellors need both general training and training for counselling in primary care. All such training must be related to accreditation.

General training for counsellors

The range and standard of training for counsellors varies from area to area, resulting in a confusing muddle of qualifications. Courses range from brief introductions to counselling skills, which may be mistaken for a professional qualification by the layman, to intensive three-year diplomas leading directly to BAC accreditation. A short course in basic counselling skills may help someone to become a better nurse, but it is not a qualification for a post as a counsellor. At present, there is no overall consistency between training courses at different institutions, and selection for courses may be minimal and influenced by an ability to pay the fees.

End-point measurement of competency also varies from course to course and may not even be assessed.

The above may seem an excessively gloomy exaggeration. There are undoubtedly excellent courses available at all levels for counselling training throughout the United Kingdom. The development of National Vocational Qualifications may provide another avenue for assessment of competence. However, what is needed is standardization of training, qualifications, and possibly career structure for counsellors, so that the public (who fund the services and who come as clients to see counsellors), counsellors themselves, would-be counsellors, and those who wish to employ counsellors can all be confident that a certain level of competence has been attained by any one counsellor.

A start on this has been made by the BAC. First, training courses are being recognized as suitable for accreditation purposes, though, as yet, few courses have been approved. Secondly, individual accreditation is available through the BAC, though this is not yet widely recognized by employers and the public as a benchmark for counselling competence. BAC accreditation is demanding, requiring the completion of an approved training course (of at least 450 hours) and a minimum of 450 hours of counselling practice under supervision. Accreditation is given for a five-year period, during which the counsellor must continue to receive supervision and adhere to the Association's Code of Ethics and Practice.

Any training leading to accreditation must involve a theoretical framework allied to concurrent supervised clinical practice, demonstrating an ability to work competently with a wide range of issues. Personal development, in a group or individually, needs to be part of this.

At present, there is no regulation of counsellors in the United Kingdom. Anyone, with or without training, can call themselves a counsellor and set up in practice. This is in contrast to the rest of the European Community and the United States of America where a licence is required in order to practise. There is also, to the outsider, a confusing overlap in language and professional bodies between counselling and psychotherapy.

A national accreditation/licencing scheme for counsellors is needed, demonstrating fitness to practise. This would ensure comparability of training and selection along with continuing monitoring of standards. It would mean that the GP (or any other employer) wishing to appoint a counsellor could be certain of a basic level of competence.

Training for counsellors in primary care

A recent survey (Einzig *et al.* 1994) has suggested that counsellors working in primary care feel that their basic training has been adequate, but that they need further specific training. Many of them felt unprepared for the content of their work in primary care and for the range of problems and specific disorders they encountered. A desire to have more training in these areas and to learn effective ways of coping with them (particularly brief therapy training and referral networks) was frequently mentioned. Other training areas considered important were the medical model of illness and health, pharmacology, health service structure, collaboration, and issues of referral. In addition, it was felt that some shared training between GPs and counsellors would be helpful.

The Counselling in Primary Care Trust is currently exploring two areas relating to quality and training (Curtis Jenkins, personal communication). The first is the development of a counselling in primary health care diploma. This is to be a one-year course for qualified and experienced counsellors. Areas to be covered in the syllabus include working in a multidisciplinary PHCT, developing referral networks, working with models of illness and health, and acquiring skills in brief counselling interventions. There can be no doubt that if such a diploma becomes a requirement for employment as a counsellor in primary health care, it will lead to improvements in the quality of service offered to the public.

The second area being explored is that of quality of counsellor competence along with methods of assessment. There are parallels here with the training/reaccreditation of GPs and the difficulty of assessing competence once basic qualifications have been obtained. These issues need further thought and development.

Training needs of other PHCT members

The assertion of the Toronto Consensus Statement that counselling/communication skills must be taught and assessed in the training of doctors (Simpson *et al.* 1991) surely applies to all members of the PHCT. Communication is at the heart of good quality health care and is of central importance, both for the professional staff (nurses, midwives, health visitors, CPNs, social workers, etc.) and for the non-clinical staff (receptionists, secretaries, practice manager).

What is important is that each team member is equipped with counselling/communication skills appropriate to their role. These will obviously be very different, for example, for the district nurse and the practice receptionist. However, both must be able to 'hear' and respond adequately, but neither needs full counselling training. Such skills need to be developed throughout training and must be appropriate to the individual's role and level of responsibility.

To take nurses as an example, with the advent of Project 2000 and the development of a new core curriculum, counselling skills are being taught as part of their basic training. This may help to raise levels of self-awareness, at an early stage in a professional career, concerning the possibilities open to the alert, listening nurse. Many nurses, through the 'hands on' nature of their work, receive confidences and hear about problems which might otherwise go untold. The nurse needs to be able to respond to such communications adequately, either personally or through discussion with, and referral to, other members of the PHCT.

Qualified social workers are required to be able to demonstrate competence in counselling skills. However, their training in this area is generally brief and founded more on theoretical knowledge than on practice.

GPs ignore, at their peril, the skills and training needs of their non-clinical ancillary staff. The reputation of a practice may be made or broken by the quality of the reception staff. There are many short courses on counselling skills which may improve relationships at the 'shop window' of a practice. Practice managers need to gain similar experience. They are in the front line in dealing with any complaints from patients, as well as having a managerial role both inside and outside the practice, for which good counselling skills are essential.

There will thus be training needs related to each individual member of the PHCT. However, it may also be helpful to train the team with an eye to multidisciplinary factors and overall team function. Communicating in a productive and supportive way with other members of the PHCT is as important as communicating with patients.

Other carers

Passing mention must be made to other skilled 'listeners' in the community. Ministers of religion, Citizens Advice Bureaux, and other agencies (such as Alcoholics Anonymous, hospice bereavement support teams, drug addiction agencies, the Samaritans) will offer support and befriending if required. The level of training undertaken may vary from the rudimentary to the highly qualified and experienced. Even those whose training is minimal, however, may give useful help, providing they have been well selected.

Conclusions

If quality primary care is to be given to local communities (as discussed in the first half of this chapter), then all members of the PHCT must be trained and assessed in basic counselling skills.

GPs are central to primary care, and GP training and assessment at all levels must provide the skills to allow attention to the psychosocial as well as the purely physical problems. The training of GPs should also involve continuing support and personal development (akin to the supervision that counsellors are required to receive) which should be continued once a career post is achieved.

A national register of counsellors is needed, preferably with a licencing/registration system as a requirement of fitness to practise. This would mean that anyone wishing to appoint a counsellor would know that training and assessment of adequate quality (that is to BAC accreditation level, or equivalent) had taken place. Specific training in counselling in a primary care setting must continue to be developed if high standards and national consistency are to be achieved.

REFERENCES

British Association for Counselling (Counselling in Medical Settings) (1993). *Guidelines for the employment of counsellors in general practice*. British Association for Counselling, 1 Regent Place, Rugby CV21 2PJ.

British Psychological Society (1993). *Regulations for the diploma in counselling psychology*. The British Psychological Society, St. Andrews House, 48 Princess Road East, Leicester LE1 7DR.

Consumer's Association (1992). GPs: your verdict. *Which?*, April, 202–5.

Corney, R. H. (1990). A survey of professional help sought by patients for psychosocial problems. *British Journal of General Practice*, **40**, 365–8.

Einzig, H., Curtis Jenkins, G., and Basharan, H. (1994). The training needs of counsellors working in primary medical care. *Journal of Mental Health*. (In press.)

Goldberg, D. and Huxley, P. (1992). *Common mental disorders*. Routledge, London.

Pendleton, D., Schofield, T., Tate, P., and Havelock, P. (1984). *The consultation: an approach to learning and teaching*. Oxford University Press, Oxford.

Royal College of General Practitioners (1993). *The quality of hospital-based education for general practice*. Royal College of General Practitioners, 14 Princes Gate, Hyde Park, London SW7 1PU.

Sibbald, B., Addington-Hall, J., Brenneman, D., and Freeling, P. (1993). Counsellors in English and Welsh general practices: their nature and distribution. *British Medical Journal*, **306**, 29–33.

Simpson, M., Buckman, R., Stewart, M., Maguire, P., Lipkin, M., Novack, D., *et al.* (1991). Doctor–patient communication: the Toronto consensus statement. *British Medical Journal*, **303**, 1385–7.

Part II
Counselling problems

5 Interpersonal relationship and psychological problems

Jill Irving

INTRODUCTION

Over two thousand years ago the physician Galen pointed out that 60 per cent of people visiting their doctor suffered from symptoms that had an emotional rather than a physical cause. The twentieth century has seen little change; a 1971 survey found that the incidence of stress-related patient attendances ranged between 50 and 80 per cent (Shapiro 1971) It seems that now, as then, patients tend to somatize unhappiness. Today the discerning GP can help a patient understand the link between the presenting symptom and underlying distress, and those who regard counselling as a viable treatment option for people experiencing difficulties in their personal lives are employing counsellors to work as members of the primary health care team.

Early schemes tended to use counsellors from voluntary organizations. Relate (formerly Marriage Guidance), a movement that gained credibility through its work and training schemes, provided one of the first sources from which counsellors were drawn to work in doctors' surgeries. Probably as a result, the referrals made in the early years of my work as a practice counsellor were more concerned with marital and partnership problems, whereas latterly they have included difficulties encountered at work, with children, gender, stress, the effects of progressive illness, bereavement, infertility, and many others. However, the majority of referrals could still be classified as interpersonal, relationship, and psychological problems—the subject of this chapter.

Throughout the text I will use the terms 'interpersonal' and 'relationship' when referring to the transactions between people, for instance between employer and employee, or husband and wife. The term 'psychological' will refer to an individual's intrapersonal relationships, that is how he or she relates to a part of the psyche, say the conscience. But it will also refer to the interaction between different parts of the psyche, such as a conflict between dependency needs and the drive towards independence.

The first part of this chapter will explore the complexities inherent in the referral process, discuss the reasons for referral, outline the form of assessment procedures, and specify the problems that bring people to counselling. The second part will use anonymized case material to illustrate the counselling process when working with clients with a range of interpersonal, relationship, and psychological problems. The cases are recounted in a way that endeavours to trace the links between theory, practice, and outcome. However, this can only reflect the framework developed and used by myself and colleagues. Given the variety of conceptual approaches that have evolved in the counselling field, others may use a different frame of reference.

PART 1

Referrals and the referral process

When two people engage in a counselling relationship there is usually a third involved—the person who makes the referral. The next few sections will look at the influence that individual expectations and the three-way relationship between client, counsellor, and the referring GP have on the counselling process.

Patients and clients share similar views about the qualities they find helpful and unhelpful in their doctors and counsellors (Oldfield 1983; Treadway 1983). Satisfaction is associated with feeling understood and being able to verbalize requests (for patients) and with feeling able to say what they like (for clients); dissatisfaction occurs when doctors or counsellors are perceived as paying more attention to their own concerns than to those of their patients or clients.

Furthermore, the emphasis placed on the use of counselling skills, such as attentive listening, empathy and rapport, whether consulting or counselling, can blur the boundary between the two activities (see Chapter 1)

Why refer?

If the skilled and responsive doctor is similar to the skilled and responsive counsellor, then why refer? As supporters of counsellor attachments to the primary care team are quick to point out, the effective use of counselling skills in the counsellor/client relationship or the doctor/patient relationship is not sufficient in itself to make a person into an effective counsellor (Rowland 1992). Counsellors need to be sensitized to their own biases, prejudices, and any predilection they have to identify with their clients in order to remain as objective as possible in their work. Doctors seldom have the opportunity for this type of self-scrutiny and, even if they did, they may eschew it as unsuitable. One GP, an ardent believer in the benefits of counselling in primary care, goes so far as to suggest that a doctor's training and experience can foster the development of personal defences that are the very antithesis to the informed personal awareness that is crucial to the counselling process (Feinmann 1991). Others, less convinced about the benefits of counselling, have expressed their concerns. Harris (1987) argues that counselling has become a vogue word covering a range of techniques and treatment procedures so wide as to be almost absurd and that these can confuse doctors rather than help them to make accurate referrals. Courtney (1989) fears that the trend to have counsellors attached to general practice may prove counterproductive, as specialization could impair the GP's ability to help patients with problems that are not traditionally medical. He suggests that only cases which present special difficulties should be referred to counsellors.

The attitudes of GPs towards counselling can range between 'seeing counselling as an antidote to misery' (Feinmann 1991) to regarding counsellors as undermining their skills and fragmenting their role. While such a diversity of opinions is unlikely to be housed in one practice, differences will exist. The comment, 'each doctor has a different idea of how useful I am', made by a counsellor attached to a busy South London practice probably sums up the situation in many surgeries fairly accurately (Grosser 1988).

Interpersonal aspects of the referral process

The complexities of the referral triangle of doctor, counsellor, and patient soon become obvious once a counsellor joins a practice. Differences in professional attitudes, ambivalent feelings about treatment procedures, false expectations of roles, and professional rivalry are ingredients for potential conflict (see Chapters 2 and 14). Brook and Temperley's (1976), study of the attachment of a psychotherapist to general practice was one of the first to point out the difficulties that can occur if professionals ignore or fail to give proper consideration to the interpersonal aspects of their relationships. Harmonious relationships can be difficult to achieve and successful liaisons require colleagues to risk challenging each others' perspective and professional philosophy. As one GP pointed out, referral to a counsellor can be useful when a doctor is at loggerheads with a patient (McLeod 1988), but it is unlikely to be so if the doctor is at loggerheads with the counsellor. Another GP (Newnes 1990) writing about the benefits of good communication between doctor and counsellor commented:

Being open to counselling attitudes allows me to recognise what I call a 'flash', a moment where I understand that the patient's problem may be emotional rather than medical.

He stressed that this didn't happen at once:

Our early experience of integrating S . . . into the practice was disturbing. We all had preconceived ideas and it took a long time for us to understand what the relationship between GPs and counsellors could become. What we have learned is that the 'tack-on' counsellor doesn't work . . . counselling must be part of the fundamental attitude of the whole practice.

The counsellor too felt that full integration was essential to the success of counselling and that his expectations of working in general practice underwent change:

I came here thinking GPs could become psychotherapists. Now I think they should simply incorporate counselling skills and attitudes into their consultations.

If integration takes time and requires change in attitudes and perceptions for both doctors and counsellors, some misconceptions are bound to linger. Sometimes, these can form the cornerstone for discussion, leading to better communication.

Sometimes, even when doctor and counsellor work closely together, a referral can present difficulties if the patient is already enmeshed in a complex emotional relationship with the GP that has not been taken into consideration.

Leslie, a man with a long history of depression, came to his GP with a request to keep him alive long enough for him to see his children through their education, when he would then feel free to take his own life. The GP's pragmatic response of 'I think we can do that for you' astonished him, as he was expecting the doctor to try and persuade him to change his attitude. By treating the request as valid and taking a non-judgmental attitude, the GP gave Leslie the space to reflect on the feelings that had brought him to this desperate decision. They immediately formed a therapeutic relationship which enabled Leslie to work through many of the feelings that had bedevilled him for years in a more adult and constructive manner. He was referred to the counsellor for help with some loose ends which seemed to prevent him from making the changes that he clearly needed to do.

On seeing Leslie the counsellor noted that although he claimed to understand the need for the referral perfectly well and fully agreed with the GP's decision, he seemed tired and unenthusiastic and distant to the counsellor. She felt that he had 'idealized' the GP to the extent that he was unable to acknowledge the mixture of feelings he experienced at being 'passed on'. By assuming that Leslie could continue to work in the same co-operative manner with the counsellor as he had with the GP, all three had got caught up in the unrealistic expectation that the quality of one relationship could be transferred, with relative ease, to another. Why should this have been so? Both doctor and counsellor were experienced, psychologically sophisticated, and regarded themselves as good communicators. Yet, on reflection the referral seemed naive. Had the GP hung on to the patient too long, unaware of transference feelings that can block progress and with which he was untrained to deal? Had the counsellor failed to acknowledge rivalrous feelings that might ruffle their working relationship? Was Leslie's behaviour an over-determined response against the anxiety of loss too complex to fully comprehend or verbalize? Or, with time at a premium in a busy practice, had the referral been too hurried? Whether or not one or all of these questions could provide the key to his behaviour is open to conjecture—he failed to turn up for his second appointment and left the area soon after. What they do highlight is that even when there is good communication between GP and counsellor, there are other factors that can adversely affect a referral.

The above are only some of the influences that have a bearing on the dynamics of the referral triangle, the significance of which is that the interpersonal relationships of all parties involved—GP, patient, and counsellor—make an important contribution to the effectiveness of the referral process and in turn to the outcome of counselling itself.

When to refer

As Morrell (1992) observes:

Doctors working in primary care are the first line for those who are bereaved, anxious, depressed and stressed or who have the sexual, marital and family problems that often accompany these conditions.

Yet research suggests there is a mismatch between the prevalence of emotional disorder in general practice and the ability of doctors to identify patients who have emotional problems (Chancellor *et al.* 1977; Marks *et al.* 1979). How then can doctors know when and how best to refer a patient for counselling? In practice, doctors have expressed surprise at the wide range of problems they have been able to refer to counsellors (personal communication). While there is a need for more comprehensive research into which types of patient problems are best treated by which types of psychological intervention (Sibbald *et al.* 1993) there is evidence to suggest that many psychosocial problems respond to counselling (Gray 1988), and that prominent amongst these are anxiety, stress, and malaise provoked by difficulties in marriage, the family, and other relationships.

The importance of making appropriate referrals has been well documented (McLeod 1992; Rowland and Hurd 1989). The knowledge and skills the GP needs to do so have also received a good deal of attention (McLeod 1992; Morgan *et al.* 1990; Thomas 1993). Those who have an informed understanding of the counselling process, are skilled in picking up emotional problems and maintain good communication with the counsellor seem well equipped to assess which patients might benefit from counselling.

In practice, gaining information about a patient's emotional well-being and suitability for counselling is often achieved by asking 'feeling type' questions such as; Are you worried about anything? How are you in yourself? Could you put that feeling into words or have you mixed feelings about the situation? What is your mood like these days? How patients answer can be as informative as the answer itself in assessing their capacity for insight and their ability to explore thoughts, feelings, attitudes, and behaviour in a counselling setting.

Many patients are anxious about revealing their personal concerns to a stranger or admitting that they are finding it difficult to cope. Doctors who understand the aims, objectives, and process of counselling are in a better position to encourage patients to use the service. By explaining that, in counselling, people are regarded with respect whatever their problem or distress, complete confidentiality is observed, and no judgements are made, they are able to give their patients a clearer understanding of the type of help they can expect. If time permits, a brief meeting with the counsellor can be arranged prior to commencement of counselling. This provides a personal touch that has been found to work well (Rowland and Hurd 1989).

Assessment procedures

Once a patient with an interpersonal or intrapersonal problem is referred for counselling there are several issues that need clarifying if it is to be a useful experience for that person. Balancing a client's needs with the resources available requires careful consideration when making an assessment. The amount of long-term work (that is from several months to several years) which it is possible to take on in general practice is usually more limited than in other settings (McLeod 1988). Contractual, short-term focused work with a specific number of sessions is more straightforward in theory than in practice, as it may take time before the extent of a client's needs become clear. To allow for this, contracts are usually renewable and many counsellors, including myself, have found their case-load includes some long-term work. However, if too much of such work is taken on, waiting lists can soon develop. When it seems likely that a client needs lengthy and frequent treatment it is probably advisable to refer them elsewhere.

Counsellors need to elicit information for assessment purposes. Some feel that a formal mode of questioning interferes with the ability of their clients to present their own ideas as to what their difficulties are about and they will adopt an informal framework. The information they require includes:

- whether there are changes the client wishes to make, and if so what they are;
- whether the client and counsellor can work effectively together, and what sort of 'contract' to offer the client (number of sessions etc);
- whether the referral is appropriate;
- how clients view their relationships with important figures in their lives: at home, school, work, etc.;
- their attitudes to sex, marriage, partnerships;
- any significant illnesses;
- whether a pattern or a theme or a life problem is evident;
- whether the problem envelops their whole personality;
- any previous similar episodes.

Observations about the client's way of relating to the counsellor are useful when trying to understand the dynamics of that person's relationships. They may appear anxious, demanding, passive, detached, hostile, dependent, co-operative, etc. Whether this response is particular to the counselling situation, or to the counsellor, or is part of the client's life pattern is something on which they can both reflect.

What brings people to counselling?

What are the personal and relationship difficulties that bring people to counselling? Many of them occur at particular points in the life or social cycle, such as going to school, leaving home, starting work, getting married, having children, splitting up, changing jobs, retirement, and bereavement. At these times ideas about one's own status/abilities and relationships with others are likely to need some revision. Many people cope on their own— looking upon any problems as 'normal'. Some, however, need the opportunity to talk through their anxieties, uncertainties, and mixed feelings with someone who is familiar with and understands the psychological tensions. 'Experienced' friends or relatives are often all that are needed.

However, for some these crisis points are more difficult to negotiate, making them aware that they lack some kind of understanding of themselves or others that is contributing to their distress. Usually this can be traced to something that the families or the environments in which they grew up were unable to provide. For instance, the loss of a parent may make a child feel, out of concern for the surviving parent, the need to take on an adult role. Its own dependency needs are thus suppressed to the extent of being unable to fully engage in a give and take relationship later on. A longed-for only child may grow up in an over-protective atmosphere and so become ill-equipped to cope with the competitive cut and thrust of adult life. Children of parents who have severe problems of their own, may suffer from abusive behaviour or have little experience of the affection and security needed for healthy psychological development and become emotionally depleted themselves. Any of these events can affect the way people live their lives; some people are able to seek out experiences and relationships that heal these gaps and deficiencies and enable them to leave their difficulties behind them. Others, less fortunate, because of circumstances or aspects of their personalities— usually a combination of both—may find themselves unable to 'move on' and make meaningful relationships or be creative in their lives. When this happens, professional help—such as counselling, psychotherapy, sex therapy—can provide the framework within which people can work on their problems.

PART 2

How counselling helps in relationship and psychological problems

Counselling is concerned with development and change and a 'successful' outcome can be seen in these terms. Yet change is not synonymous with development as it is possible for a person to change in a way that inhibits development and to develop in a situation that remains unchanged (Woolfe and Sugarman 1989). The notion of individuals becoming more 'self-empowered', that is more in charge of themselves and their lives, is a concept in greater harmony with the goals of counselling (Hopson and Scally 1980). Whilst Woolfe and Sugarman (1989) define self-empowered living as being able to identify the alternatives available in a given situation, 'to choose between them on the basis of personal values, priorities, and commitments and to act on these choices and implement them', they also stress that making a committed choice is not in itself a sufficient indicator of self-empowered living, if not underpinned by values such as self-respect and respect for others.

Although many counsellors would, in the main, agree with Woolfe and Sugarman's criteria for a successful outcome, they represent the existential shifts people make that are so difficult to categorize in concrete terms and translate into outcome measures (Chapter 17). However, in practice, these shifts seem less ethereal and are more easily linked to greater well-being. One client found counselling enabled her to relinquish the role of 'victim' she had played throughout marriage and, as a result, her relationship with her husband became more tolerable. The choice of whether or not to stay in what still constituted an unhappy marriage remained hers, but she felt this could now be assessed on a more realistic basis. Another client claimed, 'nothing on the outside has really changed but I just feel differently inside about it all!' A third found his psychosomatic symptoms abated when he 'chose' to change career, after counselling helped him realize how his fear of taking risks had held him back.

Examining client feedback can help counsellors evaluate their work and assess when and how positive change occurs. When effective, counselling usually fosters the client's ability to examine, make, and implement realistic choices based on self-awareness.

Working with clients

Counselling is an activity which entails a complex coming together of the counsellor's personality, theoretical knowledge, skills, and experience. The counsellor is engaged in a continual process of response decisions, whether it be silence or interpretation, confrontation or reflection, where the impetus for the choice of response is based on a theoretical and intuitive understanding of human emotions and reactions. The language used is jargon-free and the timing of the interventions guided by rapport and the ability of the counsellor to empathize with the feelings expressed by the client. Research on counsellor performance and outcome show that counsellors are most effective when functioning at optimal levels of empathy, warmth, and sincerity (Truax and Carkuff 1967). In practice, client and counsellor need an atmosphere of trust in which they can work together on resolving the client's problems—in essence a 'therapeutic alliance'.

The initial session

The initial session is often exploratory. Summarizing, with the client, what has been communicated during this session can form a bridge between the presenting problem and the focus for subsequent work.

Case history 1. An infertile woman: the initial session

Barbara had been referred to the counsellor because of her unhappiness at not being able to conceive. She had a history of infrequent periods for which she was undergoing medical investigations. The previous year she had married, at the age of thirty-seven, a man six years her senior and because of their ages they wanted to have a baby as soon as possible. During the sessions Barbara related that she felt the stressful events in her life over the last five years were more responsible for her infertility than any physical cause, but she had not been able to say to her GP, a woman for whom she had a great deal of liking and respect, that she thought the tests she was having were rather a waste of time. The first of these grave incidents started with the death of her father who was killed when the car he was in, driven by her only sister, overturned. This was followed by the loss of a beloved aunt and uncle who died in quick succession to each other. Finally, her sister's fiancé died of cancer shortly before they were due to get married. During all this time she had been a 'pillar of support' to her mother and sister, but when she felt she could no longer cope and took a fortnight's leave, her mother collapsed during the first few days of her holiday and she nursed her until she returned to work. The only bright spot that stood out for her in all this tragedy was her courtship and subsequent marriage, in which she felt she and her husband had established an affectionate and supportive relationship.

Her story roused a strong sense of compassion in her listener who suggested that perhaps Barbara's own emotional needs got lost in the more obvious and demanding ones of others. She responded by saying that at the moment she really wanted to stay at home and sort her feelings out, but wondered if her husband would disapprove and see her as acting in an irresponsible manner—she had vaguely suggested to him that she gave up her job, but when he said he thought she would get bored, she became uncertain and had not brought the subject up again. She went on to say that she had often experienced a sense of uncertainty about her own feelings and described how during her childhood she considered that her sister, because of frequent bouts of ill-health, had been pampered and spoilt by her parents. On the one occasion when she had passionately vented these thoughts her parents, particularly her father, a kindly man, reacted to her outburst with a shocked reminder to her of her own good health. She had been left feeling guilty and selfish and wondered if this incident had been at the root of her becoming hesitant about expressing her feelings.

It became clear during the first session that a baby, although very welcome in its own right, was also seen as providing the means for Barbara to have the time she needed for herself without anyone's disapproval. At this point the counsellor had to decide whether or not to confront Barbara with the indirect method she was using to answer her own needs. Confrontation in counselling involves risks; it is the skill of honestly pointing out to the client that their view of a situation differs from the counsellor's perception. When effective it can facilitate insight and pave the way for change, but if untimely it can raise the client's defences and may precipitate a termination of the sessions. Successful confrontation, like many interventions in counselling, rests on the quality of the relationship between client and counsellor; if it lacks sufficient empathy and rapport, confrontation, however 'right' will, more likely than not, seem unacceptable.

In Barbara's case, the counsellor intuitively felt able to link Barbara's desire for a baby to the way it would provide the 'time off' she felt she needed. Putting this to her enabled her to separate and clarify the two issues and she realized that she had become entrenched in a self-sacrificing role that wasn't necessary or desirable in her present circumstances. Drawing together the salient points that had emerged in the session helped her to recognize how her own behaviour had contributed to her difficulties. She decided that her relationship with her husband was strong enough for her to 'speak up', and that even if he did disapprove of her actions they could work something out together.

At her next appointment she related that she had managed, not without difficulty, to gain her husband's understanding of her need to consider a change of direction and they decided she should take some time off to look around. They were both surprised at the speed she sought, and found, a completely different occupation. She used the rest of the sessions to prepare herself to face the painful possibility that she might be unable to have a family and to discuss how she and her husband would cope with this together.

The above example illustrates how, during the initial session, the focus for work emerged. Although Barbara spoke about her grief at the loss of her father and aunt and the jealousy and anger she had felt towards her sister, it seemed more helpful to concentrate on her current circumstances and feelings than those experienced in the past. However, many clients are less ready or able than Barbara to acknowledge that, at the very least, some of the problem resides in the self. Until this happens it is unlikely that the counselling process can begin (see Chapter 1).

Low self-esteem

Identifying their own part in their difficulties, particularly interpersonal ones, presents a problem for those many clients with poor self-esteem, as they often feel themselves to be far too worthless to have any appreciable influence on others. Phrases such as, 'I feel inadequate'; 'I feel inferior'; 'nobody thinks I'm worth listening to', are commonly used to describe themselves. Malan (1979) considers that the growth of normal self-confidence and healthy self-regard in adult life rest on good early experiences that are taken in and held inside as part of the self. If for one reason or another this fails to happen feelings of worthlessness and emptiness tend to be internalized and any good experience there has been in the past is often seen as inadequate and disregarded. Good experiences in the present are usually 'spoilt' in the same way and so become useless as a means of modifying internal feelings of inadequacy. The extent that this self-destructive behaviour becomes generalized will depend on the amount of deprivation experienced, and aggressive tendencies within the individual.

Case history 2. A young man with low self-esteem

Andrew, a young man of twenty-five, was referred to the counsellor because he was unhappy and angry about his lack of friends of both sexes. He was the only child of a 'chilly' mother, and of a father who was hospitalized several times during his childhood because of episodes of depression. He had been sent to boarding school at the age of seven where he had always felt himself to be a 'fish out of water', as an unsporty, musical child in a sport-orientated school. In his late teens the family moved to London from their home in Cornwall. In Cornwall, although he had no friends of his own age, a neighbour had taken him under her wing and given him a good deal of substitute mothering. The move upset him and he failed to keep in touch with the neighbour, yet at the same time enshrined the kindness he had received from her by attributing it to 'the Cornish way of life'. In the sessions he was adamant that his present lack of friends was due to differences in values and attitudes between Cornish people and Londoners, for whom he had not a good word and to whom he made no attempt to hide his feelings. He was still living at home because he said he couldn't afford to do otherwise, although he felt very unhappy at the restrictions this imposed on the amount of independence he considered his adult status implied.

During the sessions the counsellor noticed that, although Andrew turned up early for his appointments and seemed reluctant to leave, he discounted or disagreed with whatever she said. She began to feel like a woman with a child who is protesting and screaming about where it is going, whilst holding on to its mother's hand as tightly as possible. When she linked the lack of help he appeared to be getting from the sessions to other dissatisfactions in his life, by suggesting that perhaps he found it difficult to 'let go' of what he had, even though he found it unsatisfactory, he agreed. He went on to say that 'the devils' he knew (his parents in this case!) were preferable to the ones he did not, adding that he was anxious that he might feel even lonelier if he left home. Although this marked a change in attitude, the counsellor suggested that because of the limited number of sessions she could offer him he was more likely to benefit from working with someone who could give him more time. She was in a difficult situation, because she guessed this would activate a feeling of rejection in him. Yet his history of poor interpersonal relationships and lack of supportive figures in his life, indicated a need for a therapeutic relationship with more flexible time boundaries. Without this, she felt he was unlikely to work through and modify the aggressive defence he had erected to protect his vulnerability and which in everyday life would feel 'chilly' to those attempting to offer him friendship.

Low self-esteem isn't always accompanied by such a strongly developed defence system of a 'bite the hand that feeds' nature, although there is usually some anger that needs to be recognized and worked through if a more confident attitude is to develop.

Case history 3. A young woman with low self-esteem

Sandra asked her GP to refer her for counselling because she wanted to 'sort herself out', as she felt totally lacking in energy and confidence. She had just given up her job as an unqualified assistant in an adolescent unit for emotionally disturbed girls because of 'burn-out'. Her reasons for choosing this type of work in the first place were unclear, until she explained that it had been a means of getting away from home and hesitantly added that it had also been a way of getting back at her father. Although she knew her father hated all forms of social work and wanted her to go to university, she thought at the time that she genuinely wished to work with under-privileged teenagers. To begin with she enjoyed the work, but as time went on she began to find it 'too heavy'. At the third session it became clear that her reason for joining the unit had been a form of identification as she herself felt deprived. Moreover, she now realized it had also served the purpose of expressing the anger she had not known she felt so strongly towards her father. His ambitions for her had always seemed beyond her ability, and although she knew this to be connected with his own rather deprived youth, most of the time she felt a failure in his eyes. The thought of going to university was the last straw, so when a residential job turned up she jumped at the chance. As the sessions progressed Sandra was amazed, and sometimes frightened, by the strength of the resentment she had bottled up for so long. Gradually, as her feelings became more manageable, she began to consider her future. Never having allowed herself to do this before—her responses had been so heavily influenced by her relationship with her father—she found it both hard and exciting. By the time she left counselling she had decided on a career in the business world and she was in the process of looking at courses that would qualify her to work in this area. Although her relationship with her father did not improve, she seemed less troubled by it.

Casework themes

Barbara, Andrew, and Sandra had all experienced difficulties in separating psychologically from their families of origin. The drive towards autonomy, which usually asserts itself in the strivings and struggles of adolescence had, for all three, engendered inner conflicts that inhibited the separation process and deprived them of a confident independent outlook. Barbara was 'deprived' of her ability to express her feelings because of the fear of parental disapproval, Andrew was 'deprived' of a warm and affectionate home life, and Sandra was 'deprived' of her own ambitions by an overriding father. As they probably knew all this, mere confirmation of existing knowledge was unlikely to be of much help. So how can counselling work? One way is for the counsellor to put together a number of observations that enable the client to gain insight into hitherto hidden feelings embedded in the problem. As they emerge and are accepted, they become 'contained' by the counselling process and a change in attitudes and behaviour can occur. Feelings often get suppressed or 'lost' when they are perceived to be unacceptable to loved ones and, not uncommonly, clients in this position will say that they never feel angry, anxious, sentimental . . . or even that they do not have feelings at all, only logic! Yet hidden feelings can undermine a person's ability to function well although the reason may be unclear— the phrase 'the right hand never seems to know what the left is doing' is the common parlance expression of this phenomenon. How did this apply in the cases outlined above? Once Barbara was able to acknowledge and explore how negative feelings made her feel guilty she began to change. Recognition that her self-sacrificing behaviour and uncertain feelings were a form of self-deprivation, aimed to ward off disapproval from those she loved (her parents, her husband, and even her GP), helped her to relinquish them. By facing her anger with her father, Sandra was able to see how anxiety about containing the intensity of her feelings had led her to hide them even from herself. This became particularly apparent when, in one session, she became angry with the counsellor. She had felt frightened and anxious by her loss of control, but when her anger was met with a calm, accepting and interested attitude, she had felt able to deal with it more effectively. Although this had been a disturbing experience for her, she had also felt 'released' and that represented a significant turning point. As she became more confident about handling ambivalent feelings her vitality and ability to look forward reasserted itself, despite the lack of improvement in her relationship with her father.

Unlike the two women, Andrew was less able to recognize the part his own feelings played in his relationships. By projecting all his hostility into others, he remained unaware of his own and became entrenched in the role of victim. To try to help him move towards a more healthy appraisal of his own feelings was likely to take more time than the confines of general practice would permit, so he was referred for psychotherapy.

Depression

Low self-esteem and depression are like siblings bonded by background and akin in appearance and behaviour. Like most close relatives, they can be distinguished by their differences and identified by their similarities. Dorothy Rowe (1983) a leading figure in the treatment of depression, cites isolation as a distinguishing factor. She stresses that it is this that singles out depressives and makes the love and concern of others unavailable to them. Other characteristics like constantly striving to be good, feeling unwanted, being harshly self-critical, and disturbance in early relationships are common to both conditions. So can a clear-cut distinction be made? As Markus *et al.* (1989) point out, whilst depression can be viewed as a continuum between 'sadness', being 'depressed', and having a 'clinical depression', classification into reactive, endogenous, bipolar, and psychotic categories is useful as some depressives may need more urgent treatment than others. However, he stresses that in the aetiology of all types there is a mixture of causes: 'genetic, past experience, current experience, family, environmental, and physical'. From a counselling perspective both low self-esteem and depression are linked with several of these factors and both conditions require working with the mixed and often distressing feelings with which they are associated.

As suicidal feelings or intent often accompany depression, counsellors find they need to be alert to any hint of self-destruction in the sessions. Following up accounts of previous self-harm; noting any tendency to dwell on death; monitoring any extreme changes in behaviour; assessing the degree of past and present disturbance with questions such as 'what is it like when you feel at your lowest?' are all ways of picking up the danger signs, as well as more direct questions about suicidal feelings. My own observation has been that depressives vary in their ability to use a counselling approach, so that counselling is not always the most appropriate form of help. However, there seems no hard and fast rule about who will respond well and who will not, and sometimes clients whose depression is severe and includes endogenous features work well with counsellors, whilst others with less chronic symptoms do not. With such a varied response, working in conjunction with the GP offers an 'all-round' supportive structure and the option of combining treatments such as a course of antidepressants with counselling, if and when appropriate. In my own practice, I found this was a form of care that worked well and was particularly effective in cases of delayed mourning, where depression persists as a result of grief that has somehow miscarried and not been worked through.

Much has been written about the relationship between depression and unresolved, ambivalent feelings about a lost person. As Malan (1979) comments;

At best these can be brought into consciousness and worked through in the therapeutic setting, at worst they can lead to suicide or even homicide . . . the mixture of love and hate towards the same person is one of the deepest and most painful conflicts that human beings suffer from, and depressive patients will do everything in their power to avoid it.

As such, the counselling of depressives needs considerable skill, and in my experience I have found it is best conducted in a setting of shared care. It requires the formation of a strong therapeutic alliance and the counsellor needs to have a well-developed capacity to encourage and contain the expression and impact of intense feelings. Sometimes, though, remarkable change can be achieved in a short space of time.

Case history 4. A deserted wife

Angela had become depressed after her husband of two years left her with large debts and was threatening to reinstate himself in their joint home without her consent. Her intelligence, capacity for insight, and underlying sunny nature seemed in sharp contrast to the way she was letting her husband ride roughshod over her— she was finding it almost impossible to put up any fight, preferring to turn a blind eye to the whole business. However, she realized she was running out of funds, could lose her home, and found she was avoiding friends who urged her to assert herself. The counsellor was mystified by the woman's behaviour until she started talking about her mentally handicapped brother who died when she was still single and living at home. Although his death had been expected, she became very distraught when talking about it and seemed to blame herself in some way. She had, in fact been alone with him when he was taken ill, but had done everything she could to get help as soon as possible. As the mixture of love, compassion, guilt, and resentment she felt towards him emerged she realized how much her feelings towards her brother had influenced her choice of male companions—her husband had been one of a series of 'lame ducks' she had befriended. After making this link for herself, she made an astonishing recovery, confronted her husband, sought legal advice, put the house on the market, and generally re-engaged with the friends and activities she had dropped. Contrary to theoretical supposition she didn't mourn her brother at this stage, but two years later she was still in good health and seemed to have made a satisfactory relationship with a new partner. However, she clearly possessed an unusual capacity for insight, could bear feelings of a distressing nature, and formed a strong therapeutic alliance with the counsellor.

Loss

Loss of an important figure in a person's life is only one form of bereavement that can trigger depression. Psychic loss of ideas, identity, or hopes can feel equally devastating, but these are losses that are often less comprehended by others. If sympathy is short-lived, it can intensify the negative effect for the 'bereaved' individual who may already feel confused and guilty about his or her inability to come to terms with the situation. The company of others may then be avoided for fear of being burdensome, and isolation is then added to loss. Two such examples spring to mind.

Case history 5. A redundant teacher

Harold, a talented teacher in his mid-forties, became deeply depressed after he was made redundant. He felt his dismissal had been manipulated by the headmaster; a man who was disliked by his staff because of his unfair and inadequate behaviour. The previous year Harold had acted as figure-head when the staff put in an official complaint about the head to the governors. Due to bureaucratic changes, nothing came of it and Harold felt his dismissal was entirely due to the acrimony the head felt towards him. He had been offered a similar position in another school, but was reluctant to take it, explaining that he felt he would never be able to engage in his profession in the way he had done before—teaching had been the mainspring of his life and his success was obvious from the illustrations he gave of his interaction with pupils. He judged his bitterness as being completely justified, yet at the same time blamed it for his feelings of lethargy and guilt. He had avoided his colleagues and friends for some time, because he felt they were fed-up with his inability to put his bad fortune behind him.

Case history 6. *The mother of a homosexual girl*

Helen, a 55-year-old Australian undergoing treatment for depression from her GP, came for counselling because she desperately wanted to come to terms with her daughter's homosexuality, about which she felt very disturbed. She was a woman of strong principles and a committed Christian, as was her daughter. She knew that her children were slightly in awe of her, albeit there was also abundant evidence of their love and respect. She was angry that her daughter, now twenty-eight, had kept her sexuality a secret until recently as she felt she had brought her family up to be truthful. Her anger had been fuelled by the attitude of some of her friends and relations, who failed to understand how she felt and disapproved of her distress.

Both Harold and Helen had by their own efforts, intelligence, and fortitude overcome the effects of some very scarring experiences in their youth. Helen had been sexually abused by her father in her early teens and Harold, whose parents divorced when he was two, had a series of 'step-mothers' to whom he was unable or unwilling to make any sort of significant attachment as they changed too frequently. Each felt the satisfying lives they had managed to build up, despite their unhappy beginnings, had suffered a shattering blow. Helen was determined to rebuild hers, but felt undermined by the feelings of anger and disappointment with which she was struggling, whilst Harold was less certain of his ability and willingness to start again. Limited space only permits a brief account here of the outcome of the work they did.

During counselling Helen was given the freedom to voice anything that was troubling her without judgement or disapproval. This encouraged her naturally courageous nature to explore and challenge some of her most dearly held assumptions and develop a more objective and accepting attitude towards her daughter, for whom she had a deep affection. Realizing that the discovery of the woman's homosexuality had reactivated her anger at her father's abusive sexual behaviour and added to her distress, helped her to deal with it more effectively.

Harold was less able to come to terms with his feelings about the loss of the place he had put so much effort into establishing and from which he felt so unjustly dismissed. At an intellectual level, he connected it to the casual way his father repeatedly replaced his mother, but as he didn't seem to wish to develop this theme the counsellor, although she thought it to be relevant, didn't 'push it'. If clients, when given the opportunity, do not respond to exploring emotionally charged material, it seldom works to do so. In Harold's case, the counsellor was aware that he had a very supportive relationship with his wife and that he found it helpful to develop his insights and feelings with her. By the time he left, although he was still undecided about his career prospects, he felt more buoyant about the future. Like Helen, he found the time and objectivity the counselling sessions offered to be helpful.

So far, in the cases discussed, the problems addressed have highlighted the nature of the interplay between the intrapersonal and interpersonal aspect of people's difficulties. Most of the clients, with the exception of Andrew and possibly Harold, were able to see how conflicts within themselves contributed to their problems and from this new perspective make changes that enabled them to 'move on'. If much of what has been written sounds artificial and contrived, it is because of the difficulty of conveying how the 'here and now' exchange between client and counsellor affects the counselling process. For example, a change in voice, posture, expression, or eye contact can have as much, or even more influence on this process than the words spoken. In my experience, efficacy rests on this interchange, without which counselling can become an intellectual discussion of limited value.

Before moving on to the next section there are two groups of clients that need to be mentioned: adolescents and the elderly, as they illustrate transitional stages in the life cycle that can feel very uncomfortable or even traumatic for all those involved.

Counselling adolescents

Few adolescents weave their way along the path from childhood to adulthood without encountering some difficulties along the way, and those that do so may be avoiding the challenges and demands of the physical and psychological changes taking place.

For most it is a period of time where, faced with bodily and emotional sensations that can make them uncertain of their own resources and coping abilities, they swing between excitement and dejection. This can produce strange behaviour, such as withdrawal, depression, inconsistency, and belligerence, and many GPs are faced with parents seeking advice on how to cope on the one hand, and teenagers seeking support on the other. Often, basic counselling skills and an educative approach are all that is needed to see both parties through. As one GP recalled, although he found dealing with adolescents and their families difficult, just sitting it through, inviting them to think about their roles and resisting the temptation to jump in with a lot of advice, was the support they later said they found the most helpful (personal communication).

Are adolescents difficult to counsel, and if so why should this be? First, it is not always easy to distinguish the 'normal' turmoil of adolescence from more severe clinical problems; secondly, many of the problems that arise during the long transition from child to adult often closely resemble those experienced by the helpers themselves. This can result in an over-identification with the client which, if not fully understood, can distort the worker's perception of the case. As one counsellor recounted, sitting listening to the angry father of a 17-year-old berate his son for his rude and inconsiderate behaviour, so reminded him of his own father that he felt quite childlike and helpless in the face of the man's rage (personal communication). Fortunately, the counsellor was well aware of the significance of his reactions and was able to adopt the objective response needed instead of getting caught up in feelings relating to his own past and letting them interfere with his observation of the interaction of the man and boy in front of him.

When counselling adolescents, the issue of autonomy from parents is often central to the work. Counsellors are only too familiar with teenagers who use their sexuality and flout family standards as a means of stating their independence.

Case history 7. An adolescent girl

Linda, a girl of sixteen, was finding it difficult to settle in a job after leaving school with only two O levels. Unlike her clever brother who had his sights on a career in law, she had never had any clear idea of what she wanted to do. When she started work at a local restaurant her behaviour astonished and dismayed her parents. She began to stay out very late, acquired a boyfriend whose influence on her they disliked, was often late for work or didn't turn up unless it suited her, and they suspected she might be experimenting with drugs. Until then, they felt she had been a helpful and agreeable girl, always happy to fit in with the family's arrangements. As they considered themselves to be a particularly close-knit family they could not understand what had gone wrong. They approached their GP for help and he suggested that Linda might benefit from counselling. Although her parents were doubtful about whether she would agree, Linda turned up for her appointment on time.

On discussing the rift that had occurred in the family, Linda said she could understand why her parents. felt so upset and did not really know why she behaved as she did. However, she also said she had told them that she enjoyed the company of her new friends, as she was not clever and ambitious like her brother. The counsellor's reply, 'who said you should be?' was the start of their exploration of the origins of her beliefs about herself, what she felt she should be like and how realistic this was. Helping Linda to sort out the confusion about her role in the family and her own identity enabled her to begin clarifying her position, first of all to herself and then to her family.

Counselling the elderly

Growing older, like growing up, requires adjustments from those around the one who is ageing, as well as from the person involved. For many, the transition from middle to old age is harmonious, as adjustments in behaviour, attitudes, and expectations occur almost imperceptibly. Others can find this period of their lives far from satisfactory, particularly when they are jolted into a sudden realization that life will never be the same again through illness, bereavement, having to move home, or simply a narrowing down of opportunities. Changes in the older person's personality can take place and someone who has previously been regarded with affection can become a source of guilt and despair for their relatives and friends. Helping all involved to mourn psychic losses, such as personality traits, and lost opportunities, as well as the current implications of physical and material losses, can ease some of the burden they feel.

Case history 8. Mrs V., a widow

When counselling the elderly it can be helpful to think about the life cycle in terms of Erikson's (1950) eight stages where the transition from one stage to the next depends on the resolution of the crisis inherent in the previous one. If resolution is not achieved, or only partially so, problems occurring in a later stage will be linked to those in an earlier one. When viewed from this perspective, the possible nature and origins of emotional problems in later life can become clearer. For instance, if the feelings around early psychical losses (or any other losses for that matter) are not resolved they can complicate the grieving process when a subsequent loss occurs, as in the case of Mrs V.

A practice counsellor was asked to see Mrs V. because her family felt she needed some help in re-adjusting after the death of her husband six months previously. They felt she should be 'picking up' by now and had endeavoured to engage her in a range of activities, none of which she showed any interest in pursuing. Mrs V. herself was not keen to see the counsellor but agreed to come along 'just once'. At the start of the session Mrs V. said her family did not realize that since her husband died there was nothing left for her in life and she did not feel she should 'do things' just for the sake of it. She added that she thought her relatives just felt guilty about her and if they really understood how she felt they would leave her alone. The counsellor said that it was important that she understood how Mrs V. felt and asked her what it was that she thought her family did not understand. Mrs V. replied, 'the loneliness'. She went on to say that her husband had been a gregarious man and because she had a retiring nature she had relied almost totally on him for company. She confessed she had not particularly wanted to get married when she first met him, but had not known what else to do, as her mother was a widow and there was not enough money for her to follow her desire to be a teacher. Despite this, she felt the marriage had been reasonably happy, mainly because they had adopted very defined roles. For a long time she had cherished a secret hope that one day she would be able to fufil her ambition to teach, but as the years went by she lost confidence in her ability and gave up any thoughts of having a job outside the home. To her surprise, she found talking to a 'stranger' helpful and it was agreed that she should have a series of appointments.

From her history it was clear that Mrs. V. had experienced difficulty in establishing her autonomy in early life and her relationship with her husband kept her fixed in this position. Helping her express the sadness of not only her husband's death, but also of earlier hopes that 'died' during the marriage, was the understanding which the counsellor felt Mrs V. needed and to which she responded. Although Mrs V. remained something of a recluse, she subsequently developed a rewarding interest in needlework, a development that was based on her own choice rather than that of her relatives.

Counselling couples

A few decades ago couples' counselling was more or less synonymous with marriage counselling. Today this is no longer so. Due to shifts in the structure of society which challenged existing ideologies, new forms of relationships have emerged. In turn, these have reverberated through the institution of marriage which is now somewhat uneasily poised. Symbolically, this has been reflected by the change in name of the Marriage Guidance movement to Relate. As a result, couples with a relationship outside the confines of marriage, particularly those seeking an alternative to heterosexual love, now have access to help when going through difficult times. But are marital dilemmas any different from those experienced in other forms of partnerships? So far, my search for comparative studies has not been successful, so it remains an unanswered question. More information on this subject should be available shortly as Relate is currently collating the findings from a survey of clients' presenting problems.

Impressionistically though, it can be assumed that difficulties arising from the care of children will occur to a larger degree amongst heterosexual couples or single-parent families, whereas problems of unfaithfulness, power, poor communication, sexual disharmony, illness, and finance are not so likely to be influenced by the nature of the partnership. Statistical evidence reveals that only 15 per cent of the people seeking help from the Tavistock Institute of Marital Studies were unmarried in 1989 and 11 per cent of couples coming to Relate were cohabiting in 1991. On balance then, the majority of couples coming for help to these agencies are heterosexual and married, but this should not be taken to mean that their problems are intrinsically different from those of unmarried or gay partners. All in all, the basic principles of 'couples' counselling' will apply equally to all forms of adult partnerships. Hence, for purposes of expediency the following section on marital counselling will be taken to apply generally, as the commonalities of couples' work far outweigh the special issues that arise for partnerships that have minority status. Because of variation in partnership systems and the wide range of problems met in clinical work, only vignettes from case studies will be used.

Couples seeking help

Marriage is a private affair and seeking professional help for marital problems is not an easy decision for most couples to make. However, when social resources, such as family or friends, are unavailable or unable to help the advice of the GP is often sought. Whether or not they are referred for counselling is usually decided at this point and this decision alone can bring considerable relief. Most couples, if they wish to be, are seen together so that the work can focus on their interaction 'in the here and now'. Occasionally, it can be more helpful to suggest separate sessions if the couple lack a shared agenda or the acrimony between them is so great it excludes the possibility of positive intervention.

Why a relationship invested with goodwill and commitment at the outset goes wrong can be mystifying to some couples, as they are unable to identify any particular point or event when they felt things began to deteriorate. Others may have a much clearer picture in their minds. However, as partners bring all their experience of life to marriage, a myriad of problems can become encapsulated in their relationship. Negotiating different stages in the normal life cycle can act as a catalyst for conflicts hitherto contained. Setting up home together, coping with the birth of a baby, gaining more responsibility at work, having adolescent children, seeing the last child leave home, or dealing with changes brought about by retirement can upset the balance of a partnership. Adultery, bitter rows, withdrawal, and even desertion and cruelty are not uncommon responses to these developmental milestones. In any of these events one partner may mature more quickly than the other, leaving both feeling unsupported in their roles.

Marital therapy

The approach developed by the Tavistock Institute of Marital Studies (TIMS) has had a considerable influence on marital therapy in Britain and America (James and Wilson 1986) and is the one that I have drawn upon most when working with couples. It is a model that focuses on the couple's interaction rather than the 'presenting problem'. For instance, if a couple were arguing about finance the counsellor would draw their attention to how, rather than why they were arguing, and may say to one, 'you seem to be dismissing J's . . . suggestion before giving it any consideration, I wonder why this is?' This is not meant to imply that current concerns are ignored, but that the focus is on helping the couple gain more understanding and insight into the underlying, and largely unconscious, emotional needs, expectations, hopes, anxieties, and disappointments that govern their behaviour and influenced their choice of partner. For a fuller dicussion of the theoretical framework developed by TIMS than can be given here, the reader is referred to Dicks (1967) and Clulow (1990)

Choice of partner

Barbara Dearnley (1990), a marital therapist, maintains that an internal image of a desired partner is fashioned from 'the unfinished business of childhood . . . the unsatisfied emotional longings, unmet physical needs', carried into adult life, invested in another who is seen through the proverbial rose-coloured spectacles and with whom 'they fall in love'. Her view is challenged by Coleman (1993) who points out that falling in love is a unique experience associated with initiation into adult life so cannot be entirely derived from infantile development. If Coleman is right there may be other regressive phenomena that influence the tenacity with which these illusions are sometimes held and which inhibit the ability of individuals to engage with each other as they really are, rather than as they would like each other to be.

Case history 9. A middle-aged couple

One such couple were Betty and Roger, a pair in their late forties. At the start of counselling they quickly fell into a familiar pattern of behaviour in which Roger berated Betty for her quick and unreasonable temper, inconsistent behaviour, insistence upon having her own way, refusal to talk, selfishness, and lack of concern for him. Betty sat through this tirade with a resigned air, occasionally retaliating, but quite often agreeing with his allegations which tended to add fuel to his fury. Despite all that he said, he claimed he still loved her and that she needed him to look after her and they both professed the wish to stay together. It emerged that Roger came from a family in which the children were brought up to be kind and considerate at all costs and where 'answering back' was considered selfishly wilful and heavily frowned upon. Several times he ruefully referred to his reputation in the family for being too outspoken and how, on the day he and Betty got engaged, his mother warned her about his sharp tongue; at the time he had been warmed by Betty's cheerful response of 'I like a little bit of spice in my food'.

This was the first indication the counsellor had that Roger's behaviour might be driven by an intense need and hope for the acceptance that had been lacking in his childhood to be remedied in his relationship with Betty. Marriage can often provide a forum for this type of healing, but there are limits to what one partner can give without getting anything in return. Betty also had hidden needs, which like Roger's had been rekindled in the early part of their relationship. Both expected more than the other could give and had been sadly disappointed when this failed to happen. It took much patience on the counsellor's part to help them see how laden their marriage had been with expectations that properly belonged to past relationships.

Marital fit

What other factors besides falling in love prompt people to feel they could be compatible as life partners? Social and financial pressures that instigate a more contractual type of marriage spring to mind. Nevertheless, whatever determines choice of partner, marriage usually contains a wish for growth and development. It may be a desire to start again and escape the frustrations and disappointments of the past, or repeat and continue the satisfactions experienced in the family of origin.

Psychodynamic theorists suggest that a couple's 'marital fit' is based on an attempt to reunite lost or suppressed aspects of a person's own personality seen in that of the partner, and that it is this drive towards unity or wholeness that at first attracts individuals to one another (Dicks 1967). Difficulties occur when one or both are 'blind' to these aspects of their own personalities, aspects that may be unacceptable or guilt laden so do not exist as part of their conscious image of themselves. Unless re-integration takes place, the qualities that at first attracted can become unacceptable and may then be treated in the partner as they were in the self by earlier figures in the person's life. However, the sense of the spouse as part of the self remains and couples locked in an acrimonious marriage, unable to change or part, often appear compelled to constantly relate to the part of themselves projected into the other—as if to make sure it is still there; a divided self that hates, but needs its other half.

Helping couples see that what they complain of in each other is an unwanted part of themselves is precarious, as it requires considerable modification of the personal identity, including sexual identity, that they have built up during their lives. Those that manage to assimilate a change in perception of themselves and consequently each other are rewarded with an increased sense of 'wholeness' and the ability to engage in a more mature form of interaction. However, as Woodhouse (1990) points out, in some marriages conflict between the partners has a 'fight to death quality, that reflects the tenacity with which the internal image of the self is liable to be defended when it is felt to be under threat'; such couples can acquire 'heart-sink' status all too easily. Others may be helped by building on established areas of co-operation, with agreed goals that are contingent on the partner's response, and some can use the containing environment of the counselling sessions to begin the process of separation; more often than not this happens when one partner has begun to outgrow the collusive psychological pattern of the marriage.

Case history 10. Separation

Throughout their marriage Mary had behaved like a punitive mother to her husband Simon, who adopted the role of 'naughty boy' by constantly testing her patience and blaming her for his childish compliance with her wishes. The children sympathized with their father, viewing their mother in much the same light as he did. Promotion at work for Mary developed her confidence and she began to adopt a more relaxed, assertive, but less domineering attitude, which upset the equilibrium of the marital relationship. Simon reacted by having an affair and a year later, when the last child left home, both parents had become emotionally distant. They came for counselling to discuss their future.

During the course of the sessions, Simon said that he felt they were like two people who had caught the same train, travelled a long distance together but now had different destinations. They had been drawn to each other because of shared interests, compatible values, and sexual attraction. Both had come into marriage with unresolved internal anxieties and conflicts relating to power and authority. At first this increased their sense of togetherness, and they felt comfortable with Mary taking the lead in most things, as this avoided arguments and unpleasantness. However, the stresses and strains of family life re-evoked in each of them a pre-occupation with authority issues which were externalized into their partnership and acted out in a fruitless interplay of dominance and submission. By the time they came to counselling, they had become emotionally detached and lacked motivation to try and save the marriage. After several sessions they decided to part, which they did on an amicable basis.

From a developmental viewpoint, personal growth for Mary and Simon culminated in separation. However, many couples live their lives within the protection of the emotional cotton wool that a collusive marital fit provides, although it may be at considerable cost to the development of one or both partners and their relationship. For instance, an agoraphobic man may provide his insecure wife with someone who is always there for her without either of them facing the challenges that independence might pose. When the containing function of marriage is threatened, perhaps when one partner matures more quickly than the other, and help is sought, counselling can offer an environment within which the couple feel safe to explore the implications of change.

Case history 11. A developing relationship

Annette and Rob, a 'workaholic', got married when Annette was anorexic. After two years, they decided she should seek treatment because they wanted a baby. Their sex life had been rather spasmodic but they both assumed this was due to Annette's 'illness'. As she began to get better and put on weight she also found herself becoming more confident, sociable, and active in areas she had previously avoided because of her condition. Strangely, she and Rob began to quarrel and their relationship, which had always been agreeable because they were so alike in their views and attitudes, began to deteriorate and sex became less, rather than more, frequent. They were disturbed and concerned by this development and, coupled with their distress, was a sense of guilt at not enjoying themselves at a time they considered they should feel overjoyed by the improvement in Annette's health. They were pleased when it was suggested that they might benefit from joint counselling.

The anxiety that Annette's more mature emotional and sexual demands introduced into a relationship that bore more resemblance to that of aimiable, undemanding chums rather than husband and wife, was considerable. In counselling, their attention was drawn to how Rob's work and Annette's health had kept differences at bay—they had never quarrelled for fear of adding to the other's stress. They began to see how they had colluded in establishing a 'safe' pattern of relating to each other by avoiding confrontation. At first they were amazed to think that their 'alikeness', which they saw as intimacy, was much more concerned with avoiding individuality. Their arguments became less aggressive and less worrying when viewed as a means of expressing their different perspectives as individuals and husband and wife, and they even began to enjoy them.

The question of how much you can be yourself in a relationship can arise for many couples on marriage, but it held a particular significance for Annette and Rob who had both experienced difficulties in establishing separateness from their families prior to meeting. Their relationship illustrates how issues revolving around health, work, and patterns of relating can mirror how a couple's intrapersonal conflicts become enmeshed, externalized, and acted out in the partnership.

Extramarital affairs

The extramarital affair is probably the most common presenting problem, symptomatic of underlying difficulties, that brings couples (or one partner) to counselling. Yet, more often than not one or both partners fail, or wish not to recognize the existence of problematic issues prior to a third party coming on the scene, who is then cast in the role of evil predator by the 'wronged' spouse and blamed for the breakdown of the marital relationship. However, it is unusual for an affair to happen in a vacuum and if the couple are able to see it as the culmination of their own emotionally charged interactions, the third party often becomes unimportant, leaving the partners free to work on their relationship. When this happens, the marriage often survives and the couple may even feel closer as a result of the experience. For others, an affair can prove too wounding for the marriage to recover or may be the last straw that decides a couple to part. So can counselling help a couple whose relationship has been threatened by an affair? Dicks (1967) classified adultery as being either benign or malignant; when benign, the boundary of the marriage is preserved, a self-healing element is present, the partners are receptive to therapeutic interventions, and the affair represents an attempt to stimulate growth in a flagging relationship. Malignant adultery, as the word implies, is characterized by more destructive behaviour, where the affair is used to belittle and hurt the partner, and an uncooperative attitude is adopted towards those approached for help. Marriages that fall into this latter category offer few opportunities for effective mitigation and frequently end up in the divorce courts. Sadly, the acrimony experienced in the first marriage often reappears in a successive one, or there is a reshuffle of roles and the first spouse is recast as the bad object in wrangles over money, property, or children that can often go on for years. However, marriages in which adultery has a more benign underlying motive, or even ones that fall between the two categories outlined by Dicks, are more likely to remain open to retrieval measures. It can be a poignant experience in counselling to witness the moment a couple become aware of how the interactional pattern of their relationship contributed to the infidelity of one partner.

Case history 12. A jealous husband

During the course of their 25 years of marriage Sally, who had been shy and retiring as a young girl, became more outgoing and confident, whereas Frank, her husband, always somewhat of a loner, withdrew more and more into his own shell. When, at the age of fifty-five, Frank was told of redundancy plans that included him, he opted for early retirement. Sally, who was ten years younger than Frank, became upset at the prospect, particularly as he seemed to think she would reduce her hours at work to be at home with him. When she tried to voice her fears, Frank reacted with his customary reluctance to discuss anything emotional. At first, she renewed her efforts to try and get through to him, but gave up when his continued lack of response started to make her tearful and depressed. She found she could confide in her boss Gordon, a man her own age and a friend of both of them. Gordon and Sally became passionately involved with each other, but parted when they decided their relationship had no future, as neither felt able to leave their respective partners. Sally found a new job and threw herself into the work, in which she became very interested and proficient. By chance, several months after it had finished, Frank found out about the affair and became consumed by jealousy and anger, the violence of which threatened the marriage. By the time they came for help, Sally was uncertain that they had a future together and Frank felt she had unnecessarily smashed everything he held dear.

In counselling Frank slowly realized that an underlying fear of intimacy had been responsible for his withdrawal from Sally as she changed from the shy, undemanding girl he married to a woman whose emotional needs seemed excessive to him. By remaining oblivious to her changing needs (so incidentally to his own) the emotional satisfactions in their marriage drained away. Once Frank acknowledged his own contribution to their difficulties, Sally was able to see that falling in love with Gordon, although emotionally warming, was also an angry reaction to the icy control Frank wielded in the relationship. Their confidence in their ability to rebuild a more emotionally satisfying marriage grew as their understanding of their interactional pattern increased and they became almost grateful for the crisis that had at first seemed so devastating.

Although retirement was only one factor that contributed to the exposure of the negative chain of reactions that prompted Sally and Frank to seek help, the transition from work to retirement can be a difficult one for many couples to assimilate. As the advice and help of GPs is often sought at this time (Markus *et al.* 1989), it may be appropriate for counsellors and other members of the primary care team to provide a group setting for those approaching retirement, in which they can explore the personal, social, and health issues it raises.

Retirement seems an appropriate note on which to conclude this chapter on the interpersonal, relationship, and psychological problems people bring to practice counsellors. Choosing material has been a difficult task as it is a vast area and much has had to be left out. Choice has also been determined by my and my colleagues' clinical experience which, in turn, has been shaped by the referrals received and the geographical location from which the examples were drawn. I am particularly aware of certain aspects that have not been included, such as sexuality in marriage, transcultural counselling, and the effects of illness, divorce, and re-marriage on people's relationships. However, much of this is covered in other chapters.

REFERENCES

Brook, A. and Temperley, J. (1976). The contribution of a psychotherapist to general practice. *Journal of the Royal College of General Practitioners*, **26**, 86–94.

Chancellor, A., Mont, A., and Andrews, G. (1977). The general practitioner's identification and management of emotional disorders. *Australia Family Physician*, **6**, 1137–43.

Clulow, C. (ed.) (1990). *Marriage: disillusion and hope*. Karnac Books, London.

Coleman, W. (1993). Love, desire and infatuation: encountering the erotic spirit. Unpublished paper.

Courtney, M. (1989) Counselling and general practitioners. *The Practitioner*, **233**, 1049.

Dearnley, B. (1990). Changing marriage. In *Marriage: disillusion and hope* (ed. C. Clulow), pp. 43–5. Karnac Books, London.

Dicks, H. V. (1967). *Marital tensions*. Routledge and Kegan Paul, London.

Erikson, E. H. (1950). *Childhood and society*. Norton, New York.

Feinmann, J. (1991). When doctor and counsellor fall out. *General Practitioner*, December 6, 46.

Gray, D. P. (1988). Counsellors in general practice. *Journal of the Royal College of General Practitioners*, **38**, 50–1.

Grosser, V. (1988). How a counsellor can work for you. *General Practitioner*, September 9, 33.

Harris, C. M. (1987). Let's do away with counselling. In *The medical annual* (ed. D. J. P. Gray), pp. 105–11. Wright, Bristol.

Hopson, B. and Scally, M. (1980). Change and development in adult life: some implications for helpers. *British Journal of Guidance and Counselling*, **8**, 175–87.

James, A. L., and Wilson, K. (1986). *Couples, conflict and change*. Tavistock, London.

Malan, D. H. (1979). *Individual psychotherapy and the science of psychodynamics*. Butterworths, London

Marks, J. N. Goldberg, D. P., and Hillier V. F. (1979). Determinants of the ability of general practitioners to detect psychiatric illness. *Psychological Medicine*, **9**, 337–53.

Markus, A. C., Murray-Parkes, C., Tomson, P., and Johnston, M. (1989). *Psychological problems in general practice*. Oxford University Press, Oxford.

McLeod, J. (1988). *The work of counsellors in general practice*. Occasional paper, 37. Royal College of General Practitioners, Exeter.

McLeod, J. (1992). The general practitioner's role. In *Counselling in general practice* (ed. M. Sheldon) p. 11. Royal College of General Practitioners, Exeter.

Morgan, G., Wallace, B., and Houston, H. (1990). How to assess a patient who is unhappy. *MIMS*, January 15, pp. 39–41.

Morrell, V. (1992). Developing counselling skills. In *Counselling in general practice* (ed. M. Sheldon) p. 5. Royal College of General Practitioners, Exeter.

Newnes, G. (1990). Bodyguards may be better therapy. *General Practitioner*, January 15, 54.

Oldfield, S. (1983). *The counselling relationship: a study of the client's experience*. Routledge and Kegan Paul, London.

Rowe, D. (1983). *Depression: the way out of your prison*. Routledge and Kegan Paul, London.

Rowland, N. (1992). Counselling and counselling skills. In *Counselling in general practice* (ed. M. Sheldon) p. 2. Royal College of General Practitioners, Exeter.

Rowland, N. and Hurd, J. (1989). *Counselling in general practice: a guide for counsellors*. British Association for Counselling, Rugby.

Shapiro, A. K. (1971). Placebo effects in medicine, psychotherapy and psychoanalysis. In *Handbook of psychotherapy and behavioural change* (ed. S. L. Garfield, and A. E. Bergin).

Sibbald, B., Addington-Hall, J., Brenneman, D., and Freeling, P. (1993). Counsellors in English and Welsh general practices: their nature and distribution. *British Medical Journal*, **306**, 29–33.

Storr, A. (1964). *Sexual deviation*. Penguin, England.

Thomas, P. (1993). An exploration of patients' perceptions of counselling with particular reference to counselling in general practice. *Counselling*, **4**, 24–30.

Treadway, J. (1983). Patient satisfaction and the content of general practice consultations. *Journal of the Royal College of General Practitioners*, **33**, 769–71.

Truax, C. B. and Carkhuff, R. R. (1967). *Toward effective counselling and psychotherapy training and practice*. Aldine, Chicago.

Woodhouse, D. (1990). Theoretical development. In *Marriage disillusionment and hope*. (ed. C. Clulow) p. 103. Karnae Books, London.

Woolfe, R. and Sugarman, S. (1989). Counselling and the life cycle. In *Handbook of counselling in Britain* (ed. W. Dryden, D. Charles-Edwards, and R. Woolfe,) p. 35. Routledge, London.

6 Psychiatric disorders

Colin Forth

INTRODUCTION

As community care develops and fewer people remain in hospitals for the mentally ill, the involvement of primary health care teams in psychiatric care will increase. Many general practitioners feel poorly equipped or too busy to treat mental health problems as well as they would like. To remedy this, the availability of a community psychiatric nurse—a 'specialist'—who is able to respond fairly quickly and can see a patient in the surgery or at home has proved to be a big advantage. The use of counselling in treating patients with mental health problems is becoming prevalent in primary care settings, and can be used to complement or replace other established treatments, for example treatment with drugs.

This chapter outlines how psychiatric nursing care developed in the community and how it utilizes counselling skills. The way of determining the most appropriate person to counsel the patients, together with outlining the skills needed for the different types of psychiatric disorders is discussed. The value of using primary care settings instead of the hospital when carrying out such treatments is emphasized.

DEVELOPMENT OF THE COMMUNITY PSYCHIATRIC NURSING SERVICE AND ITS MOVEMENT TOWARDS GENERAL PRACTICE

The first community psychiatric nursing (CPN) service was established in 1954 at Warlingham Park Hospital in Surrey. May and Moore (1963) described the service as:

Two hospital based nurses who were seconded to carry out part-time community duties. The service was organised for two main reasons. Firstly there was a shortage of psychiatric social workers and secondly there was recognition of the need for continued supervision of patients following discharge from hospital.

Green (1968) described a service which had been organized at Moorhaven Hospital in 1957. The service used nurses in the hospital setting thus giving them a dual role of hospital/community nurse. Green went on to say that, 'The community psychiatric nurses (CPNs) had something special to offer in the way of nursing and were not substitute social workers.'

From then onwards, the CPN service steadily grew. The Local Authorities

Table 6.1 *Distribution of sources of client referral to community psychiatric nurses, over time*[a]

| Referral agent | Proportion of referrals | | % change (1985–1990) |
	1985	1990	
Psychiatrist	59.2	42.7	−16.5
General Practitioner	23.3	35.8	+12.5
District Nurse/HV	5.0	3.9	− 1.1
Other hospital staff	5.0	5.5	+ 0.5
Social Services	3.2	3.6	+ 0.4
Relatives/self	2.2	4.4	+ 2.2
Other	2.2	4.1	+ 1.9
Total	100%	100%	

[a] Taken from the 3rd Quinquennial National Community Psychiatric Nursing Survey, White 1990

Act, 1968, which implemented some recommendations of the Seebohm Report, was an important factor. This Act absorbed local authority mental health departments and mental welfare offices into general social services departments. Paykel *et al.* (1982) reported that:

Specialised workers were temporarily replaced by relatively inexperienced generalist social workers with different skills and priorities, leaving a vacuum in follow-up care. This vacuum was filled by the CPN service.

Initially CPNs were based in psychiatric hospitals and accepted referrals solely from psychiatrists. This closed referral system, however, has changed. Leopoldt and Hurn (1973) described the first attachment of CPNs to a general practice in the Oxford area. They raised two major issues. Firstly, the change in base led to a change in role for the CPNs who began working in relatively unsupported environments as independent practitioners. Secondly, general practitioners readily referred patients to a CPN before a crisis occurred, thus possibly avoiding the need for hospital admission. If an admission did occur, however, the eventual discharge was not so difficult as CPNs had a good working knowledge of local services.

As well as giving supportive care to those patients who were discharged from hospital or who had longstanding chronic mental problems, the CPN is now involved in other treatment, including counselling, behaviour therapy, and psychotherapy. Changes have also taken place in the bases from where CPNs operate: there has been a gradual shift from psychiatric hospital to GP/health centre and community mental health centre. This change can be linked to the proportion of referrals that the CPN receives from different sources. Between 1985 and 1990, there was a 16 per cent decrease in referrals from the psychiatrist matched by a 12 per cent increase in referrals from GPs (see Table 6.1).

The success of a CPN attachment in primary health care teams depends largely upon the individuals involved. If there is good CPN–GP face-to-face contact, there is likely to be a better understanding of the nature and type of work taken. White (1986) has suggested that an individually negotiated relationship between a CPN and GP is the most important factor affecting the number and appropriateness of referrals.

COUNSELLING PEOPLE WITH PSYCHIATRIC DISORDERS

In primary care settings, there are many opportunities for counselling. Counselling aims 'to help people accept and come to terms with their difficulties and identify ways of coping more effectively' (Irving and Heath 1991). In recent years, the use of counselling skills has increased when helping patients with psychiatric disorders. Ironbar and Hooper (1989) listed the appropriate objectives when counselling in mental health practice. These include:

- promoting insight and self-awareness;
- increasing self-confidence and self-esteem;
- developing social understanding;
- enhancing decision-making, problem-solving, and coping skills;
- increasing personal responsibility and autonomy;
- resolving emotional stress;
- facilitating and supporting change;
- developing healthier and more effective relationship-making skills;
- improving social and communication skills;
- maintaining hope and motivation.

The term 'counselling', when treating patients with psychiatric disorders has sometimes been confused with psychotherapy. Burnard (1992), however, defined psychotherapy as:

An umbrella term for the wide range of therapies that are usually used to help people who are suffering from mental ill health, who want to solve some fairly deep-seated personal problem, or who feel that they want to develop themselves through a therapeutic relationship.

Burnard went on to say that examples of the varieties of psychotherapy include psychoanalysis, behaviour therapy, gestalt therapy, transactional analysis, and group therapy (see also discussion in Chapter 1).

Counselling is normally considered appropriate for people going through difficult life events, such as bereavement or relationship problems, and who are becoming anxious or depressed as a result (Dowrick 1992). Counselling may be less effective, although sometimes still of value, in the more chronic, psychotic illnesses. The severity of the illness should indicate to the practitioner if counselling is appropriate. This is supported by Dryden and Feltham (1992) who suggest that seriously psychiatrically disturbed patients or those preoccupied with metaphysical questions about the meaning of life may need referral for alternative therapy.

A GP is normally the first person to assess the problems of someone who is suffering from a psychiatric disorder. The GP will then decide on the most suitable intervention at this primary stage. If the choice is counselling, the counsellor may come from a differing background. Independent counsellors who work in general practice are normally expected to have a recognized qualification (although see findings of Sibbald *et al.* 1993). The British Association for Counselling has produced guidelines for accreditation as a recognition of training, supervision, and breadth of experience. Irving and Heath (1991) state that the training need not be taken in one course, as long as there is a balance between theory and practice and the overall training is coherent. Evidence is also required of supervised practice over a period of at least three years, as well as a serious commitment to continuing professional and personal development. By contrast, the basic qualification for a CPN who may counsel a patient is a three-year, full-time course to qualify as a Registered Mental Nurse. They may also have additional, post-basic qualifications in community psychiatric nursing. Within this training, counselling skills and techniques are practised. Many CPNs undertake additional specialist counselling courses to increase their abilities in this form of therapy. The range of skills a CPN has will vary from one individual to another, but a good basic knowledge of psychiatry will be assured. As well as using specific counselling skills, the CPN will use a systematic 'problem solving' approach, or the 'psychiatric nursing process'. The publication of Yura and Walsh's book in 1967 introduced the 'nursing process' as a tool for clinical nurses. It has four clear stages of assessment, planning, implementation, and evaluation.

Although there are many variations of the nursing process in use, Pollock (1989) commented that 'this approach to care remains the main prescriptive model used by most nurses'. It is often stated that counselling requires a non-directive approach; however for psychiatric disorders a more structured approach may be necessary. The nursing process is used to help the patient develop coping mechanisms that may be a solution to their problem.

When a GP selects counselling as an appropriate form of treatment, there are various decisions to be taken. First, will the GP counsel the patient or will another person be chosen, for example practice counsellor, nurse, CPN? Secondly, what will influence the choice of counsellor? This may depend upon the GP's assessment of the severity of the (mental) problem, the availability of the appropriate counsellor, or even the financial implications of using a counsellor. Thirdly, how can the chosen counselling be evaluated? Will it be by consumer satisfaction, by easing the GP's workload, by reduction of prescribing and hospital costs, or evidence to show that the patient's mental state has improved. Corney's (1990) review of studies of counselling in primary care found some benefit to patients, but reckoned that the evaluation techniques had to be questioned because of the difficulty in assessing effectiveness and improvement especially when judged against other forms of treatment (see also Chapter 17). There are no simple answers to the above questions. However, the outcome would seem to depend heavily on the initial individual judgement of each GP, his expertise in the field of mental illness, his choice of counsellor, and that counsellor's training and experience.

The following sections describe examples of how various counselling skills can be used when treating specific types of psychiatric disorder. They are based on the writer's experience in a primary health care setting.

DEPRESSION

Sadness and depression are common emotional experiences in everyday life. These moods may arise from within and be without apparent cause, or can be a reaction to a disappointment, stress, or loss. When people seek to alleviate the pain and suffering that a depressive episode may bring, it is to their GP that they are most likely to turn. It is then the decision of the GP as to which avenue of therapy will be appropriate. This can range from the prescription of medication and/or limited counselling from the GP, to the involvement of 'specialists', such as a practice counsellor, CPN, or hospital psychiatrist. The choice will depend on the severity of the depression, the interest and expertise of the GP, the availability of 'specialists', and the wishes of the patient.

Once the individual is referred, the counsellor will observe the patient's posture, grooming, facial expression, movement, and vocal physical qualities. These often rapidly reveal the severity of the problem. Counsellors believe that each patient's needs are unique and have to be assessed individually. Allowing a patient to ventilate his/her feelings is an important component of the process. By careful listening, paraphrasing, and reflecting, the counsellor can communicate to the patient that the situation is understood, and establish a structure from which to explore the problem. This therapeutic relationship between the counsellor and the patient permits deeper and more sensitive issues to be explored.

When counselling a depressed patient, the counsellor needs to be aware of the frequently poor concentration span. Hence complicating or confusing an issue by using intricate language must be avoided. With a depressed patient, the counsellor needs to be constantly aware of potential risks, in particular suicidal ideas; so any past history could well be important. If suicidal thoughts are present, the patient must be allowed to talk freely about them. By reflecting and paraphrasing, the counsellor will decide whether the patient is truly at risk and whether additional intervention from the family, GP, or hospital-based psychiatric services is necessary. When counselling a depressed patient, the counsellor must not forget the pain he/she may be experiencing. In the words of Dexter and Wash (1986):

By using sensitivity, warmth and understanding, it is possible to enter into a patient's world. In doing so you must be strong enough to withstand the enveloping nature of the patient's mood and stand back to respond with empathy. This will help you to lead the patient out to look forward to the future where he can value his life.

Case history 1

Mr J., a 47-year-old man, was referred to the counsellor, a CPN, by his GP. He had attended the surgery complaining of having disagreements with his wife, poor sleep, and difficulty in concentrating in his work as a bricklayer. He was also worried about his elderly father.

The counsellor carried out a detailed assessment. Mr J. had been married for 23 years and had no children; His wife had had several miscarriages. His father lived alone in a flat, but was becoming increasingly demanding after suffering a recent heart attack. Although Mr J. had two other brothers, he felt that being the eldest and without the commitment of children, it was his responsibility to care for his father; this took up a lot of his time. This responsibility for himself and his wife, plus his inability to see how the problem could be resolved, had precipitated his depression.

During counselling, Mr J. was offered opportunities for exploring his feelings regarding the relationship with his wife, his feelings about her miscarriages, his employment, and the responsibility of caring for his father. After five sessions, Mr J. was able to pluck up enough courage to ask his younger brother to help him with the care of their father. To his surprise, his brother was happy to oblige, and in turn asked their other brother. This mutual involvement has now strengthened the relationship between the brothers who share the responsibility of giving care and support to their father. A social worker was also contacted to organize additional community benefits.

After seven sessions, Mr J. has recovered from his depressive episode and is back to normal. During this process Mr J. required no medication, was not referred to hospital, and the counsellor discussed Mr J.'s progress regularly with his GP.

ANXIETY

Chronic anxiety is one of the commoner psychiatric disorders that the GP may refer for counselling. It can be seen as a response to potentially threatening situations. Initially the individual may mobilize resources to cope with these threats, which may be of a physical, psychological, or social nature. Ultimately, however, there is a point at which the anxiety ceases to facilitate adequate responses and becomes a problem in itself. This point will be dependent on the person's memory, perception, and understanding of previous experiences. Symptoms of an anxiety state can include palpitations, tension, rigidity, dizziness, headache, hyperventilation, and tremor.

Counsellors must remain calm and confident, despite the patients' ability to make them feel uneasy, since this in itself can be reassuring. Counsellors must be aware of their own anxiety levels. The skills required to help anxious patients are mainly associated with stimulating them to enquire into their feelings in order to identify more specifically the areas in their life that are instrumental in causing an anxious state. One of these skills is to divert their attention from dwelling too long on their fears. Despite this, the counsellor must be able to acknowledge and show understanding of how the patient feels. From an identification of feelings and problems, coping strategies can emerge. As well as counselling skills, relaxation techniques can prove valuable. By including these techniques, counselling leads on to psychotherapy. Early use of counselling and relaxation techniques in primary care has been found to lower the incidence of referrals for specialist treatment at a later stage (Power *et al.* 1990).

Case history 2

Mr E., a 55-year-old teacher, was referred to a counsellor by his GP after presenting himself as being anxious and irritable, especially in the classroom. He also felt uneasy at home, could not relax, and experienced difficulty in getting off to sleep. He worried constantly about his work.

When the counsellor interviewed Mr E., they talked of his changing role and the additional responsibilities that reorganization at his school had brought. As well as teaching his specialist subject, history, Mr E. was undertaking a new task of preparing and developing lessons on economics and associated subjects. Mr E. had always taken pride in his work, and had reached a high standard. However, this additional commitment was too much for him, necessitating him working late into the evening in order to maintain his standards. During his sessions with the counsellor, Mr E. revealed two basic needs: first, to be able to relax and secondly, to lessen the additional commitment he had undertaken. Even before being counselled, Mr E. had considered early retirement, but was unsure whether he should pursue this. By using the counselling process, Mr E. explored this avenue further and discussed how it could affect his life. He also considered the alternative of lowering his standards in order to fulfil the commitments placed upon him at his school and how this might affect him psychologically.

After exploring all aspects, he considered that early retirement would be the best possible option. This was facilitated by his sound financial situation and the agreement of his wife. For the first month, Mr E. saw the counsellor weekly, but this reduced to once a month for the next eight months. During this period Mr E. negotiated his early retirement, restructured his lifestyle to occupy his time constructively, and learnt relaxation techniques. He did not require any medication to help him cope. His sleep improved and his irritability disappeared. Currently he does some supply teaching when he wishes. He is in total control of his life once again.

OBSESSIVE COMPULSIVE STATE

A person suffering from an obsessional compulsive state has the persistent intrusion of contrived thoughts and ideas into his awareness. These thoughts are accompanied by the need to carry out specific ritualistic behaviour. It becomes impossible for them to ignore their irrational and sometimes absurd thoughts and compulsions; severe anxiety follows until the ritualistic behaviour is complete. If the behaviour is not completed, the person will be in fear of imagined consequences. If it is completed, then this can act as a positive reinforcement to the obsessional thoughts, thus allowing the cycle to repeat itself.

When counselling a patient suffering from an obsessive compulsive state, the counsellor must have a sound knowledge of this specific type of disorder. Initially anxiety must be lessened. By using the skills of listening, non-verbal sensitivity, and careful questioning, the counsellor will be able to collect information that will provide a plan of management. They will also create a trusting relationship between counsellor and patient, which will lead to a therapeutic understanding.

In the early stages of therapy, it is important to carry out a baseline assessment against which any improvement or regression can be measured. It is important to include the family if possible, as this gives a picture of any domestic disruption. Family support is also valuable, since the patient may be extremely troubled by his obsessional behaviour and could be at risk of suicide if depression ensued. The counsellor will allow the patient to ventilate thoughts and feelings regarding their behaviour. Underlying conflicts can be unearthed and the patient encouraged to develop ways of limiting their compulsive behaviour. To complement general counselling techniques, behavioural therapies have proved to be effective in this condition, but they need to be fully explained to the patient. Relaxation techniques are often needed in preparing people for behavioural therapies. If a patient is reluctant to co-operate, the counsellor may need to use challenging skills and possibly involve the family. In such cases, the nurse would be instrumental in encouraging the family to talk, if necessary conducting family therapy alongside individual counselling sessions (Dexter and Wash 1986). The following case history shows the relevance of family resources when treating a patient with this type of psychiatric disorder.

Case history 3

Mr A., a 37-year-old man, was referred to the CPN by his GP because he was becoming increasingly troubled by his repetitive and obsessional actions of checking the locking of doors and windows, and the repetitive washing of his hands. If he did not carry out these actions he would feel panicky, but could not explain what the fear was. He worked as a process operator in a chemical factory and lived with his wife and two children in a smart, semi-detached house. The CPN used counselling skills to explore the area of personal conflict. It became apparent that Mr A.'s ritualistic behaviour was connected with the fear of not reaching the standards of perfection set by his own father. The CPN also learned that Mr A.'s father had tried to dissuade him from joining the chemical company, because of the fear of infection. The therapeutic rapport established by the CPN enabled Mr A. to speak about his fear, something he had not been able to do before.

The CPN commenced behaviour therapy. During this Mr A. became more aware of his own qualities and ceased comparing his accomplishments with those of his father. Mr A. was also able to rationalize the safety procedures that he used in his employment as a process operator, which made his father's fear of infection invalid. Relaxation therapy proved useful at this time. During this period Mr A. agreed that his wife should be made aware of his problems and the CPN involved her in monitoring his progress and assessing his improvement. His wife was also able to shed other light on her husband's problems.

After twelve, weekly sessions with the CPN, Mr A. had ceased his ritualistic behaviour. The CPN reported briefly on a weekly basis to the GP and, during his period of treatment, Mr A. needed neither sick leave nor medication.

SCHIZOPHRENIA

The schizophrenias are considered by many authorities to be a related group of disorders of thought, emotion, behaviour, and perception. These psychotic disturbances hamper a person's ability to interact with others. This isolation often leads to progressive deterioration and further difficulties.

Most people with schizophrenia are not in hospital, but are trying to cope alone or are being looked after by their family, sometimes at great cost to themselves and their carers. Of those schizophrenics living in the community, Ironbar and Hooper (1989) estimated that 71 per cent lived with relatives, 17 per cent lived alone, 9 per cent lived in a hostel, and the remaining 3 per cent lived under supervision.

The success of counselling for a schizophrenic patient will depend on the severity of the psychosis. If the patient is being treated with medication which reduces the florid symptoms, it is then possible to form a trusting relationship. This enables the counsellor to explore areas of fear and anxiety that may be causing great pain and which could eventually lead to relapse. Thus counselling can help to prevent further episodes of the illness. When counselling the schizophrenic patient, unrealistic goals must be avoided. However, Wing (1977) believes that skilled counselling is at the heart of good management in schizophrenic patients. The management of the schizophrenic in the community should not only be about the patient but also about his/her family since relatives are often the major carers. The counsellor can encourage them to adopt a more tolerant and supportive attitude towards the patient. CPNs are often chosen as the most appropriate person to counsel the schizophrenic patient in the community, because of their expertise when dealing with this psychotic disorder (Falloon *et al.* 1990).

The deluded patient

There are many forms of delusional thinking. Patients can feel grandiose, nihilistic, paranoid, unworthy, etc. When counselling deluded patients, non-verbal communication is important and a direct and open approach, reinforced by positive eye contact, is advisable. This lessens any suspicion that the patient has of the counsellor. The counsellor's speech should be clear and loud, hence avoiding misunderstanding which could reinforce the delusions. The delusions themselves should neither be agreed with, nor argued against. Using the skills of reflection, the counsellor aims to develop an empathy with the patient, in order to focus upon feelings rather than the delusional thoughts and ideas. By establishing a trusting relationship, it is more likely that the counsellor will learn about other problems and worries. Relieving these can lessen the delusions. As they recede the counsellor should give positive acknowledgement and encouragement. By counselling, the deluded patient can be encouraged towards positive actions, varying from changes in behaviour to taking appropriate medication.

Disturbances of perception

Of the perceptual disturbances, auditory hallucinations are relatively common. They often manifest by inappropriate behaviour, laughing to oneself, transient grimacing, etc. Trust between counsellor and patient in order to create a therapeutic environment is essential. Hallucinating patients are often in great distress. This distress can be alleviated when the counsellor reinforces reality and thoughts can be diverted from the hallucinations. Methods of distraction include talking about current interests and hobbies and how the patient may feel about them. The more a trusting relationship develops, the more the patient will accept advice and make appropriate changes for his/her overall mental well-being.

The counsellor must never underestimate the patient's distress, confront the individual with negative reactions, nor be judgemental; this will merely undermine trust. In schizophrenia, counselling is frequently used only for short periods, but it is a valid method of developing a trusting and beneficial relationship in a difficult, organic, mental disease.

Case history 4

Mr S., a 53-year-old man, was referred to the CPN by the GP after refusing to accept his Depo antipsychotic medication from the practice nurse at the surgery. Mr S. had been diagnosed as having paranoid schizophrenia 16 years earlier whilst in the Army. Since that time he had had two further relapses, both episodes being precipitated by non-compliance with treatment. When the CPN assessed Mr S., there was still no evidence of a recurrence of any psychosis. By the use of counselling skills, the CPN was able to uncover feelings of anger in Mr S. dating back to his wife leaving him two years earlier. He did not blame his wife for leaving home, but complained that the diagnosis of him as having a psychotic illness, which precipitated her departure, was incorrect. The CPN neither agreed nor disagreed with Mr S.'s feelings but, by listening to him and forming a trusting and therapeutic relationship, he was able to persuade Mr S. to accept his medication once more, thus avoiding his customary relapse.

The CPN now administers the Depo antipsychotic medication on a three-weekly basis. During his regular contacts with Mr S., the CPN has arranged for him to attend a local Social Services day centre two days a week—he had previously refused this. During this episode, the hospital psychiatric services have not been required.

THE ADVANTAGES OF TREATING PSYCHIATRIC DISORDERS IN THE COMMUNITY

Treating patients suffering from psychiatric disorders in the community has reduced the stigma associated with such illnesses. Simmons and Brooker (1986) state that: 'people may be much more willing to see someone who works from a local health centre than they would be to attend the psychiatric hospital, since there is no inherent stigma with the former'. Robertson and Scott (1985) supported this view: 'easy access to the CPNs removed the potential stigma of a psychiatric label for some clients by preventing the need for a psychiatric referral'. In 1977, Corser and Ryce described the work of a small psychiatric team attached to a health centre. They reported a 97 per cent attendance rate for appointments for mental health problems and claimed that this high level was because of accessibility and lack of stigma. The need to minimise stigma was also highlighted by Ironbar and Hooper (1989), who commented:

Once a person has a diagnosis or a label attached to them, there are a number of consequences. The person's self-perception and that of others towards them undergoes a significant change. Behaviour, emotions and thought, past and present, are re-interpreted in terms of illness. The stigma of mental illness also tends to isolate the person and their family from other people. These reactions serve to reinforce the patient's image and their role as an ill person and tend to inhibit their return to normal life.

Another advantage a counsellor has in helping patients in the community is the possibility of easier contact with their families. Once a referral has been received, the counsellor can arrange by mutual agreement to see the patient, either in the surgery or health centre or in their own home. If the patient lives with relatives, the entire family unit may be engaged in the support and care which is required. The counsellor can offer regular sessions to family members, in order to bring an awareness of interpersonal communication skills essential to the conduct of an open, constructive, problem-solving framework which will enhance recovery. Once this framework has been established, it is important for the family to take responsibility by taking part in all decisions, and possibly continuing the therapeutic direction in the absence of the professional. The family will then hopefully learn not to depend too much upon the counsellor (Butterworth and Skidmore 1981). Corney (1985) supports the concept of supporting the resource of family carers:

The effect of psychological disorder and distress are likely to place extra strains on a relationship within the family and on outsiders, as well as the individual's performance and management of his or her affairs. Support needs not only to be given to the suffering individual, but also to the family members in order to reduce any resulting disharmony.

SUMMARY

In the disorders that have been discussed, the success of any counselling depends to a large degree on the psychotic gravity of the problem. However, to totally rule out the opportunity for counselling in any psychiatric disorder, including severe schizophrenia, is not justified. Assessment of the patient before deciding on his/her suitability will normally be the task of the GP. This assessment will largely depend on the expertise and knowledge the GP has of the various psychiatric interventions that are available in the community.

The need for counselling of psychiatric disorders in primary health care settings is increasing now that the large psychiatric hospitals are discharging many of their patients. In addition, the traditional reliance on pharmacological treatment is lessening because of concern about side effects, habituation, and addiction. The success of counselling as compared with other traditional psychiatric interventions has yet to be proved, research is being undertaken but there are difficulties in measuring effectiveness.

Increased care in the community has lessened, although not eliminated, the stigma of mental illness. The families of patients, who are often the main carers, welcome the community support and often benefit from counselling themselves.

Although this chapter has concentrated on the CPN as the person who can deliver counselling care to psychiatric patients, the writer would point out there are other skilled practitioners who are part of the community mental health teams who can also offer this service. These include psychologists, psychiatric social workers, occupational therapists, and practice nurses. As well as workers in statutory agencies, mention must also be made of the invaluable contributions of the voluntary agencies (such as the National Schizophrenic Fellowship).

REFERENCES

Burnard, P. (1992). *Counselling—a guide to practice in nursing.* Butterworth-Heinemann Ltd, Oxford.

Butterworth, C.A. and Skidmore, D. (1981). *Caring for the mentally ill in the community.* Croom Helm, London.

Corney, R. (1985). Social factors, psychological distress and mental ill health. In *Responding to mental illness.* (ed. G. Horobin), pp. 27–42. Kogan Page, London.

Corney, R. (1990). Counselling in general practice—does it work? *Journal of the Royal Society of Medicine*, **83**, 253–7.

Corser, C. M. and Ryce, S. W. (1977). Community mental health care—a model based on the primary care team. *British Medical Journal*, **2**, 936–8.

Dexter, G. and Wash, M. (1986). *Psychiatric nursing skills—a practice centred approach.* Croom Helm, London.

Dowrick, C. (1992). Improving mental health through primary care. *British Journal of General Practice*, **42**, 382–6.

Dryden, W. and Feltham, C. (1992). *Brief counselling.* Open University Press, Buckingham, Philadelphia.

Falloon, I., Shanahan, W., Laporta, M., and Krekorian, H. (1990). Integrated family, general practice and mental health care in the management of schizophrenia. *Journal of the Royal Society of Medicine*, **83**, 225–8.

Green, J. (1968). The psychiatric nurse in the community. *The International Journal of Nursing Studies*, **5**, 175–83.

Ironbar, N. and Hooper, A. (1989). *Self instruction in mental health nursing* (2nd edn). Ballière Tindall, London.

Irving, J. and Heath, V. (1991). *Counselling in general practice* (revised edn). British Association for Counselling, Rugby.

Leopoldt, H. and Hurn, R. (1973). Towards integration. *Nursing Mirror*, **136**, 38–42.

May, A. R. and Moore, S. (1963). The mental nurse in the community. *The Lancet*, **i**, 213–14.

Paykel, E. S., Mangen, S. P., Griffith, S. H., and Burns, T. P. (1982). Community psychiatric nursing for neurotic patients. *British Journal of Psychiatry*, **140**, 573–81.

Pollock, L. C. (1989). *Community psychiatric nurses—myth or reality*. Scutari Press, Middlesex.

Power, K. G., Simpson, R. J., Swanson, V., and Wallace, L. A. (1990). Controlled comparison of pharmacological and psychological treatment of generalised anxiety disorder in primary care. *British Journal of General Practice*, **40**, 289–94.

Robertson, H. and Scott, D. J. (1985). Community psychiatric nursing: a survey of patients and problems. *Journal of the Royal College of General Practitioners*, **35**, 130–2.

Sibbald, B. Addington-Hall, J., Brenneman, D., and Freeling, P. (1993). Counsellors in English and Welsh General Practices: their nature and distribution. *British Medical Journal*, **306**, 29–33.

Simmons, A. and Brooker, C. (1986). *Community psychiatric nursing: a social perspective*. Heinemann Nursing, London.

White, E. (1986). Factors which influence general practitioners to refer to CPNs. In *Reading in psychiatric nursing research* (ed. J. Brooking), pp. 215–32. John Wiley, Chichester.

Wing, J. K. (1977). *Schizophrenia and its management in the community*. National Schizophrenic Fellowship, Surbiton, Surrey.

Yura, R. and Walsh, M. B. (1967). *The nursing process*. Appleton Century Crofts, Norwalk, NJ.

7 Fertility

Sue Jennings

> O wind of Tizoula, O wind of Amsoud!
> Blow over the plains and over the sea,
> Carry, O, carry my thoughts
> To him who is so far, so far,
> And who has left me without a little child.
> O wind! remind him that I have no child.
>
> O wind of Tizoula, O wind of Amsoud!
> Blow away that desire for riches
> That sends our young men away
> And makes them forget the girls they've married,
> Their mothers, and the old ones left in the village.
> O wind! remind him that I have no child.
>
> (Berber woman's song, Ancient)

BACKGROUND AND CONTEXT

Although this chapter addresses the counselling needs of people who are experiencing problems with their fertility as well as those who wish to limit their fertility, more attention will be paid to the former, that is those people, numbering some one-in-six couples, who experience problems with conception. It is a matter of individual choice whether general practitioners choose to offer preliminary fertility counselling themselves or to use a counsellor if they have one in their primary health care team (PHCT). In both situations, there is a need for medical knowledge regarding treatments for subfertility and a basic understanding of the new legislation, as well as specialist skills in fertility counselling itself. Although fertility counselling provision must be available by law in licensed centres for fertility treatments, it is my conviction that the PHCT is in a crucial position to offer a considerable amount of counselling before decisions to refer are made. In this context I am referring to the additional dimension of fertility counselling itself, as envisaged by the Human Fertilization and Embryology Authority (HFEA).

INTRODUCTION TO FERTILITY COUNSELLING

The Berber woman's song at the beginning of this chapter illustrates very poignantly the deep-rooted desire and longing experienced by most people to produce their own children. In my work over many years as a fertility counsellor, I have witnessed both the very strong grief experienced by men and women if they are unable to realize their wish for children, a grief which until recently was ignored by most professionals (Jennings 1989) and the overwhelming confusion when that grief is discharged and the longed for infant becomes a reality. Because there is now the possibility of 'high-tech' treatment for fertility problems (what might be termed the 'reproduction revolution'), public awareness has been heightened and the demand for possible treatment has accelerated. Many people are seeking advice from their general practitioners at an earlier stage, and indeed have become more knowledgeable about potential treatment on the one hand, while increasing their worry about reproductive failure on the other. I refer throughout to 'fertility' counselling rather than 'infertility' counselling; the latter already casts a sense of gloom and depression over the situation. At the London Hospital Medical College we have found that patients respond more optimistically with this change in language. Fertility counselling needs to address the uncertainty and stress of possible childlessness, as well as being able to consider the possible outcomes of treatment and their implications, particularly where there is the use of donated gametes.

There may, in some cases, be a need for more extensive therapeutic counselling or psychotherapy, when referral to another agency is more appropriate. Additionally, we must not forget the need for an awareness of different cultural attitudes to fertility problems, as well as the profound bereavement and mourning experienced by those for whom treatment has not provided children. Fertility counselling is a new specialism within counselling rather than being a discipline in its own right. I think there is a case to be argued for more development of 'counselling within reproductive medicine' to include fertility, psychosexual issues, hysterectomy, abortion, neonatal death, and multiple miscarriage (Jennings (ed.), 1994).

THE CENTRAL ROLE OF THE PHCT IN COUNSELLING FERTILITY PROBLEMS

As someone who works at the secondary and tertiary levels of health care, I see an urgent need for both increased fertility awareness and knowledge for the PHCT on the one hand, and an endorsement of existing counselling skills and experience on the other. Generalist counselling in general practice is looked at elsewhere in this book (see Chapters 1 and 2) and many of the skills—empathy, active listening, focusing, use of metaphor, for example—should all be part of the general practitioner's basic repertoire. From my own experience, most general practitioners integrate these skills into good practice, together with up-to-date information and judicious advice. An increasing number of general practices have at least one member of the group with an obstetric/gynaecological specialism who would seem the obvious person to take responsibility for pre-referral fertility counselling.

Later in this chapter I address the requirements laid down by the HFEA in relation to counselling provision; however, this only applies to those counsellors who work in the secondary/tertiary health care sectors. General practitioners need to be encouraged to develop their counselling specialisms which, in turn, enable the client/patient to see counselling as a part of health care rather than as an extra 'tacked on' which means that you are 'mad' or 'bad' or are about to have a nervous breakdown, or, specifically in relation to fertility, that you are not 'fit' to be a parent.

MAIN CAUSES OF SUBFERTILITY

Male factors

Sperm disorders are the most common single cause of subfertility (Hull 1991) and are diagnosed when sperm are either defective or absent. At the time of writing, medical treatment for sperm disorder is unproven, but the 'processing' of poor sperm can assist conception success and the reduction of tobacco and alcohol use can also improve sperm quality, (Lee, 1994).

Female factors

Tubal damage or blockage can prevent conception; decisions are made whether to use tubal surgery or assisted conception techniques which bypass the Fallopian tubes.

Ovulation failure is indicated by an absence of menstruation (amenorrhoea) or infrequent periods (oligomenorrhoea). Where there is disturbance of the HPO (hypothalamic, pituitary, ovarian) axis, some treatments can restore fertility to levels that are almost normal. Eating disorders, especially anorexia nervosa, also influence ovulation and frequently result in subfertility.

Endometriosis can result in subfertility, even when in a mild form, yet many women with endometriosis do conceive spontaneously. Surgical and medical treatments for the condition itself are disappointing.

Congenital causes

Congenital absence or maldevelopment of vas, ovaries, uterus, and testes, are all conditions which need assisted conception.

Drug damage

It must always be remembered that radiotherapy and laser treatments can damage reproductive organs and processes, and although people are usually well informed before commencing such treatments, there are times when it is not 'heard' or is forgotten.

Psychological causes

There is no conclusive evidence to suggest that there are psychological causes of infertility, or that there is such a thing as an 'infertile personality'. Most professionals are agreed that stress plays a part in fertility problems, although it is not yet clear if it is the stressful life style or the stress of the infertility that is the contributory factor, or both! The results from a pilot project suggest that certain forms of dependency could contribute to fertility problems (Jennings 1993).

UNEXPLAINED SUBFERTILITY

In 28 per cent of cases no definitive reason is found (Hull 1991). If the fertility problem is of less than three years' duration, couples are usually 'unlucky so far' and will probably conceive within two years; after three years there is a much reduced chance of natural conception, and assisted conception techniques must be considered. Long waiting lists may encourage the GP to refer earlier.

ASSISTED CONCEPTION TECHNIQUES

These include:

1. Donor insemination (DI):

- with husband's sperm; *or*
- with partner's sperm; *or*
- with donor's sperm.

2. *In vitro* fertilization and embryo transfer (IVF–ET, 'test tube method') which can include donated gametes (sperm or ovum) or embryos (surrogacy).
3. Gamete intrafallopian fertilization (GIFT)—also with donated transfer gametes (surrogacy).
4. Microsurgical epididymal sperm aspiration (MESA) for congenital absence of vas. The exudate obtained from the epididymis can be used for DI, GIFT, or IVF.

5. Ovum donations by a volunteer (OD) for congenital absence of ovaries or premature menopause. The ova may be used for GIFT or IVF.
6. A female volunteer (historically a relative or friend) elects to receive a couple's fertilized eggs (or embryos) created by IVF, through embryo transfer.

IVF–ET is currently the most commonly practised treatment, especially where there is tubal damage. In 1990 the average pregnancy rate with IVF–ET was 17 per cent (per treatment cycle), which translates into a 12 per cent maternity rate (per treatment cycle). Some clinics distort this rate by counting twins as two successes and triplets as three, whereas they should all be counted as only one.

Assisted conception techniques must be undertaken in a licensed treatment centre whose work and practice is regulated by the HFEA.

FERTILITY COUNSELLING REQUIRED BY HFEA

The recent legislation regulating medical treatments for fertility problems includes a mandatory requirement for the provision of counselling.

People seeking licensed treatment (i.e. *in vitro* fertilisation or treatment using donated gametes) or consenting to the use or storage of embryos, or to the donation or storage of embryos, must be given 'a suitable opportunity to receive proper counselling about the implications of taking the proposed steps', before they consent.

(HFEA Code of Practice, 1991, p.6.i)

The HFEA, which is the statutory body empowered to enforce the Act, has provided a Code of Practice, Guidelines and a Consultation Document to make sure that licensed centres and their staff understand their responsibilities in relation to the provision of fertility counselling. For example:

Centres must make implications counselling available to everyone. They should also provide support or therapeutic counselling in appropriate cases or refer people to sources of more specialist counselling outside the centre.

(ibid, p.6.ii)

Despite the requirement by law for licensed centres to make this counselling provision, there is still uncertainty amongst doctors about what constitutes such counselling. The Code of Practice states that:

Counselling should be distinguished from the normal relationship between the clinician and the person offering donation or seeking storage or treatment, which includes giving professional advice, . . .

(ibid, p.6.i)

However, though highlighted by HFEA, clinicians seem unable to distinguish this, and counselling appears to be confused with the giving of advice and information on the one hand, and the practice of psychotherapy on the other. Other chapters in this book clarify the definitions and practice of counselling in its several forms, and the chapters on HIV and sexual counselling are particularly relevant to the present topic (see Chapters 8 and 10).

HFEA have identified the following types of counselling which must be available for people contemplating assisted conception:

1. *Support counselling*: aims to give emotional support at times of particular stress, for example when there is a failure to achieve a pregnancy, or during the waiting time for results of tests, or even longer waiting time for treatment.
2. *Implications counselling*: where a couple reflect on the *implications* of a successful outcome of treatment, particularly where it involves the use of donated gametes.
3. *Therapeutic counselling*: which is intended to assist people to come to terms with the consequences of treatment failure and adjust to their infertility, within the context of their life as a whole. Also, failed fertility can highlight other deeper issues such as marital or sexual dysfunction.

The HFEA Code of Practice obviously considers that implications counselling, especially with donated gametes, is most important in that it devotes considerably more detail to its practice. It emphasizes that both existing and unborn children's needs must be considered. Clients and prospective donors need implications counselling in relation to both treatment decisions and gamete donation in itself. They need to consider their feelings about not being the biological parent of their child, and what they will decide to tell the child as well as their extended family (Jennings 1992).

It is generally assumed that openness with existing and future children is preferred, rather than keeping secrets for life that might be guessed at anyway. Children born from assisted conception have a right to know their biological origins if they ask, although anonymity is preserved for donors of gametes. Counsellors have sometimes to deal with the situation where a couple request the use of a known donor, and the implications counselling reveals that it is not in the best interest of all concerned. The following case history illustrates such a situation.

Case history 1

Mr and Mrs J. attended for 'implications counselling' before making treatment decisions. Mrs J. had no ovaries and wanted to accept her sister's offer of donated eggs. The couple insisted that they wanted known donorship within the family, and Mrs J. said, darkly: 'And she owes me something anyway'. I suggested a session with the sisters together, which Mrs J. refused, but said that her sister would come to see me. Ms W., the sister, came to see me in a very distressed state, saying that she wanted 'everything to be all right', and that this was why she was offering her eggs. She was a single woman with no ideas at the time of having a family. When asked about 'everything being all right', she burst into tears and said that her father had abused her and that she felt so bad that perhaps this was something good she could do. Patently more counselling was necessary before final decisions could be taken.

My own view is that more emphasis should be placed on the variations between the presenting problems of people who attend fertility clinics and assisted conception units. For example, there are a significant number of people who have a psychosexual problem and turn to fertility clinics for assistance. This, of course, raises the whole issue of whether assisted conception treatments should be used for social and psychological problems rather than medical ones. There are those who suggest that if people choose to have assisted conception rather than sexual intercourse, then it is their decision; however, with the people that I counsel, there are usually feelings of guilt and distress concerning the psychosexual problem and a lack of knowledge of where to turn for help, illustrated by case history 2.

Case history 2

Mr and Mrs S. appeared to be suffering from unexplained infertility, as preliminary investigations showed no medical problems with sperm, ovulation, or tubes. Mrs S. requested counselling and presented as very tense, attending with her husband who was loud and florid in his attempts to suggest that his wife had 'the problem'. Careful probing brought to light the fact that they did not have vaginal intercourse through to full orgasm as Mr S. had to climax orally and his wife had hoped that some semen would spill before withdrawal to enable her to conceive. Once having disclosed 'the secret', it was then possible for them to request psychosexual help rather than assisted conception.

There may be couples who need to be referred to marital therapy because of the stress of their relationship, and there are times when the presenting behaviour is so disturbed that a psychiatric referral is necessary rather than a gynaecological one.

The following are considerations for the GP before making a referral:

1. How long have the couple been trying to conceive? Up to three years may be within the normal range. However, most clinics have waiting lists of at least two years which may affect the timing of referral.

2. Are the couple having regular vaginal intercourse? Could this be a psychosexual problem in disguise?
3. Have you (the GP) excluded organic disease in either partner by referring to previous history and by appropriate examination and tests (for example for thyroid deficiency)?
4. Are there any eating disorders? In the case of anorexia, bulimia, or obesity, the Ponderal Index should be calculated to indicate the likelihood of ovulatory disorder, and an appropriate referral made.
5. Is there an assumption that it must be 'the woman's problem' and, therefore, she must have the investigation? Fertility clinics will not usually proceed with invasive investigation until there has been a sperm test.
6. What is the presenting level of distress? Anger, depression, and guilt are the most common feelings.
7. How much pressure is on the couple from their families or towards each other? What support is available to the couple before and during treatment?
8. Have the couple considered the possibilities of childlessness? The loss of the 'dream child' that never was can be as acute as losing a child that lived.
9. What is your response to single women seeking treatment? Having taken into account the HFEA's requirement for consideration of the welfare of the child, especially a child's need for a father, do you have your own personal stance?
10. How do you respond to a lesbian couple seeking assisted conception, given that some prefer to attend an assisted conception unit rather than undertake self-conception (see also 9).

SUMMARY FOR GENERAL PRACTITIONERS CONSIDERING FERTILITY COUNSELLING

There is a strong case for general practitioners, or a member of their PHCT, undertaking some fertility counselling with patients prior to referral to a fertility clinic. I suggest that this is separate from the advice and information that a general practitioner would expect to give such patients in order for people to begin to address the complex issues involved in considering 'high-tech' treatments.

Information packs on the problems of fertility and their management are available and the general practitioner can provide these (see list of Useful addresses at the end of this chapter). General practitioners are well placed to explore the many and varied reasons for the fertility problem, as well as providing support for patients embarking on a lengthy and stressful period of treatment whose results are uncertain.

Currently, there is only one training course in fertility counselling. This takes place at The London Hospital Medical College. This diploma course has been endorsed by The British Infertility Counselling Association as being an appropriate course for multidisciplinary professionals in fertility counselling skills. There are also opportunities for general practitioners to attend specialist courses in 'high-tech' fertility treatments.

However, in the new 'purchaser/provider' milieu, it is important to point out that many Health Authorities are not willing to fund assisted conception treatment. It is important for general practitioners to be aware of the policy and priorities of their Health Authority, thus avoiding undue disappointment.

COUNSELLING TO LIMIT FERTILITY

There seems a certain irony in the contrast between people who are desperate to have children and those who are desperate not to. There is also a painful reality in the fact that many hospitals run their antenatal clinic and their fertility clinic in the same space and at the same time.

With the reduction in resources for well-women centres and family planning clinics and the shift of emphasis for this work to be carried out by PHCTs, it is inevitable that the team members will undertake to give more advice and provide more information, as well as counselling, when required.

Community Health Councils and the Family Planning Association provide leaflets and posters with the latest information, and there is now a wide choice of possible methods to be used before and after childbearing. Why is it, then, that in the Chief Medical Officer's Report for 1990 it was estimated that almost half of all conceptions were in some sense unwanted or unintended? Obviously not all these pregnancies result in unwanted children; nevertheless there is a plea from government to provide better access to family planning information and advice (Department of Health 1992).

Prompted by the spread of HIV, the Government has developed a strategy within which the importance of re-education is stressed regarding unprotected sexual intercourse and the spread of AIDS-related illness and other sexually-transmitted diseases. Sexual health includes not only the control of disease, but also family planning. Family planning services play an important part in the health of children and the well-being of families.

One of the main targets is to reduce the rate of conception amongst the under-16s by at least 50 per cent by the year 2000, from 9.5 per 1000 girls aged between 13 and 15 in 1989, to no more than 4.8 (Department of Health 1992) It is now recommended that boys should be targeted as-well as girls, and there is some indication, following the high-profiling of HIV, that 'condom consciousness raising' is having some effect, both girls and boys being more likely to carry condoms.

Although the National Curriculum now requires pupils aged 11–14 to understand the processes of conception in human beings as well as the physical and emotional changes of adolescence and the responsibilities of sexual behaviour, it is left to schools' governing bodies to decide whether any further sex education should be included in the school's curriculum.

I would suggest that as well as the family planning information and counselling provided by the PHCT, more outreach work should be developed pro-actively with schools, colleges, and youth groups.

The aim of government is that by 1994/5 the full range of NHS family planning services, however provided, should be appropriate, accessible, and comprehensive. Additional fertility counselling skills could be used by a whole range of professional people, including to the general practitioner, nurse, counsellor, embryologist, and social worker.

What part should the general practitioner play in an overall strategy for family planning and fertility care?

FAMILY PLANNING AND FERTILITY CARE—THE PHCT

Although I have already suggested that there should be an identified person within the practice who specializes in fertility counselling and advice, I think that it is important that they are seen within the context of the PHCT. The team as a whole is able to integrate the 'womb to tomb' life journey, through all the stages of birth, menstruation and puberty, fertility and family planning, psychosexuality, mid-life changes and ageing. The team's counselling expertise should embrace the family doctor, the family planning nurse within the team, the health visitor, and the midwife and clients/patients of all ages should be able to find sensitive responses to any lack of information, anxiety, distress, and confusion.

The PHCT is in an ideal position to know people within their social, cultural, and domestic setting in a way that is impossible for secondary and tertiary agencies. Good counsel can be available based on local knowledge and understanding of family circumstances. Young people especially need to be encouraged to contact and increasingly use their PHCT facility and, as previously mentioned, there is a strong case for the PHCT doing outreach work in schools and communities. Some PHCTs already have counsellors attached to them who take on complementary roles to the other specialists involved. Some are also able to avail themselves of interpreters and nursing and midwifery aides who are able to discuss in greater depth both the symptoms and cultural practice in a person's first language. Orientation courses for doctors' receptionists can also assist the integrated function of the PHCT. All of these enhance good practice.

PHCTs will have greater demands put upon them in the future as other clinics close down, and I can only hope that sufficient resources are made available for any additional personnel and specialist training which may be needed.

REFLECTIONS FOR GENERAL PRACTITIONERS AND THE PHCT IN FAMILY PLANNING/CONTRACEPTIVE COUNSELLING

General practitioners have a responsibility to provide comprehensive information and advice on all forms of contraception (leaflets are available in several languages). Government targets to improve the nation's health and reduce unwanted pregnancies as well as sexually-transmitted disease, includes a more comprehensive family planning service. The attitudes of general practitioners towards underage sex or homosexual behaviour, for example, can discourage people from seeking counsel. Within the PHCT there needs to be one identified specialist to co-ordinate practice initiatives and policy. People need to know that there are several different types and choices of contraception, including 'natural methods', and to be helped to take responsibility for their choices. For example:

1. Are people being made aware of the wide range of choices of contraception including the advances made in 'natural methods'?
2. Is contraception or 'safe sex' the prime reason for consultation?
3. Within the couple relationship is one person taking responsibility for avoiding pregnancy?
4. How can people's autonomy be encouraged in family planning?
5. What are the team's assumptions about homosexuals and regular drug users?
6. What are the team's attitudes towards underage intercourse?
7. Is contraception seen as the woman's or the man's responsibility?
8. Is it possible that more explicit sex education is required in order for people to understand contraception?

CONCLUSIONS

In this chapter I have addressed the importance of general practitioners and their team in relation to fertility treatment as well as fertility regulation, and of recognising the key role of the PHCT in helping, wherever possible, all pregnancies to be welcome ones and all to become parents who wish to do so. I have suggested some key issues for consideration which include both accessibility of knowledge (such as the HFEA's legislation and *The health of the nation*) as well as a confrontation of our own prejudices and assumptions.

A fertility counsellor is supportive to people undergoing treatment at any stage of the procedures—before, during, or after treatment. This may be akin to grief and bereavement counselling as people come to terms with the loss of the child they have never had.

Perhaps, most importantly, the counsellor is there to assist people to come to terms with the likelihood of treatment not resulting in a take-home baby. As GPs are probably the first medical port-of-call for fertility problems, it is hoped that the complexity of these issues is now a little clearer. Similarly family planning needs to be seen within the context of the individual on the one hand and the society as whole on the other, and decisions made for a positive and responsible outcome for all concerned.

DEDICATION

This chapter is dedicated to Professor Gedis Grudzinskas who has supported and encouraged all my counselling work.

ACKNOWLEDGEMENT

I am indebted to Dr Sammy Lee for the technical aspects of this chapter.

REFERENCES

Burnard, P. (1989). *Counselling skills for health professionals*. Chapman and Hall, London.
BICA (1992) *Infertility counselling: guidelines for practice*. The British Infertility Counselling Association, Doncaster.
Department of Health (1992). *The health of the nation*, Cm 1986. HMSO, London.
Hull, M. (1991). *Infertility treatment: needs and effectiveness*. Dept, of Obstetrics and Gynaecology, University of Bristol.
Jennings, S. (1994). *Infertility counselling*. Blackwells Scientific Publications, Oxford.
Jennings, S. (1989). Legitimate grieving? Working with infertility. In *Children and death* (ed. D. Papadatou and C. Papadatos) Hemisphere, New York.
Jennings, S. (1992). Nurses' role in fertility counselling. *Professional Nurse*.
Jennings, S. (1993). The drama in counsel: the counsel in drama. *Counselling*, **4**, No. 3.

Lee, S. (1994). Male factor infertility. In *Infertility Counselling*. Blackwell Scientific Publications, Oxford.
The Human Fertilisation and Embryology Authority (HFEA).
—— (1991). *Code of practice: consultation document.* London.
—— (1992). *Annual report.* London.
—— (1993). *Code of practice: explanation* London.
The School of Public Health (1992). *Effective health care: the management of subfertility.* University of Leeds.

USEFUL ADDRESSES

Issue
318 Summer Lane
Birmingham
BR19 3RL

London Diploma Course in Fertility Counselling (and Short Training Courses)
26 Overmead
Sidcup
Kent
DA15 8DS

London Lesbian Health Care
c/o London Women's Centre
Wesley House
4 Wild Court
London
WC2

The British Association for Infertility Counsellors (BICA)
White House
High Street
Campsall
Nr Doncaster
South Yorkshire

The Family Planning Association (FPA)
27–35 Mortimer Street
London
WIN 7RJ

The Human Fertilisation and Embryology Authority (HFEA)
Paxton House
30 Artillery Lane
London E1 7LS
Tel: 071 377 5077

8 Sexual problems

Roland Freedman

INTRODUCTION

It can be embarrassing or discomforting to talk about one's sexual feelings and functionings even when one is not particularly worried about them. How much more alarming and difficult, therefore, to reveal them when one is disabled by them. Guilt, shame, self-disgust, or the assumption of inadequacy is often associated with sexual distress; so it is not surprising that patients tend to 'test the water' when seeing a doctor and, if it feels cold, draw back saying to themselves 'this proves what I knew before: that I am guilty and deserve to be rejected'.

For the doctor there are many difficulties in unearthing sexual distress. How is the GP to extricate, from the undifferentiated conglomeration of complaints, those which are indicative of such distress? Some symptoms are frequently associated: for example, women with vaginal discharges who have negative findings on physical and laboratory examination; recurrent symptoms of cystitis, again with negative physical and laboratory results; or women who cannot find a method of contraception that suits them. In this last example it may not take too profound a discussion for such women to reveal their unhappiness at having their bodies 'messed about' by drugs or foreign bodies. However, it may be more difficult to elicit a loss of excitement associated with taking a contraceptive which is virtually 100 per cent effective, and even greater sensitivity will be required to reveal and discuss feelings of sexual disappointment, inadequacy, antipathy, or even non-consummation.

OFFERS AND ACCEPTANCES

But even vaguer symptoms such as headaches, backaches, 'tired all the time', recurrent virus infections may be tentative offers which signify sexual distress. On the other hand, they may not, and if the doctor makes assumptions leading to direct rather than to open questions an embarrassing outcome could result. But even when the doctor is correct, the patient may be unprepared for the approach at that time and may deny or rebut it angrily. This will cause considerable discomfiture to the doctor as well as to the patient. In addition, an opportunity of ventilating a major source of distress will have been missed.

So the approach always needs to be tentative, creating an atmosphere of acceptance and avoiding direct questions. Nebulous, open-ended comments as to how the patient seems to be feeling, coupled with silences—comfortable or uncomfortable—have to be tolerated. This approach frees the patient to reveal their problem if they feel the time is ripe. 'If you ask questions you only get answers' is a consistently valid dictum (Balint 1964).

Having discovered that there is a sexual problem, what is to be done about it. A laughing dismissal of the problem by the patient should be ignored as mere subterfuge. In fact the patient is sharing with the doctor an intimate problem which affects the whole person and which may previously have never been disclosed. He/she must not be dismissed lightly, nor referred elsewhere too readily. For the doctor the impact may be wideranging. Embarrassment, being 'out of my depth', and helplessness are commonly experienced feelings. The doctor may even experience anger at having to shoulder such a heavy load of distress.

But above all, most doctors will experience a feeling of ignorance. Let me put this in perspective. Conventional medical school teaching is that the doctor is the expert, knows the answers, and can give advice; none of that is true for GPs dealing with sexual problems, for every patient is unique and the range and diversity of problems is encyclopaedic. By capitalizing on this uniqueness, doctor and patient together can explore the problem, gain insights and learn how it impacts on the whole person. It must also be borne in mind that many patients are extremely ignorant of their sexual physiology and a very large number of sexual problems brought to doctors are extremely simple to deal with and extremely simple to explain. If GPs think about the degree of illness in many other areas of patients' lives—minor blemishes, coughs and colds, sore throats, transient aches and pains—they will know that many, many problems are extremely minor and sexual problems are no exception to this rule.

Having taken the patient's history, a physical examination usually follows; this very frequently reveals no positive findings. It is tempting to reassure him/her that there is no abnormality and that all is well. However, such reassurance is not only unhelpful, but even counterproductive if it precludes uncovering the fears and fantasies that underlie the problem.

Sometimes the patient's behaviour when consulting the doctor gives early clues as to the nature of the problem.

Case history 1

Hurrying into the consulting room, David seemed desperate. Aged 25, a successful insurance agent, he was unable to get the sexual side 'right' of what was otherwise an excellent relationship with a woman with whom he was in love. Intercourse was unsatisfactory because of either premature ejaculation or an unsustained erection. This had not been a problem in previous casual relationships. In his despair he had tried to break off the affair, but she would not let him. Although his partner was calm, reassuring, and uncomplaining, he urged the doctor to do something or give him something quickly. The doctor explored the possibility that David's 'hurry' into the consulting room was the symbolic equivalent of premature ejaculation; he suggested that he was focusing too much on performance rather than on sharing feelings and communicating fears. He also counselled less haste to regain what he had previously taken for granted—his sexual athleticism—and that impatience would be counterproductive.

David returned a few weeks later, delighted with himself. He had gradually improved following the consultation. Previously he reckoned he had had a good understanding of financial matters, but now he understood about feelings.

PROBLEMS AND RESPONSES

Significant sexual difficulties cover a wide range of problems—loss of libido, non-consummation, frigidity, impotence, dyspareunia, premature ejaculation, failure of orgasm, etc., etc. But these are mere labels, perhaps useful for providing medical students with an elementary classification. When counselling patients with such problems, they are much less clearly categorized and the aetiology is frequently confused.

Case history 2

Susan has not only lost interest in sex since the birth of her baby a year ago, but cannot even bear her husband to touch her. She is also tired all the time. Is this all the result of looking after the baby so that she has no time for herself or her husband, or is it that her self-image has become so depreciated that she can no longer visualize herself as an exciting sexual partner? Or is she harbouring some suppressed, unrealized anger or anxiety regarding her pregnancy or labour: was her labour so traumatic that she assumes her vagina has been irretrievably damaged, or is she harbouring a fantasy of having been 'stitched up too tight' because attempts at penetrative sex have been impossible? Conversely, is she feeling 'nothing' and attributing this to having been stretched too much, or is she modelling herself on her own mother for whom sex was only acceptable for 'girls' but not for mothers? Or was she at one time the victim of sexual abuse, or is she suffering from post-natal depression? Or perhaps the sexual problem is a manifestation of a disturbed marital relationship? Analysis of these complexities is an essential part of counselling.

Sometimes a consultation about contraception may reveal, with little or no prompting from the doctor, that intercourse is disappointing, to the extent that the woman is having to make excuses to avoid it. And yet she becomes sexually aroused with her boyfriend and cannot explain what goes wrong.

Case history 3

Marie, aged 19, attributed such a problem to her upbringing and avoidance of any mention of sex by her parents. Had this made her feel it was dirty or wrong? Perhaps not entirely, but it had contributed to ambivalent feelings about it. Marie was projecting a problem away from herself and into the past, and indeed this was relevant; but during the consultation it became clear that her theorizing was a painless subterfuge to avoid confronting her own self doubts. The doctor was able to point this out to her and she then revealed that she felt 'too small'. The symbolism here appeared to be that she was declaring herself unready for sex and using her 'small vagina' as an excuse. She was surprised at the ease of an internal examination, then admitted that she had felt she was 'undersexed', this reinforced by an inability to use tampons. A few weeks later Marie reported that since realizing the problem had nothing to do with her upbringing, but rather with herself and her misconceptions, it had disappeared.

The male patient who reveals casually, as he leaves the consulting room, that one testicle is larger than the other and asks whether it matters may be describing a simple and normal finding, but he may be expressing an anxiety about his sexual ability. Has he been worrying that his sexual performance has not seemed to be as fulfilling as previously and that he is becoming impotent? Is he alarmed that he doesn't seem to be as sexually aroused by an attractive woman or a pornographic video? Is his perceived decline in sexual performance the consequence or the cause of his other anxieties? Is one anxiety to do with problems in his relationship with his partner and is he feeling that 'better sex' would put things right?

Case history 4

Barry, a tall, well-built, close-cropped man in his late twenties, stormed into the consulting room. He looked very tough and fierce. He was a new patient to the doctor. He announced angrily and without preliminaries that he couldn't ejaculate and that it had now gone on for five years. He had been with his wife for nine years and had one child aged 7. He said he was very fit and did construction work during the day and was a part-time doorman bouncer at night.

The suggestion from the doctor that the problem might have something to do with the relationship was angrily rejected—it had happened when he was with other women and he was sure there must be something wrong with 'the mechanism'. The doctor's suggestion that his disability might have something to do with feelings was even more angrily rebutted, with the comment that if it was being suggested that it was all in his head then he had no idea why. He said he nearly hadn't come to the surgery but his wife had pressured him and they were fighting a lot. He said he had been trying desperately to 'come', but it wasn't happening, despite having no problems with masturbation. The doctor replied that he seemed insecure in letting go except when by himself; and 'the mechanism' worked then. The patient responded that he did feel insecure, looked very sad and thoughtful, and then looked about to weep. The doctor suggested that Barry seemed to have very strong and sensitive feelings; he started to weep openly. The doctor paid tribute to these feelings and remarked that perhaps Barry was ashamed at giving way, needing to present a macho image. He responded that he certainly did so as a bouncer. 'How about with your wife, Barry?' He looked surprised and then admitted that he had always hidden his despair from her. He began to see things differently, realizing that there was no need to hide his distress but that he could share it. He felt glad he had come to the surgery and that he had not cancelled his appointment.

These case studies give some flavour of the complexity of the problems which may be presented. It would be misleading to suggest that they are typical, nor can they be clearly categorized. Nor do all patients demonstrate the capacity for understanding or the rapid improvements of those in the above examples. Every problem and each individual is unique and special and however many examples were given they would do no more than emphasize that rules cannot, and should not, be laid down.

Yet some doctors say they never have patients with sexual problems. Others encounter several in a month, or even in a week. However, it is not the patients of these doctors who are different; it is the doctors themselves. Faced with signals (powerful or weak) from patients who are distressed yet often ashamed and guilt-ridden, or perhaps not even recognizing the real cause of their distress, doctors whose antennae are incapable of, or are reluctant to pick these up continue to believe that they are never consulted by patients with sexual problems.

When assessing sexual dysfunction, doctors must be on the alert for physical causes such as diabetes, alcoholism, neurological disease, or hypertension and the drugs used to treat them. Hormonal deficiencies can also be important; for example androgen lack, or oestrogen lack in menopausal women leading to vaginal dryness and soreness. As well as what might be regarded as a loss of normal functions, patients experience fears of 'sexual differentness' such as homosexuality, transvestism, transexuality, etc.

THE COUNSELLING PROCESS

Having indicated the wide range of sexual problems and how they may present to the general practitioner, let us consider what may be the appropriate response and from whom. The GP's involvement has so far been mandatory—the patient made the appointment. Is he now willing to participate in the way indicated at the beginning of the chapter? Assuming he has not been put off by his personal feelings or assumed lack of expertise, how does he proceed?

Sometimes all that is required is listening—the sympathetic, and frequently, therapeutic ear. But often rather more is needed, requiring skills which vary greatly and can be enhanced by suitable training.

To return to Susan, who cannot bear her husband to touch her. The doctor has considered the various possible causes of her problem. The 'here and now' consultation can also be used to elucidate matters. What are the GP's feelings at this time and how do they reflect this patient's feelings about, and behaviour towards, her partner? The doctor begins to get some inkling of the negative feelings which she is currently focusing on her vagina. Perhaps this reflects negative feelings about herself. Possibly in the process of a vaginal examination more will be revealed than merely its physical state. The response to the suggestion of an examination is noted. Is there reluctance or an expression of distaste, or is there a detachment? On the couch there may be non-verbal behaviour to which the doctor 'listens'. Is there fear and associated vaginismus or is there a detachment, an implied 'get on with what needs to be done to this part of me' accompanied by an apparent lack of ownership and turning of her face to the wall? Or does she weep for what she may assume is lost?

The origins of Susan's problem are reflected in her behaviour at the time of the examination. The doctor notes the varying responses, for later discussion with her. Various, widely differing diagnoses are possible. Perhaps the commonest is post-natal depression which the doctor, in conjunction with the health visitor, needs to treat appropriately. Also common would be an emerging relationship problem requiring counselling. It might be more appropriate for this to be provided by the counsellor in the primary health care team rather than the doctor. Relationship counselling may require a considerable input of time both in duration and in frequency of sessions and may not fit easily into the pattern of busy general practice. Furthermore, the specialized training of counsellors may provide different, more appropriate skills.

So far only the patient has been involved—but what of their partner? What about behaviour therapy—Masters and Johnson for example. The omission is intentional. My experience is that in sexual problems one patient is usually better than two. To send for a partner not only precludes perceiving that partner through the revelations of the patient—this is far more significant than an 'objective' assessment—but it also complicates unnecessarily an already difficult process. There are exceptions. Patently, when two partners come together they have both elected to be patients and are accepted as such. But an individual who presents has adopted the role of patient. Not infrequently they may complain about their partner, since projecting the problem away from themselves is often less painful than confronting their real problem; for example when it is to do with sublimated self-dislike. It is, therefore, incumbent on the doctor to go along with the presenter's 'patient role' and study it thoughtfully, carefully, and critically rather than involving the partner who has not opted to be 'a patient'. Observing these guidelines will often be more productive and lead to a better outcome.

The practice of behaviour therapy and 'couple therapy' for sexual problems is probably more suited to trained counsellors and community psychiatric nurses, or sometimes health visitors, than it is to GPs. Occasionally two members of the team may act as co-therapists.

Finally in this section on problems and responses, mention must be made of sexual abuse. This has been revealed to be far more prevalent than was ever imagined and its effects have overshadowed many people's lives. Those members of the primary health care team with special training and interest in this field have an ever increasing part to play. Currently the GP's major role is to be alert to the symptoms and behaviour, often bizarre and unrecognized, that indicate child sexual abuse. The common ones are aggressive behaviour, 'don't care' attitudes, 'watchfulness' (especially in small children), happiness only in school, poor socializing, tummy pain, eating problems, disturbed nights and bedwetting, absconding, self-inflicted injury, withdrawal, and depression.

SPECIALIST REFERRAL

The quality and quantity of services available in any one primary health care team will vary greatly; currently their growth is considerable. Nevertheless, there are occasions when it would be inappropriate for the patient to be treated by members of the primary health care team. The patient him/herself may have decided this is a problem for a specialist, or may wish to avoid revealing an 'intimate problem' to his/her usual carers. Such preferences should be respected and the appropriate referral made. Alternatively, the problem may be of such complexity or may seem to be a mask for such severe psychiatric disturbance that specialist referral may be sought by the GP at the time of first presentation or, more commonly, as the problem unfolds.

DISABILITY

People with disabilities of widely differing forms may need help. Direct confrontation of a putative sexual problem associated with disability is often best avoided, but non-verbal messages do pass, between the known doctor and his patient, from which sensitive queries can be made which will eventually lead to a full discussion of the problem. Less well-known patients will take longer to come to the point. As a simple example, when is it safe to resume sex after a myocardial infarction? Whether this question is posed directly or elicited indirectly, the response can be somewhat categoric: when running up one flight of stairs can be achieved without undue breathlessness. For musculoskeletal conditions affecting posture or mobility and associated with pain, the physiotherapist in the team, using appropriate counselling skills along with specialist therapy, can be the person with most to offer. Patients with 'disfigurement' following mutilating operations, such as mastectomies, ileocolostomies, etc., where there is fear of loss of desirability by the patient, and fear of damage by the partner, frequently require supportive counselling and encouragement in order to return to their previous sex life. Anxieties concerning functioning after hysterectomy, or the menopause, frequently require positive reassurance, or occasionally more prolonged, interpretative psychotherapy.

OUTCOMES

Outcomes depend on a number of factors, but primarily on the primary health care team of doctors, nurses, health visitors, CPNs, counsellors, and so on, proffering help to patients with problems in this sphere of sexual difficulty. It may transpire that one or more members of the team will be, or will become, particularly receptive and skilled in dealing with them. Once the patients with such difficulties have approached the team and have been identified, the vast majority of them can be helped very significantly; some are going to achieve a resolution of their problems through the counselling process, almost all are going to attain some benefit, few are going to be disappointed. An example of the latter, however, is the obese, heavy-drinking, hypertensive man in his fifties or sixties, who has entered a new relationship and has been disappointed in his inability to achieve coitus. No amount of counselling is going to help to overcome this problem, but there are physical methods of treatment which can be effective. Not infrequently a combination of physical treatment and counselling can produce excellent outcomes.

It is difficult to measure the success or otherwise of counselling. Such an emotionally charged topic does not lend itself to statistical analysis. Follow-up can be difficult as many patients wish to forget what has been a painful and distressing episode and some resent being reminded of it. Nevertheless, enormous benefits ensue quite frequently. Such remarks as, 'I am a different person, no longer irritable, and I am happier in every way, even the children have noticed a change', or 'How is it that just talking can have made such an enormous difference?'; or 'I wish I had been able to talk about this years ago, all those wasted years'; or similar conversational fragments suggest that enormous benefits can ensue from sexual counselling.

TRAINING

Training is discussed in Chapter 4. Nevertheless, some mention needs to be made of the only training organization specifically and exclusively for doctors, which is the Institute of Psychosexual Medicine. To quote from the prospectus:

The Institute of Psychosexual Medicine is a learned body for promotion of psychosexual medicine through seminar training and research. It offers training to doctors to improve their skills with patients who seek help with sexual difficulties and related marital or psychosomatic problems, which may present openly or in the guise of other symptoms. Doctors who are suitable for this training thus work in general practice, family planning, community health, gynaecology, venereology, or psychiatry. The training aims to increase skill rather than knowledge, and the method of training is concerned with practice rather than theory.

It involves:

(1) an ability to understand the general examination as a psychosomatic event and to use the findings therapeutically;
(2) an ability to understand the contribution of both doctor and patient to the doctor–patient relationship;
(3) sensitivity to unconscious elements in the patients' communications;
(4) Some understanding of the dynamics of emotional development.

Other organizations train members of a number of professions including doctors—The Association of Sexual and Marital Therapists, Relate, The London Marriage Guidance Council, The Institute of Family Therapy, The Institute of Group Analysis, The Tavistock Institute of Marital Studies, and so on. Their approach is less medical or clinical and the physical examination is of lesser significance.

COUNSELLING OR ADVICE

Counselling about sexual problems must be a two-way process. The pressure on the counsellor to give advice—to tell a patient what to do—must be resisted if the outcome is to be totally successful. Giving advice to a receptive patient may be easier than making him/her aware of the necessity for personally being involved in the work of resolving his/her problems; it is not, however, matched by the enhanced sexual life which can emanate from the latter approach.

REFERENCE AND FURTHER READING

Balint, M. (1964). *The doctor, his patient and the illness* (2nd edn). Pitman, London.

Bancroft, J. (1983). *Human sexuality and its problems*. Churchill Livingstone, Edinburgh.

Courtenay, M. (1968). *Sexual discord in marriage*. Tavistock Publications, London.

Draper, K. (1983). *The practice of psychosexual medicine*. John Libbey, London.

Elstein, M. (ed.) (1980). *Sexual medicine*, W. B. Saunders, Eastbourne.

Freedman, G. R. (1983). *Sexual medicine* Churchill Livingstone, Edinburgh.

Kaplan, H. S. (1974). *The new sex therapy*. Ballière Tindall, London.

Kaplan, H. S. (1979). *Disorders of sexual desire*. Ballière Tindall, London.

Main, T. F. (1977). *On female sexuality. Journal of National Association of Family Planning Doctors*, London.

Masters, W. H. and Johnson, V. E. (1970). *Human sexual inadequacy*. Little Brown and Co., Boston.

Skrine, R. L. (ed.) (1987). *Psychosexual medicine and the doctor/patient relationship*. Montana Press, Carlisle.

Tunnadine, P. (1970). *Contraception and sexual life*. Tavistock Publications, London.

Tunnadine, P. (1983). *The making of love*. Jonathan Cape, London.

9 Substance misuse

Pip Mason

INTRODUCTION

In primary health care the health professional will encounter a wide range of problems relating to the misuse of substances, and counselling is an important part of managing such situations. The drugs used or misused will include cigarettes, alcohol, solvents, prescribed drugs, over-the-counter medication, and illicit drugs.

About 30 per cent of adults smoke. One in four men and one in twelve women drink more than the sensible amount (21 units per week for men and 14 for women); 6 per cent of men and 1 per cent of women are 'high-risk' drinkers with consumption over 50 units per week for men and over 35 for women. (Smythe and Browne 1992).

The incidence of drink-related problems varies across ethnic groups with Whites and Sikh Asians experiencing more problems than other groups (Cochrane and Bal 1990).

Statistics on the misuse of prescribed drugs and illicit drugs are much more difficult to obtain and vary enormously geographically. There are varying local patterns of illicit drug use and solvent abuse and these change over time as the availability of each drug changes. Local drug agencies can advise on local patterns.

'Poly-drug-use' is very common, that is many people both drink excessively and smoke, or use a combination of licit and illicit substances.

The health problems related to each drug will vary as will the patterns of associated social problems. However, the same principles underlie the counselling regardless of the drug or drugs involved. This chapter does not address the specific issues around detoxification, or reduction, or maintenance programmes, but considers how people change 'addictive' behaviours and the types of counselling intervention that assist in the process. There are three main categories of situations regarding substance misuse counselling.

The first is when a patient requests help for a substance misuse problem because s/he believes it to be a problem and wants to reduce the harm and/or change the drug use. This category is most suitable for a traditional person-centred counselling approach as the patient has defined the problem and is actively seeking change. Resolution of the difficulty will probably involve a mixture of counselling, advice, medical treatment, and education.

In the second type of situation a health professional wants the patient to change the substance use because it is contributing to a health problem or concern. In such situations, although the counsellor has the client's best interests at heart, the starting point of the intervention is the counsellor's wish for the client to change, not the client's wish to do so. Again a cocktail of counselling, advice, medical treatment, and education may be appropriate, but with different measures of each, with an initial goal not of changing the behaviour but of engaging some motivation to consider change.

In the third type of situation a patient asks for help in dealing with a family member's substance misuse. The patient is requesting help to change not his or her own behaviour, but someone else's. The first stage of such an intervention will be to reframe the goals to make them realistic. Counselling to help the patient cope with or change his/her own responses to the substance misuser will be appropriate and may be accompanied by advice on coping strategies. Education about substance misuse may help to inform the development of coping strategies.

DEPENDENCE--WORKING ASSUMPTIONS

There is considerable academic debate around the concept of dependence or addiction. There is not space in this chapter to go into the debate, and it is not necessary to resolve it in order to be able to work effectively with substance misusers. Below are some working assumptions that are helpful in considering the type of help someone will need in order to change a substance misuse habit and the role counselling can play.

Sometimes a person's nervous system adapts to the continued presence of a psycho-active drug

This process is sometimes referred to as 'physical addiction'. Some drugs have a greater potential for this type of 'addiction' than others. For example, it is rarely, if ever, seen in cannabis users and is far more frequently a factor in smoking or benzodiazepine use. Withdrawing from a drug to which one's body has adapted can produce a variety of symptoms, ranging from the merely unpleasant (such as the irritability and loss of concentration people experience when giving up smoking) to the dangerous (such as delirium tremens when withdrawing from alcohol). Where withdrawal symptoms are a major problem, medical detoxification is appropriate. Counselling is not a substitute for medical treatment in such circumstances.

Human beings are purposeful and use substances to meet needs and fulfil functions in their lives

Reducing substance use can expose otherwise unmet needs in a person's life. For example, a person who uses alcohol to relax, may find it difficult—on cutting down—to unwind at the end of a day without a drink. Counselling is a very appropriate way to help people identify the functions of their drug use and the new skills and activities they will need to develop to maintain change. Sometimes drugs are used to mask deep-seated difficulties and counselling around the function of the drug use will lead into other counselling areas, such as bereavement, sexual abuse, or relationship problems. Occasionally drug use masks mental illness, and the need for medical or other treatment is only discovered when the drug use changes.

Changing habits is difficult

Aside from the chemical properties of the substance, the associated pattern of behaviour can be difficult to change. Substance use may also be an established part of group behaviour or of social rituals. Cognitive-behavioural counselling can be useful in learning to break habits or to replace 'bad' habits with harmless ones. Assertion skills may be required to resist pressure from others.

THE PROCESS OF CHANGE

Regardless of the nature or degree of dependence on the substance, people changing addictive behaviours go through certain stages. Prochaska and DiClemente (1986) have described the process of change and Fig. 9.1 is adapted from their work.

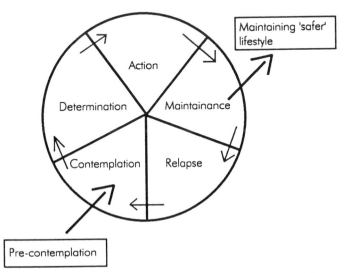

Fig. 9.1. The process of change (adapted from Prochaska and DiClemente 1986).

Pre-contemplation

This describes the stage when a person either has never considered changing or has considered it, but is really not interested. The pre-contemplator can see plenty of reasons for continuing drug use and not enough reasons for changing. Possibly there are, as yet, no problems resulting from the drug use. If there are problems, the pre-contemplator does not recognize that they are linked with or resulting from the drug use. Sometimes there are severe problems, clearly linked with the drug use, but the benefits the drug use confers or the functions it fulfils are too important to pass up.

Contemplation

Contemplators are aware that there would be benefits from changing and/or that their current behaviour is harmful. However, they are not yet ready to make the decision to change. At this stage people are weighing up what they would gain by changing against what they would lose.

Determination

People in 'determination' are poised on the brink of change, preparing for change and ready for suggestions on how to go about it.

Action

This stage is dynamic and may include detoxification, finding alternative ways to meet needs, and changing other habits that are associated with the drug use.

Maintenance

It is an old adage that anyone can stop drinking or smoking, but 'staying stopped' is more difficult. The maintenance stage can be a struggle for years before the person begins to feel that the substance misuse is no longer a problem lurking in the wings, waiting to make a comeback.

Relapse

Most people who change an addictive behaviour have at least one relapse. People commonly relapse several times on the way to resolving the problem.

THE PLACE OF COUNSELLING IN THE PROCESS OF CHANGE

Counselling is clearly appropriate for supporting and empowering clients who are in the stages of determination, action, or maintenance. In relapse, counselling may be helpful in enabling the client to come to terms with the 'failure' and to start again. Other forms of counselling can help engage and maintain motivation or facilitate problem-solving and these may be appropriate for contemplators or pre-contemplators.

As has been discussed earlier, after the action stage it may emerge that counselling is indicated to deal with underlying problems, such as stress or bereavement. Techniques for such work are discussed in other chapters. Below are some techniques and frameworks for providing counselling to specifically address the substance misuse.

MOTIVATION AND MOTIVATIONAL INTERVIEWING

A helpful way of conceptualizing motivation is as a set of scales, weighing the pros and cons of changing. There is no such thing as an unmotivated person, but some are more strongly motivated to stay as they are than they are to change. Continuing any sort of substance misuse involves the person taking action, and it frequently also costs them money and effort. Therefore, it is not appropriate to see pre-contemplators as passive or apathetic. Rather, as they see it they have too many reasons to continue as they are and do not consider change worthwhile. Motivation changes over time and between situations, as the scales are seen to tip one way and then the other. Factors that give more weight to the reasons to change include:

(1) receiving new information about the damage substance misuse causes or the benefits of change;
(2) being able to see the personal relevance of general information about substance misuse;
(3) changes in a person's personal value system or priorities;
(4) being able to see that change is really possible as well as desirable.

Motivational interviewing is a style of counselling first described as such by William R. Miller (1983) in a description of his work with problem drinkers. He describes it as (p. 147):

. . . an approach based upon principles of experimental social psychology, applying processes such as attribution, cognitive dissonance and self efficacy.

In order to use this technique effectively, the counsellor requires all the basic skills of active listening, empathy, and a non-judgemental approach. The counsellor also needs to be able to use these skills within a framework of specific deliberate strategies to engage motivation. Motivational interviewing is a sophisticated technique best learnt from a skilled practitioner and trainer, and most alcohol and drug training units provide courses. Miller and Rollnick (1991) is a good source for reading about motivational interviewing. Some key concepts are:

1. The conceptualization of motivation not as a personality trait, but as an interpersonal process. Denial is seen not as 'inherent in the alcoholic individual' but as a product of the confrontative ways in which counsellors sometimes choose to interact with problem drinkers.
2. The balance metaphor for motivation. People feel two ways about changing drug use, recognizing some drug-related problems but also having reservations about doing something about it. The process of motivational interviewing can be seen as tipping this balance in the desired direction.
3. The creation of an 'affirming atmosphere' to enable the individual to feel empowered and motivated towards positive action to take care of him/herself,
4. Strategies to increase awareness of the process and effects of drug-taking in the context of the client's life and overall intentions. Increasing the dissonance between the drug use and the individual's beliefs and knowledge is a key strategy.

Motivational interviewing is primarily useful with people who have not yet reached the action stage, but it may also be of use at other times.

COGNITIVE–BEHAVIOURAL APPROACHES

Frequently people continue using substances in order to change the way they feel. Maintaining change in the substance use will depend on finding alternative cognitive or behavioural ways to change their feelings.

Cognitive-behavioural counselling approaches in this context will include.

1. Analysing the patterns of events, thoughts, and feelings that are associated with the substance use.
2. Identifying where the possibilities are for change in these patterns.
3. Exploring the options with the client.
4. Helping the client learn techniques to modify *beliefs* or irrational thought processes in order to change feelings.
5. Development of *behavioural* techniques and skills to change feelings.

AN EXAMPLE MAY SERVE TO ILLUSTRATE:

Case history 1

Mr J. drinks and smokes heavily. He would like to give up smoking and to drink moderately. He is able to go through the week without drinking or smoking but on Friday nights goes to the pub straight from work with his workmates. Although he starts out intending to drink only two or three pints and not to smoke, he soon accepts a cigarette and spends the rest of the evening in the pub, drinking and smoking. This sets a pattern for the weekend. The events associated with this pattern (which he wants to break) are:

It is Friday night.

- His friends assume that he will go along as usual.
- He has money in his pocket.
- He has no other plans for the evening.
- He does not drive to work, so has no constraints on his drinking with regard to drink/driving.

He thinks:

- 'I've had a hard week and I deserve a good night out.'
- 'The lads will think I'm being miserable if I don't go with them.'
- 'It's a poor sort of night out if you can't have a few drinks and a smoke.'
- 'I'll worry about my health when the weekend's over.'
- 'Right now I deserve to let my hair down and have fun.'

He feels:

- tired (after the week);
- relaxed (especially after the first couple of drinks);
- resentful if he does not accept drinks and cigarettes.

It can be seen that there are any number of options, such as:

1. Changing jobs to break the pattern.
2. Leaving his money at home on Fridays so that he cannot go out after work.
3. Changing his group of friends to a crowd who know how to have a good time without drink and cigarettes.
4. Planning to go away at weekends straight from work as an alternative reward for a week's work.
5. Learning to be more assertive, refusing drinks/cigarettes.
6. Taking disulfiram so he cannot drink at all, so that the relaxation of his self-control after a couple of drinks is avoided.
7. Reading more to frighten himself about the health risks, to strengthen his resolve.
8. Developing a positive self-image of himself as a non-smoker and light drinker.

We may consider some of these to be clearly easier or more likely to succeed than others. Mr J. will have his own views on which are most compatible with his self-image and his views on what is possible. The counselling task is to generate options, explore them, assist Mr J. in choosing between them and then to support him as necessary in taking action.

It is clear from this example that this type of technique will only work with clients who want to change, are ready to explore their difficulties in doing so, and are keen to find strategies for changing.

REINFORCING BELIEFS THAT ARE CONDUCIVE TO CHANGE

This approach (Raw 1992) is particularly appropriate where the health professional wants to get the person to change as part of a health promotion initiative. A typical example might be someone who, at a health check, is found to be a regular smoker. Both health professional and patient know that smoking is a health risk but the patient continues to smoke. In order to change, people need to hold three key health beliefs:

1. The behaviour is bad for me.
2. I will be better off if I change.
3. If I try to change, I can succeed.

This approach to counselling involves exploring to what extent the client holds each of these three beliefs, and working to develop such beliefs. It can be seen as a mixture of counselling and information-giving with an underlying agenda that the professional wants the client to change.

The behaviour is bad for me

Information can be exchanged relating to this. To reduce resistance it can be given as neutrally as possible with an invitation to the patient to consider the personal relevance of it (Rollnick *et al.* 1992). Very often people already hold this particular belief and it is more appropriate to check existing knowledge by asking:

'What do you know about the risks of . . . ?'
or
'Is there anything you'd like to know about . . . ?

rather than immediately offering facts and figures.

I will be better off if I change

The hope of avoiding negative consequences is sometimes a weaker motivator for change than the promise of positive consequences. Frequently people believe that if they have drunk/smoked/taken drugs for a long period of time 'the damage is already done' and there is nothing to be gained by changing now. This may apply to health risks. For example, a smoker may believe his/her lungs to be irreparably damaged, a male drinker whose wife has left him may already know she will not come back now even if he does change, or an unemployed glue sniffer may see no hope of a job regardless of a change in drug use. Exploration of the client's belief about the consequences of change may show up some misconceptions or false information that can be replaced by accurate information.

Alternatively, this exploration may give the counsellor more empathy with the client's ambivalence about change, which will at least strengthen the relationship and form a realistic base for further work.

If I try to change I can succeed

Obstacles to the client believing this include:

- previous experiences of failure or relapse;
- a generally poor self-image or feelings of powerlessness;
- a feeling of loss of control over the substance use;
- lack of knowledge of techniques to effect change;
- a tendency to 'externally attribute' the substance use.

If someone does not recognize that they have control over their substance-use it is difficult for them to see that they could take responsibility for changing it.

Developing this belief will include affirming and helping the person to recognize and give themselves credit for previous successes in making lifestyle changes (not necessarily those connected with substance-use). However, this needs to be done with some gentleness and subtlety or the client may feel they are being 'jollied along' and are not having their anxieties or fears heard properly. Looking at relapse as a useful learning experience (while acknowledging the disappointment and problems that may accompany it) can be helpful, as can focusing on the previous successful weeks/days/hours rather than the unsuccessful ones. There is a technique in solution-focused brief therapy (George *et al.*, 1990) which emphasizes successes rather than failures ('you tell me you often feel depressed—tell me about the times you don't feel depressed', or 'you get drunk most days—tell me about one of the recent days when you did not get drunk'). This can be useful in creating an affirming atmosphere.

These three beliefs need to be present for the client to move into 'determination' and 'action', and exploration of the client's beliefs in these areas can be a useful assessment framework, showing up the biggest current obstacles to change.

THE TWELVE STEPS MODEL

This approach, used by Alcoholics Anonymous and Narcotics Anonymous, amongst others, is most appropriate for people who have recognized that their substance use has become a major problem in their lives and are experiencing some loss of control over it. Counsellors who use this approach are usually people who have themselves had problems of 'chemical dependence' and have been trained to help others to use the methods that they themselves found helpful. A twelve steps approach has some aspects in common with all approaches to substance-misuse counselling, for example 'one day at a time' is widely accepted as a useful attitude to adopt when trying to change behaviour, as is the importance of peer support. Other aspects such as learning to accept one's 'powerlessness' over the substance contrast quite sharply with other approaches that seek to strengthen the client's belief that they do make decisions at every stage in their substance use and can make different choices. More information on this approach is available from Hazelden Europe, PO Box 616, Cork, Ireland.

EVIDENCE TO SUPPORT SUBSTANCE MISUSE COUNSELLING IN PRIMARY CARE

Over the last couple of decades it has been increasingly recognized that problems relating to substance-misuse can often be effectively managed by community-based services. Potamianos *et al.* (1986) conducted a randomized trial of community-based versus conventional hospital management of 151 problem drinkers, and concluded that treatment at a community day centre is 'at least as cost-effective as hospital treatment of alcohol abuse'. Babor *et al.* (1986) reviewed early intervention strategies for managing alcohol problems in the primary health care setting and concluded that 'low intensity, brief interventions have much to recommend as the first approach to the problem drinker in the primary care setting'. Drummond *et al.*, (1990) randomly allocated problem drinkers to a specialist clinic or to a GP for treatment and found that (p. 915):

After an initial detailed assessment and advice session, the treatment provided by GPs is at least as effective as that from a specialist clinic with respect to improvements in drinking behaviour and alcohol-related problems.

Community-based or primary health care services have the advantage of being able to recognize substance-misuse problems at an early stage and thus to intervene before the drug use has irreparably damaged the client's health, social support systems, housing, or employment situations.

There have been a great many randomized trials examining the effects of GP-administered smoking cessation interventions. Richmond and Heather (1990) review these and conclude that 'most studies found a superiority of GPs' brief advice over non-intervention and other control conditions', and 'the greater investment of the GP's time, the greater intensity of counselling, and more frequent contacts were worthwhile in producing higher abstention rates.' (p. 111).

Minimal interventions by GPs to reduce drinking have repeatedly been shown to be worthwhile (Wallace *et al.* 1988; Anderson and Scott 1992). Currently further research projects are exploring to what extent brief counselling is more effective than very brief advice.

The evaluation of the Scottish Health Education Group's DRAMS Scheme (Heather 1988) concluded that the intervention would be more appropriate if redesigned to take into account Prochaska and DiClemente's model of the change process and the principles of motivational interviewing, and that this more sophisticated type of intervention would better meet the needs of the majority of patients concerned. The scheme has now been redesigned accordingly and GPs trained to use it.

So there is certainly good evidence to suggest that primary health care is an appropriate setting for intervening to change patients' use of substances. Smoking research has led this field of enquiry and alcohol studies are producing similar results. Within the general area of 'brief interventions', counselling and follow-up have been shown to be important components and to lead to better outcomes than just brief advice. The process of change and motivational interviewing are key principles underlying most current work to evaluate brief counselling in the area of substance misuse.

WHO, IN THE PRIMARY HEALTH CARE TEAM, SHOULD UNDERTAKE SUBSTANCE MISUSE COUNSELLING?

Briefly, anyone with enough time and the necessary expertise may be involved in this type of counselling.

Counselling on substance misuse is very likely to lead into other counselling areas and the counsellor needs to be prepared for this and, within reason, to be able to work with the other issues that may be related to the substance misuse. As with other areas, the counsellor needs to be able to empathize fully with the client and to understand his or her views about the substance misuse. There are differences in the ways men and women see drugs, and in the ways they are judged for using various substances. There are also major cultural differences in attitudes to all substances, depending on religious beliefs, and social customs. The counsellor will need an understanding of such issues and an ability to work with people of the opposite gender and transculturally as required. Where the client is being prescribed drugs (either the drugs of misuse, or the drugs to help cope with withdrawal) then close liaison between the counsellor, client, and the prescriber (if the counsellor is not the prescriber) is crucial, as is clear agreement on each other's limits and boundaries on the issue.

Practice nurses are likely to pick up the need for substance-misuse counselling through their health promotion role. Health checks provide an ideal opportunity for asking about drinking and smoking. Doctors are more likely to recognize when substance misuse is causing actual presenting health problems. In either case nurses or doctors may embark on appropriate counselling themselves or refer to a colleague.

Some practices have specialist substance-misuse counsellors either dealing with one specific substance (for example smoking counsellors, alcohol counsellors) or with a broader brief. Such counsellors, as well as seeing referred clients, can help primary health care teams to develop their own skills and knowledge of substance misuse and help to forge stronger links with specialist agencies outside the practice. The support that specialists provide can enable primary health care professionals to offer a more comprehensive counselling service within the practice using specialists for consultancy and for counselling supervision.

PHILOSOPHICAL ISSUES

The following questions are posed for the primary health care professional to consider with regard to substance-misuse. We all have our own views on the rights and wrongs of substance *use* and our own definitions of substance *misuse*. As in many other areas in counselling, it is important to be clear about the rules we make for our own personal lives and the extent to which it is ethical or professional to impose these rules on others.

The counsellor in primary care might like to consider the following.

Is self-inflicted illness a right?

Is it acceptable for someone, knowing a behaviour is potentially dangerous, to make a deliberate and well-considered decision to continue the behaviour? As health professionals is it ethical for us to accept and even support such a decision? Client-centred counselling has to be based on the client's right to choose to continue the substance use. An example may highlight the issues.

Mr S. smokes 60 cigarettes a day and drinks 60 units of alcohol a week. He is already experiencing chest problems and has very high blood pressure. These problems lead to him being a frequent attender at surgery, he is prescribed regular medication and will, if he continues to smoke and drink, eventually take up a hospital bed as his health deteriorates. He has a high chance of dying prematurely.

How far can the health professional maintain a true client-centred approach with Mr S.? How can this be made compatible with responsibilities to actively promote health? How does it fit with our responsibilities to ration scarce resources in an economic climate of cash-limited budgets?

Client-centred counselling on substance-use can only be undertaken by members of the team who can honestly work from the premise that we all have the right to choose to take risks, at least with our own health if not with the health of others.

Harm reduction and the doctor's role in the drug market

Since the spread of HIV infection it has increasingly become acceptable to pursue a harm-reduction role. Users of illicit drugs, who choose not to stop using, are encouraged to obtain safer drug supplies and safer equipment from doctors and pharmacists. Doctors who prescribe their patients methadone, valium, temazepam, etc. are protecting them from the dangers of the illicit drug market and the risks of adulterated supplies and unreliable dosages. They are also protecting society as a whole from the spread of HIV infection through unsafe intravenous drug use.

However, this does put doctors in an interesting position of supplying drugs that would otherwise be illegal and that are not supplied for medicinal reasons. In effect doctors are part of a state-run monopoly for the legal recreational use of certain drugs. This is a peculiar position to be in, and a better way of resolving both the needs of individuals and the public health issues may one day be found. Meanwhile it is important that people counselling illicit drug users have come to terms with their own or their colleagues' position as drug suppliers in a way that does not damage the counselling relationship.

CONCLUSIONS

Substance misuse is a complex area. The drugs used, the circumstances, methods of use, social structures surrounding use, and many other factors impinge on the issue. The substance-misuse itself may be a 'symptom' of other problems.

Many types of intervention can be helpful, including advice, information, prescription of other drugs, education, and counselling. Many schools of counselling have something to offer to working with substance-misuse problems. An understanding of the process of change and the nature of motivation helps to provide a structure for such complexity and eclecticism.

REFERENCES

Anderson, P. and Scott, E. (1992). The effect of general practitioners' advice to heavy drinking men. *British Journal of Addiction*, **87**, 891–900.

Babor, T. F., Ritson, E. B., and Hodgson, R. J. (1986). Alcohol-related problems in the primary health care setting: a review of early intervention strategies. *British Journal of Addiction*, **81**, 23–46.

Cochrane, R. and Bal, S. S. (1990). Patterns of alcohol consumption by Sikh, Hindu and Muslim men in the West Midlands. *British Journal of Addiction*, **85**, 759–69.

Drummond, D. C., Thom, B., Brown, C., Edwards, G., and Mullan, M. J. (1990). Specialist versus general practitioner treatment of problem drinkers. *Lancet*, **336**, 915–18.

George, E., Iveson, C., and Ratner, H. (1990). *Brief therapy with individuals and families*. Brief Therapy Press, London.

Heather, N. (1988). Lessons from a controlled evaluation of a general practice minimal intervention for problem drinking. *Australian Drug and Alcohol Review*, **7**, 317–28.

Miller, W. R. (1983). Motivational interviewing with problem drinkers. *Behaviour Psychotherapy*, **11**, 147–72.

Miller, W. R. and Rollnick, S. (1991). *Motivational interviewing—preparing people to change addictive behaviour*. Guilford Press, New York.

Potamianos, G., Meade, T. W., North, W. R. S., Townsend, J., and Peters, T. J. (1986). Randomised trial of community-based centre versus conventional hospital management in treatment of alcoholism. *Lancet*, October 4, 797–9.

Prochaska, J. O. and DiClemente, C. C. (1986). Towards a comprehensive model of change. In *Treating addictive behaviours, processes of change* (ed. R. Miller and N. Heather) pp. 3–27, Plenum Press, New York.

Raw, M. (1992). The role of doctors in tobacco control. Paper read to symposium on *Tobacco and other risk factors in coronary disease*, 27–31 July 1992, University of Complutense, El Escorial, Spain.

Richmond, R. and Heather, N. (1990). General practitioner interventions for smoking cessation: Past results and future prospects. *Behaviour Change*, **7**, 110–19.

Rollnick, S., Heather, N., and Bell, A. (1992). Negotiating behaviour change in medical settings: The development of brief motivational interviewing. *Journal of Mental Health*, **1**, 25–37.

Smythe, M. and Browne, F. (1992). *General household survey 1990* (ed. E. Goddard) HMSO/OPCS, London.

Wallace, P., Cutler, S., and Haines, A. (1988). Randomised controlled trial of general practitioner intervention in patients with excessive alcohol consumption. *British Medical Journal*, **297**, 663–8.

10 HIV counselling in primary health care

Tim Bond

INTRODUCTION

Since the early 1980s, counselling has been an important component in the services to people concerned about infection with the human immunodeficiency virus (HIV). The opportunities for providing this service and the obstacles which face the provision of HIV counselling in primary health care will be explored later in this chapter, followed by some practical suggestions on how to provide counselling to patients in different circumstances. First, it is important to explore what is meant by HIV counselling.

WHAT IS HIV COUNSELLING?

There is a continuing debate amongst practitioners about whether HIV counselling is different from counselling, as it is understood, in other settings. At the core of this debate is the assumption amongst non-counsellors that HIV counselling is primarily about HIV prevention and only secondarily about psychosocial support. For example the World Health Organization (1990) defines HIV counselling as:

An ongoing dialogue and relationship between client or patient and counsellor, with the aims of: (1) preventing transmission of HIV infection and (2) providing psychosocial support to those affected.

This seems to set HIV counselling apart from counselling as I have described it in Chapter 1. It is fundamental to counselling that respect for the client's capacity for self-determination is paramount (BAC 1992). If this view is applied to HIV counselling then the order of priority in the WHO definition would have to be reversed, with psychosocial care as the primary objective in HIV counselling and prevention as secondary. This was the overwhelming view of 142 HIV counsellors and 38 of their managers participating in the consultations about good practice in HIV counselling sponsored by the Department of Health (Bond 1991). It is a point of view about the values which are the basis of HIV counselling and that also has implications for the way counselling is actually provided.

First, there is general agreement about the potential importance of HIV counselling in HIV prevention. More information is not sufficient (Aggleton 1989; Greenblat *et al.*, 1989; Stoller and Rutherford 1989). Most people are afraid of HIV infection, but fear-arousal appears to be insufficient to motivate behavioural changes. The ineffectiveness of fear-arousal alone appears to be an international finding. The 1989 Montreal AIDS Conference received papers demonstrating that fear was insufficient to overcome resistance to using condoms and to prevent the conversion from nasal to intravenous use of drugs (Sherr 1989). My experience as a counsellor would suggest that the high levels of fear aroused by the possibility of HIV infection fades quite quickly. Fear may be an important initiator of change, but other factors often need to be taken into account in order to sustain social and behavioural change. For example, a lack of social skills to negotiate safer sex may frustrate someone's intentions to avoid infection. The comparative powerlessness of the receptive partner in both heterosexual and homosexual sex may also be a factor. Low self-esteem, dispiritment, social isolation, and peer group pressure may contribute to someone's difficulty in sustaining the desired changes. The obstacles people encounter which reduce their ability to avoid infection are often quite individual to them and are too personal to be satisfied by general information programmes. Therefore, despite a great deal of uncertainty about how best to enable people to change their behaviour, counselling is seen as having an important role. The House of Commons Social Services Committee considering 'Problems Associated with AIDS' were:

Repeatedly told that the most effective means of providing information and enabling individuals to understand that information and relate it to their own life is through one-to-one discussion. People coming forward for counselling represent the next stage in the educational process (after public education by leaflets, advertisements and other means).

(House of Commons 1987)

For policy-makers, it may seem sensible, and certainly pragmatic, to emphasize the preventive functions of counselling in order to attract funds for a service. However, the emphasis is extremely vulnerable to misunderstanding in the face-to-face relationship between counsellor and client. In this relationship, the clients' trust in the counsellors' commitment to helping clients decide what is in their own best interests is essential. An emphasis on psychosocial care is perceived as providing this. Conversely, an emphasis on prevention raises unhelpful suspicions that the counsellor has priorities which may override the client's capacity for self-determination. This is particularly true in the context of HIV because some of the transmission routes involving sexual behaviour and injecting drugs are both socially and morally contentious. Therefore, it is essential that the counsellor avoids moralizing. Dr Anthony Pinching was adamant about the importance of distinguishing between morals and moralizing in his evidence to the House of Commons Social Services Committee:

. . . if you tell somebody what he or she has done is unnatural or bad or use any judgmental term about them, then you immediately alienate them from the community you are trying to protect . . . you put them on the defensive and they are less likely to listen to what you say next.

(House of Commons 1987)

Confidentiality is also seen by clients as extremely important if they are to feel able to discuss personally sensitive information. Once clients are satisfied that these conditions are provided within a relationship committed to respecting their own views of their psychosocial needs, then the avoidance of becoming infected or infecting others becomes an important part of the counselling agenda because this is what most people want to achieve. Therefore, in comparison to public policy makers, the actual service providers tend to emphasize psychosocial care over and above HIV prevention, even though in practice they are complementary goals for most clients.

Second, there is some evidence that a naive overemphasis on HIV prevention may have contributed to poor practice. In a study to discover what actually occurred in HIV counselling sessions, David Silverman and colleagues (1992) analysed transcripts of pre- and post-HIV test counselling sessions and found that many placed excessive reliance on the worker imparting information with minimal opportunities for the client to respond. This is contrary to what is considered good practice in both counselling and health promotion, where it is much better to have a style of interaction which encourages the client's participation and, therefore, the giving of information is restricted to a minimum and focused on the specific declared concerns of the client. These findings parallel earlier studies about the interaction between general practitioners and patients (Byrne and Long 1976) which found that in only a quarter of the interactions were patients encouraged to participate in decisions about their health care. Therefore, opportunities to encourage a patient's commitment to a particular treatment programme or to changes towards health-enhancing behaviour were being missed. I do not underestimate the difficulties of providing this level of service and will consider the practical obstacles later in this chapter.

OPPORTUNITIES FOR HIV COUNSELLING IN PRIMARY HEALTH CARE

Workers in primary health care are ideally placed and indeed cannot avoid providing services to people concerned about HIV as well as the care of people with HIV.

The role of general practitioners and their staff in health education is well established (RCGP 1983) and the Royal College of General Practitioners is committed to GPs having a key role in responses to HIV (RCGP 1988). This commitment is not merely a pious hope. Studies consistently show a relatively high frequency of consultations with people concerned about

HIV (Gallagher *et al.* 1990; Roderick *et al.* 1990). The figures extrapolated from a study of consultations in England and Wales suggests a rate of consultation (6.5 per 1000 of population) which is a higher rate than for the problematic use of alcohol (4.8 per 1000 of population) (Rhodes *et al.* 1989). It is probable that the numbers of consultations will continue to rise as public awareness increases. The role of primary health workers is also important because of a growing trend towards community care for people with HIV or AIDS, which raises the possibility of shared care schemes with hospitals or the provision of care for all aspects of HIV, which is the preferred option by GPs who already have experience of patients with HIV (Roderick *et al.* 1990). The trend towards community care is not merely a response to the increased numbers of people with HIV-related illness or a strategy for cost-effectiveness; it actually accords with patients' wishes (Adler 1987).

The provision of HIV counselling is an essential part of the service to people with concerns about HIV. It provides an opportunity in which people anxious to avoid becoming infected can be helped to achieve that goal. If the possibility of an HIV-antibody blood test is being considered, it has been Department of Health policy since 1985 that patients should be offered counselling beforehand and that post-test counselling should be available following a positive result. Once someone has developed symptomatic HIV, he or she is confronted with the life-threatening nature of their condition. The psychological and emotional difficulties this causes, especially for young people, may be best assisted by counselling, particularly as the need for secrecy, because of the public panic over AIDS, may prevent someone from seeking support from within their own social network.

OBSTACLES TO THE PROVISION OF HIV COUNSELLING

Unfortunately the provision of HIV counselling in primary health care is not straightforward, and there are significant obstacles to its provision in that setting. These relate not only to patient resistance but also to difficulties arising from within primary health care and particular problems associated with insurance.

Patient resistance

Studies of patients' attitudes to general practitioners show that fears over confidentiality, and the general practitioner's competence to deal with HIV-related illness, deter patients from informing their GP that they are HIV positive (King 1988; Mansfield and Singh 1989; Wadsworth and McCann 1992). Fear of outright rejection or a negative reaction from a

GP is also mentioned (King 1988). For these reasons there is a tendency amongst substantial numbers of people with HIV to bypass primary care and seek medical care from out-patient clinics (Helbert 1987). Some of the findings from studies of GPs' views on HIV-related work mentioned below would appear to justify some of these fears.

Confidentiality

General practitioners are divided in their attitude to confidentiality and presumably, therefore, in their actual practice. One study showed that many GPs would wish to be informed confidentially about an HIV-positive patient, even if the patient did not wish this (Boyd *et al.* 1990); or without a patient's specific consent (Rhodes *et al.* 1989; Roderick *et al.* 1990). In another study, nearly 50 per cent of GPs would contact a hospital doctor personally when making a referral. About a third would write a letter, which raises questions of confidentiality as such letters may be opened by clerical staff or others (Natin 1989). A majority of general practitioners were in favour of disclosing a patient's HIV status without consent, or even against the patient's wishes, to practice partners, practice nurses, hospital surgeons, hospital doctors, and dentists (Rhodes *et al.* 1989).

These views are not consistent with the ethical guidelines provided by the General Medical Council (1988) and the British Medical Association (1988) and conflict with the common-law duty of confidentiality. Recent guidelines on additional testing facilities, testing of women receiving antenatal care, and the issue of partner notification provided by the Department of Health assume high standards of confidentiality and that usually communications about patients will be with their consent. Even in the case of notifying partners who may be at risk of becoming infected, the importance of confidentiality is stressed and that such confidentiality helps to protect public health. Without it, patients with sexually transmitted diseases, including HIV infection, may be unwilling to seek diagnosis, treatment, and counselling. Patients, therefore, have a right to be treated sensitively and not to be put under undue pressure to notify partners, reveal the names of partners, or to agree to partners being notified by a health care worker (Department of Health 1992). The General Medical Council has issued guidance on the exceptional circumstances when partner notification without consent might be considered. Disclosure to a third party would only be justified where there is a serious and identifiable risk to a specific individual who, if not so informed, would be exposed to infection. The question of informing a partner or a spouse must have been discussed with a patient and consent to disclosure withheld in circumstances where the doctor considers it a duty to inform the sexual partner in order to safeguard such persons from infection. The General Medical Council does not require that partners are informed, it is a matter of professional judgment (General Medical Council 1991).

The United Kingdom Central Council for Nursing, Midwifery, and Health Visiting requires that its registered practitioners should:

. . . protect all confidential information concerning patients and clients obtained in the course of professional practice and make disclosures only with consent, where required by the order of a court or where you can justify disclosure in the wider public interest.

(UKCC 1992)

The vulnerability of people with HIV to prejudice and hostility has caused many practitioners to reconsider their practice of confidentiality. A survey in north and mid-Staffordshire and Wolverhampton areas found that 30 per cent of GPs would keep a record of a patient's HIV status in notes which are only available to themselves (Natin 1989). The use of a separate record-keeping system is likely to go a long way towards reassuring patients who are worried about confidentiality within the primary health care team, particularly in areas where patients, clerical staff, nurses, and doctors may all be living in reasonably close proximity.

Any records of counselling sessions may also need to be kept separately. A survey of HIV counsellors found no consistency in the way counselling records were kept or in the access of other staff members to these records (Bond 1991). This is unsatisfactory. The issue of keeping counselling records has been discussed in a different context and these practices may be transferable. The Code of Practice, authorized by the Human Fertilisation and Embryology Act, 1990, states: 'A record should be kept of all counselling offered and whether or not the offer is accepted', and 'all information obtained in the counselling should be kept confidential,' unless 'a member of the team receives information which is of such gravity that confidentiality *cannot* be maintained, he or she should use his or her own discretion, based on good professional practice, in deciding in what circumstances it should be discussed with the rest of the team' (Human Fertilisation and Embryology Authority 1990). I would recommend that these principles are applied to HIV counselling in primary health care. The record of whether counselling has been offered and accepted would be kept in the same records as the patient's HIV status, but any records of the content of counselling sessions would be kept separately.

Difficulty in discussing personal sexual behaviour

Discussions of sexual behaviour are an important part of HIV counselling because HIV is always a sexually transmittable disease although it may not have been acquired in this way. However, there is some evidence that practitioners are at most ease discussing sexuality in general terms and in the following order of patient groups: heterosexual women, heterosexual men, gay men, lesbians (Rhodes *et al.* 1989). This study found that the degree of difficulty increased substantially when discussing sexuality in personal terms and particularly with gay men and lesbians. Previous experience of HIV-related consultations reduced the reported level of difficulty. A degree of personal comfort in discussing safer practices in terms specific to the client is essential to HIV counselling.

Reservations about drug users and harm-reduction strategies

Practitioners are at greater ease discussing the use of injecting drugs than sexual behaviour (Rhodes *et al*. 1989). However, studies show that injecting drug users are the least wanted patient group (Roderick *et al*. 1990), and that someone who is known to be an injecting drug user is unlikely to be accepted on a practice list by over half of all practitioners (Rhodes *et al*. 1989). The distribution of sterile needles is an important strategy in reducing harm to injecting drug users and in the prevention of HIV. Under half of practitioners appear to be willing to distribute sterile needles whereas over 60 per cent were willing to provide condoms from the surgery (Rhodes *et al*. 1989). These figures are still representative of current practice, and they are disturbing because general practitioners are probably the main point of contact with this client group who are notoriously difficult to reach because of the illegality of their drug use. The management of drug users, including those with HIV, constitutes a major challenge for inner city practices in particular, especially as these practices also need to be able to attract other patient groups in order to maximize income (Robertson 1992). Leaver *et al*. (1992) provide a more recent analysis of the relationship between drug takers in inner London and their general practitioners, and discuss the implications for the new style of general practice.

Inadequate knowledge base and uncertainty about counselling skills

Surveys have shown that GPs doubt the adequacy of their own knowledge base about HIV (Natin 1989; Rhodes *et al*. 1989), and when tested some were shown to lack important information (Rhodes *et al*. 1989). However, young doctors and trainers are better informed (Shapiro 1989) and trainees are generally more knowledgeable than their vocational trainers (Brown-Peterside *et al*. 1991). Furthermore, it is much harder to determine whether practitioners have the counselling skills to counsel effectively. Inferences that once an adequate knowledge base has been reached, someone will be able to counsel (Brown-Peterside *et al*. 1991) need to be treated with caution. The level of counselling skills amongst those who specialize in HIV counselling in hospitals and voluntary organizations has proved surprisingly low (Silverman *et al*. 1992). In my experience, there is much to be gained by trained counsellors working as members of interdisciplinary primary health care teams. The relationship works to mutual advantage. Health professionals have opportunities to become more familiar with the skills and insights of counsellors about their way of relating to clients and encouraging their own decision-making process. Counsellors are not generally trained in conveying the volume of potential information that may be requested by patients about HIV and its implications, and can learn much from the best practice of health professionals. After completing my report on HIV counselling (Bond 1991), which involved consultancies across all the major professions, I was left with the clear impression that personal aptitude and interest was more important in deciding who would be best at providing HIV counselling and that it is not the prerogative of any particular group.

Life insurance

The current methods used by life insurance companies to limit their exposure to HIV-related risks pose particular problems for anyone seeking advice, counselling, or testing by a general practitioner. Often patients approach GPs for these services in ignorance that should they subsequently apply for life insurance, perhaps in connection with a mortgage, that on the application form they will be asked:

Have you ever been counselled or medically advised in connection with AIDS or any sexually transmitted disease?

Have you ever had an HIV/AIDS blood test—if so please give details, dates and results.

Experts in HIV counselling are extremely critical of the way these questions on the insurance application forms deter people from seeking appropriate help about how best to prevent themselves becoming infected (Bond 1991; Department of Health 1991). In particular, this wording recommended by the Association of British Insurers (above) focuses primarily on whether someone has taken the highly desirable precaution, from a health education viewpoint, of a confidential consultation rather than whether he or she has been diagnosed HIV positive. The combination of reservations over the focus of the questions and the general practitioner's role in providing reports to insurance companies has led the National AIDS Helpline and most voluntary organizations to recommend that people seek counselling and testing from genito-urinary medicine clinics with their independent confidential record-keeping rather than primary health care. It is highly probable that the current policy of insurance companies has a disproportionately deterrent effect on those realistically at risk of infection rather than those with low-risk behaviours (Department of Health 1991). Therefore, the Department of Health has sought changes in the procedures recommended by the Association of British Insurers. These have met with limited success.

In March 1993, the Department of Health received assurances that routine testing in connection with antenatal care, employment, the follow-up of patients treated by someone with HIV, or research will be disregarded. A joint statement agreed between the Department of Health and the Association of British Insurers about testing in antenatal care is illustrative:

The results of an HIV test taken as part of ante-natal care need to be declared on any future proposals for life insurance (existing policies will not be affected). If the result is negative your application for life insurance will not be affected in any way provided you make it clear that the test was taken as part of routine ante-natal care. However, where there is a serious medical condition or there are other risks unconnected with the test, normal underwriting considerations will apply and it may be that a very small percentage of those taking part will still be charged an additional rate of premium.

(Department of Health 1992)

On the other hand, all people who declare that they have been advised, counselled, or tested for other reasons will be sent a lifestyle questionnaire regardless of whether the result of any test was negative. If the replies to the questionnaire reveal behavioural risks, any insurance that is offered may be at higher cost or may even be refused.

Because it cannot be assumed that all patients who seek advice, counselling, and testing in connection with HIV from their general practitioner are aware of the future implications for life insurance, several GPs have told me that they caution patients about the risks of seeking these services from primary health care and do not make any record of this preliminary negotiation. So far as I know, this is the only situation in primary care where the GP may feel it is desirable to obtain the patient's consent prior to even starting a discussion about health education. I certainly recommend that conscientious general practitioners discuss with patients the potential implications for reports provided for life insurance and employment before the patient has incurred any disadvantage by elaborating their concerns. Patients need to know their general practitioner's policy over keeping records regarding HIV-related issues and the writing of reports in advance, if they are to make informed choices about where to obtain this kind of help. Some may prefer to seek help from a genito-urinary medicine clinic, but this is a much more desirable outcome than someone having a consultation in ignorance of the future implications for medical reports. A patient's sense of betrayal if they subsequently encounter difficulties over insurance or employment can be avoided by ensuring that they are fully informed about the consequences of requesting the consultation.

METHODS OF PROVIDING HIV COUNSELLING

Despite all the obstacles to providing HIV counselling, general practitioners have substantial contact with people with HIV infection or worries about HIV (Gallagher *et al.* 1990). These consultations take place under a variety of circumstances and, therefore, offer differing opportunities for the use of counselling skills and counselling.

Testing for visa and insurance reasons

This contact with patients is probably the briefest of all categories considered in this chapter. The reason for the test is often bureaucratic rather than that the patient is at real risk of infection, although this is not always so. Very often the patient wants the test for non-medical reasons and so the issue of consent is usually straightforward. Perhaps the most that can be achieved in the relatively brief contact is to try and reinforce the patient's knowledge of HIV and AIDS and to encourage their commitment to anything they are doing to reduce the risk of infection. A few questions and listening to the response before commenting may be the best strategy:

- What do you know about HIV and the ways it is transmitted?
- Do you consider yourself to be at risk of infection?

If the answer is 'yes', then a more extended discussion of health education and preparation for a possible positive result may be indicated.

If the answer is 'no', continue with the next question:

- What are you doing to minimize the risk of you becoming infected?

This line of questioning provides the maximum number of opportunities to correct any misinformation and to encourage any sensible precautions that are being taken. Often with people at low risk of infection, the message can be reinforced by indicating that sensible precautions against HIV also protect against other illnesses. The overall approach is preventive and, therefore, one of encouraging a healthier lifestyle.

'Worried well'

The term 'worried well' has changed in its meaning from anyone who does not know their HIV status but is concerned about it, to a more specific group who are persistently worried that they might be infected regardless of all the evidence to the contrary, that is to say there are no factors which put them at risk or they have already tested negative. Every illness, usually minor, appears to become the focus of unsubstantiated anxieties. An analysis of 33 diaries of HIV counselling sessions offered by 33 workers in statutory and voluntary agencies, including one GP, revealed that the 'worried well' used 20 per cent of the available sessions (Bond 1991). They are also the most numerous group seeking consultations about HIV in primary health care (Roderick *et al.* 1990). Finding adequate strategies for reducing their anxiety would release resources for other work. Further studies are required to give clear guidelines about how to achieve this most effectively, but it would appear that, in the first instance, a willingness to listen by using counselling skills and to offer accurate and personally-relevant information with reassurance will lower the anxiety of some enquirers. Again, it is probably better to start by encouraging the patient to discuss:

- What do you know about HIV and the ways it is transmitted?
- What makes you think you are at risk?

This should enable you to discriminate between people who are simply ill-informed and those whose anxieties have a deeper cause. Sometimes the cause becomes more apparent by exploring:

- When did these worries start?
- What major events were occurring in your life about the same time?

The death of someone significant to the patient or guilt about something, usually sexual, are common catalysts. Other people can be helped by more extended counselling sessions to address these issues more directly.

Some people become wholly absorbed into a state which combines anxiety, obsession, and hypochondria. The longer this state persists, the harder it is to treat. The following strategies are recommended by Tom Davey and John Green (1991):

- Reframe the problem. It is *not* HIV/AIDS but the *fear* of HIV/AIDS which may be exacerbated by other stresses in someone's life. It is worth exploring whether these are present and then planning to reduce them.
- Offer practical strategies including, discouragement from taking any interest in media coverage of HIV/AIDS.
- Put energy into alternative activities.
- Monitor and reduce time spent thinking about HIV/AIDS
- Address issues of guilt in order to normalize the source of the self-punitive feelings. If it is infidelity then it may be helpful to know that 30–40 per cent of men and 20–30 per cent of women have extramarital sexual relationships (Bancroft 1989).
- Teach stress-reduction techniques.

Realistically, the amount of time involved to work through a programme of this kind with some patients is considerable and may be better provided by a counsellor or clinical psychologist familiar with these methods. The challenge of alleviating the unsubstantiated anxieties of the 'worried well' is associated with many other illnesses, including heart disease and cancers.

People at risk of HIV infection

Basic questions about why someone thinks they are at risk and about their knowledge of the transmission of HIV can be useful for all the reasons already mentioned. In addition, if you listen to the language and terminology used, it gives you a vocabulary in which to discuss a person's sexual behaviour or other activities. Sometimes slang terms will be used and it is appropriate to ask what these mean. These interviews often involve:

- Risk assessment—the likelihood that someone may already be infected,
- Helping the person to plan how to reduce the risk of becoming infected or transmitting the virus; any behaviour changes have the dual action of protecting both the patient and others,
- Testing for HIV antibodies—see next section.

Pre-test counselling

Pre-test counselling is primarily to ensure the patient's consent to be tested is based on accurate information and is an opportunity to discuss any doubts and uncertainties. It also helps to establish a relationship and plan for how the results should be given, important preparations in the event of a positive result.

The work of David Silverman and colleagues (1992) has shown how hard it is to manage these sessions effectively. The tendency is for the counsellor to spend too much time giving information or keeping discussions at a general level rather than on a personal basis. It is considered much better to use questions and other counselling skills to encourage the patient to talk. A reflective style of communication is particularly helpful where the skilled repetition back to the patient of the essence of what he or she has said helps to reinforce the validity of their experience and to move the discussion forward. However, even for skilled counsellors, it is hard to conduct these sessions because of the likelihood of some inputs of essential information being required. For instance, the implications of the three-month delay between infection and the presence of detectable antibodies need to be taken into account. In other words, it may be necessary to explain that to be reasonably certain someone is not infected, the test needs to be at least three months after last being at risk of infection.

Issues which are often considered in pre-test counselling are:

- reasons for wanting the test;
- anticipating personal response to the result—positive/negative;
- anticipating the impact of having been tested on relationships with others, especially partner;
- who to tell about the test and/or result;
- planning how best to give the result and when;
- any practical consequences of being tested—sometimes these are reduced by being tested in a GUM clinic with their high levels of confidentiality;

- planning for support between being tested and receiving the result. Telephone helplines can be particularly useful—see end of chapter.

Post-test counselling

Inevitably much of the attention on post-test counselling has concentrated on the positive result, but there are also opportunities for reinforcing decisions about how to avoid becoming infected after a negative result.

In the event of a positive result, it is important to be prepared for a great variety of reactions, from relief that a period of uncertainty is over to disbelief or extreme distress. It is important to limit the aims of this session. Information is very likely to be forgotten because of the raised emotions or misheard, therefore, leaflets or writing down essential information for the patient is particularly helpful. Barbara Hedge (1991) suggests the following structure:

- Focus on the reason for the session.
- Give results in clear, simple, unambiguous language.
- Clarify what an HIV-antibody test result means.
- Address the patient's immediate concerns.
- Identify immediate difficulties: who to and who not to tell, who to use for support, safer sex, emotional reactions.
- Provide a life line, for example a 24-hour telephone number;
- Give a further appointment in four or five days.

Person with asymptomatic HIV infection

Individuals vary enormously in their capacity to cope with the uncertainties of HIV diagnosis and the associated issues, such as conception, pregnancy, safer sex, drug use, 'who to tell', and a heightened awareness of dying and bereavement. Many people, after only one or two counselling sessions, may prefer to manage on their own or with support from people close to them. For others, periodic counselling at times of major change, for example in employment or partners, may be sufficient. Some appear to require regular counselling or some other form of active psychological intervention. These sessions often require a skilled and experienced counsellor.

Person with symptomatic HIV

A time when people often seek counselling arises when either symptoms of HIV-related illness arise or there is a significant change in health. The appearance of the first symptoms is often particularly anxiety provoking and this is compounded by the ambiguity of many of the less serious symptoms which could equally indicate heightened stress or a physical illness unconnected with HIV infection. A combination of psychosocial interventions with practical help over accommodation, welfare benefits, etc., is often a considerable help as someone's health becomes erratic or degenerates to chronic poor health. The point where treatment stops and palliative care begins is also another time when counselling may be appreciated. It is a time when many people experience the losses and fears associated with dying. Partners and carers may also be experiencing similar feelings and sometimes adequate support of them considerably improves the quality of life of the person with HIV. The intensity of this kind of work can lead to burnout, so counsellors, primary care physicians, nurses, and others all need to consider their own needs for support and to monitor the impact of this kind of work on themselves. There is much in common between the terminal care of someone with HIV and other illnesses. (Terminal care is discussed in Chapter 12.)

Who should counsel?

With a modest amount of training in consultation communication skills or counselling skills and perhaps some opportunity to update and gain experience at a GUM clinic (alternatively in a haemophilia unit, drug addiction unit, or antenatal clinic in areas with a high incidence of HIV might be more appropriate), I feel it is realistic to think that most GPs and practice nurses can develop a high standard of service for people wanting to be tested for insurance or visas, the more straightforward 'worried well' and a great deal of pre-and post-test counselling. Much will depend on the level of skills, knowledge, and attitude of the person concerned. It is possible that within all these groups of patients, there will be some who will benefit from seeing a trained counsellor who is also experienced in HIV-related issues. Cost may also be a factor in deciding who provides the counselling.

Some primary health care workers already provide very high levels of pre-and post-test counselling, but it is apparent that this is not universal. The counselling of people living with the consequences of HIV infection can be much more demanding and usually requires much more extensive training in counselling. I have already mentioned that personal aptitude and interest are more important factors to be considered in who should provide this service, rather than professional background. I am struck by how the human qualities and experience of some good receptionists would suggest a natural aptitude for becoming counsellors. On the other hand, the counselling may be better provided by a nurse, doctor, or someone who is already trained and experienced, and employed by the practice for this purpose. Again, cost may be a factor in deciding who should provide counselling. When the Department of Health (1992) analysed the cost differential between pre-test counselling provided by a midwife or a GP, the latter cost an additional 36 per cent. Counselling is time consuming and, therefore, differences in pay levels are an important factor in the cost of service provision.

The outcome of counselling

There is no research which specifically considers the outcome of HIV counselling provided in primary health care. This is a subject which is worth further study. However, on the basis of counselling provided in other settings, it seems reasonable to anticipate that HIV counselling will have a demonstrable beneficial contribution to HIV prevention and the improved quality of life of people with HIV, and that it is a useful addition to the management of people with symptomatic HIV (Miller *et al.*, 1986) which may reduce the time required in some medical consultations.

CONCLUSIONS

The growing importance of primary health care as the provider of services to people with HIV, including HIV counselling, seems certain to continue. There are several reasons for this trend. The general public almost certainly finds their primary health care centre a more accessible place than an out-patient clinic in which to discuss concerns about HIV. It is the policy of the Department of Health to ensure that: 'Anyone who wishes to have an HIV antibody test should be able to do so with the minimum of inconveniences' (Department of Health 1992). GPs are already important providers of testing and they seem likely to increase this area of work. For people with HIV infection, there are several reasons why the role of primary health care seems certain to expand. Many patients with HIV prefer to be cared for at home for as long as possible. In some areas, hospital services are overstretched (Roderick *et al.* 1990), and as the disease becomes more prevalent this will worsen. For practices who already employ a counsellor, it is possible that this increasing involvement in the care of people with HIV will involve the counsellor in more extended contacts with patients. However, it cannot be assumed that all counsellors will feel competent to take on this role. In this respect, counsellors are faced by the same extension of skills and personal challenges that working with people with HIV inevitably involves for any member of staff and will need opportunities for training and experience in settings which already provide HIV counselling.

Primary health care teams without counsellors will be faced with finding additional sources of extended counselling, perhaps from specialist HIV community care teams, or counsellors attached to specialist clinics. HIV is not merely a medical problem. It is a 'social phenomenon with urgent medical issues attached' (Miller 1988). The successful and humane response to the steadily rising numbers of people with concerns about HIV will require close co-operation between counsellors and other members of the primary health care team as well as other services provided by social workers and voluntary organizations. In the 1980s the novel problems posed by HIV infection required novel solutions, including counselling which was just becoming more widely available (Phillips 1993). In the 1990s, responses to HIV are becoming more routine, and there is now a need for consolidation and maximizing the good practice of counselling skills by all members of the primary health care team involved in HIV as well as the extension of the role of the practice counsellor and others who wish to provide counselling.

REFERENCES

Adler, M. (1987). Care for patients with HIV and AIDS. *British Medical Journal*, **295**, 535–7.

Aggleton, P (1989). Evaluating health education about AIDS. In, *AIDS: social representations, social practices* (ed. P. Aggleton *et al.*), pp. 220–36. Falmer Press, Basingstoke.

BAC (1992). *Code of ethics and practice for counsellors*. British Association for Counselling , Rugby.

Bancroft, J. (1989). *Human sexuality and its problems*. Churchill Livingston, Edinburgh.

Bond, T. (1991). *HIV counselling: report on national survey and consultation 1990*. Department of Health, London/British Association for Counselling, Rugby.

Boyd, J. S., Kerr, S., Maw, R. D., Finnigan, E. A., and Kilbane, P. K. (1990). Knowledge of HIV infection and AIDS, and attitudes to testing and counselling among general practitioners in Northern Ireland. *British Journal of General Practice*, April, 158–60.

British Medical Association Foundation for AIDS (1988). *HIV infection and AIDS: ethical considerations for the medical profession*. BMA, London.

Brown-Peterside, P., Sibbald, B., and Freeling, P. (1991). AIDS: knowledge, skills and attitudes among vocational trainees and their trainers. *British Journal of General Practice*, **41**, 401–5.

Byrne, P.S. and Long, B. E. L. (1976). *Doctors talking to patients*. HMSO, London.

Davey, T. and Green, J. (1991). The worried well: ten years of a new face for an old problem. *AIDS Care*, **3**, 289–93.

Department of Health (1991). *AIDS and life insurance*. HMSO, London.

Department of Health (1992). *Department of health guidance: additional sites for HIV antibody testing; offering voluntary named HIV antibody testing to women receiving antenatal care; partner notification for HIV infection*. HMSO, London.

Gallagher, M., Foy, C., Rhodes, T., Philips, P., Setters, J., Moore, M., Nasi, S., Donaldson, C., and Bond, J. (1990). HIV infection and AIDS in England and Wales: general practitioners' workload and contact with patients. *British Journal of General Practice*, April, 154–7.

General Medical Council (1988). *HIV infection and AIDS: the ethical considerations*. GMC, London.

General Medical Council (1991). *HIV infection and AIDS: the ethical considerations*. GMC, London.

Greenblat, C. *et al.* (1989). An innovative program of counselling family members and friends of seropositive haemophiliacs. *AIDS Care* **1**, 67–75.

Hedge, B. (1991). Counselling the HIV-positive patient. *The Practitioner*, May, 418–22.

Helbert, M. (1987). AIDS and medical confidentiality. *British Medical Journal*, **295**, 552–3.

House of Commons (1987). *Third report from the Social Services Committee: session 1986–87—problems associated with AIDS*. Westminster, London.

Human Fertilisation and Embryology Authority (1990). *Code of Practice*. HFEA, London.

King, M. (1988). AIDS and the general practitioner: views of patients with HIV infection and AIDS. *British Medical Journal*, **297**, 182–4.

Leaver, E., Elford, J., Morris, J. K., and Cohen, J. (1992). Use of general practice by intravenous heroin users on a methadone programme. *British Journal of General Practice*, **42**, 465–8.

Mansfield, S. and Singh, S. (1989). The general practitioner and human immunodeficiency virus infection: an insight into patients' attitudes. *Journal of the Royal College of General Practitioners*, **39**, 104–5.

Miller, D. (1988). HIV and social psychiatry. *British Medical Bulletin*, **44**, 130–48.

Miller, D., Weber, J., and Green, J. (1986). *The management of AIDS patients*. Macmillan, London.

Natin, D. (1989). GP's attitudes to HIV. *The Practitioner*, **233**, 1372–5.

Phillips, K. (1993). AIDS and psychology. In Counselling and Psychology for Health Professionals, (ed. R. Bayne and P. Nicholson), pp. 197–208. Chapman and Hall, London.

Rhodes, T., Gallagher, M, Foy, C., Philips, P., and Bond, J. (1989). Prevention in practice: obstacles and opportunities, *AIDS Care*, **1**, 257–67.

Robertson, J. R. (1992). Drug abuse and HIV infection: general practice treatment and research agendas, *British Journal of General Practice*, November, 451–2.

Roderick, P., Victor, C. R., and Beardow, R. (1990). Developing care in the community. *AIDS Care*, **1**, 127–32.

Royal College of General Practitioners (1983). *Promoting prevention*, Occasional Paper 22. RCGP, London.

Royal College of General Practitioners (1988). Human immunodeficiency virus infection and acquired immune deficiency syndrome in general practice. *Working Party of the Royal College of General Practitioners*, **38**, 219–25.

Shapiro, J. A. (1989). General practitioners' attitudes towards AIDS and their perceived information needs. *British Medical Journal*, **298**, 1563–5.

Sherr, L. (1989). Health Education. *AIDS Care*, **1**, 188–92.

Silverman, D. Perakyla, A., and Bor, R. (1992). Discussing safer sex in HIV counselling: assessing three communication formats. *AIDS Care*, **4**, 69–82.

Stoller, E. J. and Rutherford, G. W. (1989). Evaluation of AIDS prevention and control program. *AIDS*, **3**, 5289–96.

UKCC (1992). *Code of Professional Conduct*. United Kingdom Central Council for Nursing, Midwifery and Health Visiting, London.

Wadsworth, E. and McCann, K. (1992). Attitudes towards and use of general practitioner services among homosexual men with HIV infection or AIDS. *British Journal of General Practice*, **42**, 107–10.

World Health Organization (1990). *Guidelines for counselling about HIV infection and disease*. WHO, Geneva.

11 Chronic illness and disability

Eddy Street and Jo Soldan

INTRODUCTION

Physical disease and disability present individuals and families with a particular set of psychosocial problems. The necessary practical and psychological adaptations to the demands of the illness, the changed role of the patient provoked by the illness, and the stress of caring for a chronically ill person within the family, are but a few of the difficulties encountered. Research findings support clinical experience of the importance of psychosocial factors and potential benefits of counselling for this population. Wai *et al.* (1981) found physiological variables to have little relationship to outcome in 285 dialysed patients, but psychosocial variables, particularly depression, discriminated clearly between survivors and non-survivors. Spiegel *et al.* (1989), gave weekly group counselling sessions to an experimental group of women with cancer and found increased longevity compared to the control group who received no counselling.

However, it is not just the patients themselves who are 'at risk'. Tyler *et al.* (1983) found that 82 per cent of the principal carers in their sample of sufferers with Huntington's disease reported being distressed, 39.5 per cent were depressed, and 21 per cent were currently taking sedative medication. On a more qualitative note, Nichols and Springford (1984) found that dialysed patients and their families reported stress arising from problems in communication because of poor access to staff, and in not being permitted to express normal emotional reactions. It is not surprising, therefore, that in many cases, GPs will be primarily consulted by carers and other family members, rather than by the patient. Given these considerations, illness should be conceived, not just as a task faced by the patient, but as one faced by the whole family. Within this framework, the size of the problem becomes enormous. *The Sunday Observer* and the Crossroads study 'Caring for carers' (Hart *et al.* 1990) estimated there to be six million carers in Britain. The importance of these individuals, socially, economically, and in personal terms, needs no elaboration, and the need to address their own difficulties is well emphasized in the *Ten point plan* published by the King's Fund (1989), where one of the services required by carers was counselling for the carers themselves. In terms of research, the potential preventative role played by appropriate counselling for carers has also been demonstrated. Bunn and Clarke (1979), for example, found that one-session brief intervention counselling with relatives of seriously ill patients reduced their high levels of diffused and generalized anxiety. Therefore, it is important for any counsellor, in providing services to this population, to consider the effect of any illness against the background of the family. The adage used by Nichol (1991), 'Patient home, partner now at risk' is particularly salient for those working in primary health care who are responsible for the care of patients post-discharge, (Hasler and Schofield, 1990). If services are to meet new health gain and service targets, such as: 'By 1995, reduce the number of Social Crisis admissions to hospital of people with disabilities, compared with 1993', and 'Health Authorities, with others as appropriate, should establish a system for anticipating and helping Carers in Crisis by 1994' (Welsh Office 1991), counselling clearly has an important role in an integrated package of care services.

Therefore, the preventative aspects of counselling in primary care have particular relevance in the area of chronic illness and disability, where the long-term nature of the condition requires a different form of relationship between patient and carer, and involves long contact and development of the individual and family over the course of the illness. The invasive and prolonged nature of chronic illness and disability into family life, however, mean that it is difficult to monitor the quality, efficiency, and effectiveness of any counselling service. This is especially true if one bases any monitoring mechanism on individual counselling sessions, which may be dependent on outcomes over a relatively short timespan. Clearly such time perspectives and foci do not allow for the complexity that is presented to the practitioner dealing with a large variety of differing illnesses and disabilities in families, which cover the entire spectrum of human types and conditions. How then to proceed with an evaluation of any counselling provided in this situation? In this chapter we present a view which offers a framework for understanding how chronic illness can affect families through the life cycle, as well as providing a means for understanding the specific needs of counselling service provision and the construction of appropriate monitoring of that provision. This model is elucidated below.

A CONCEPTUAL MODEL

It is clearly very important to the individual patient that the specific problems and effects of their particular disease course and the way in which these impinge on their lives, is recognized. The specific stressors and demands of individual medical regimes will clearly need careful advisory counselling from someone with the appropriate background knowledge, particularly as potential stressors in chronic conditions include those imposed by the medical organization, culture, and regimes.

The model presented here combines the acknowledgement of the specifics of a disease, with the background, developmental perspective on the whole of the patient's life. It is assumed that the reader already has an understanding of the specific illness and basic counselling skills, which represent a unique and valuable combination in promoting physical and emotional well-being. We aim to provide a conceptual model, incorporating a person-centred approach, which counsellors can use to guide and inform their work, and which can be used pragmatically at a service planning level for work with these patients. In constructing this model, three strands of (1) a psychosocial typology of chronic physical illness, (2) the time phases of illness, and (3) the family life cycle, are seen in their interplay and interaction.

The psychosocial typology of chronic illness

With each specific disease process, biological factors dictate significantly different psychosocial demands for the sick individual and family. A distinct number of categories frame the major psychosocial influences of an illness and these form a continuum in which Rolland (1984) identifies four elements:

1. *Onset*—The nature of onset, whether it is acute or gradual, dictates the speed at which the family will have to adapt to the new circumstances and whether the family will require crises management skills from their counsellor.
2. *Course*—The change in the condition over time, meaning whether the condition has a constant, progressive, or relapsing course, and the episodic or continuous nature of this will dictate the type and nature of changes that the individual and family are required to make. The input of the counsellor, with information, crises management, personal counselling, or advocacy for support services, will need to fit with the tasks presented.
3. *Outcome*—The nature of the prognosis and expectations held by the family have obvious implications. Some illness have the quality of 'an ever ticking time bomb' with family members waiting for a sudden and rapid loss of a loved one. Others more gradual bring to the fore issues of mortality in a way that involves all family members in considering the future loss of a relationship and the changes that will follow from that. The emotional problems of dealing with terminal conditions are many. Acknowledgement of this by the counsellor, whilst non-judgementally allowing individuals to explore their own feelings, can be extremely helpful in assisting in adjustment to the inevitable, and in preserving relationships within the family as this adjustment is made (see also Chapter 12).
4. *Incapacitation*—This can range from mild to severe, and can result from a variety of impairments in, for example, cognitive capacities, movement, energy production, and disfigurement. The nature of the incapacitation clearly presents differing physical and psychosocial tasks for different family members, particularly in terms of role allocation and the ability to plan

ahead. The effect of the incapacitation on a particular family will depend on the nature of the incapacitation and the pre-illness roles occupied by members, in particular the sick member.

Using the typology, the psychosocial effect of a stroke in a 50 year-old-father can be understood in terms of an acute onset, which requires very sudden adaption by the patient and family. Following rehabilitation and failing further attacks, there is typically a constant, stable course which requires no further adaption—but does demand adjustment to the chronicity of the situation, often without continuing medical input. The outcome and incapacitation vary depending on the severity of the stroke, and the psychosocial effect and necessary adjustments are likely to be very different in this scenario than, for example, in that of a 70 year-old-woman who was already dependent on her family.

In comparison, a diagnosis of rheumatoid arthritis follows a gradual onset, typified by progressive deterioration of joint function and increasing discomfort. Adjustment to this gradual onset and chronic condition is punctuated by acute periods of increased pain, that may require different temporary adjustments from patient and carers. In relation to outcome, the family have to adjust to the knowledge that the severity and degree of incapacitation is likely to increase with time.

Time phases and task is in the illness

All illnesses develop through time and, therefore, present families with different psychosocial tasks at different times over the natural history of the condition. These fall into distinct phases. The four time phases outlined below extend those originally proposed by Rolland (1984).

1. *The pre-illness phase (phase of knowledge)*—This is specific to familial conditions where the likelihood of the carrier status leading to an affected state, is known: for example, Huntington's disease or the knowledge that an individual is at risk of cardiac problems. The task of living with uncertainty, but with some knowledge of the future is the main one in this phase, and in some cases counselling may be needed to assist in future planning, involving such diverse aspects as fertility and diet.

2. *The crisis phase*—This is the initial symptomatic phase which may begin pre-or post-diagnosis. Informational counselling will play a major role at this stage, when individuals may need repeated explanations and an opportunity to ask questions of someone with extensive knowledge of the illness with which they are having to learn to live. Consideration will have to be given to the family's role and they will need to take on all the tasks that relate to coping with and integrating with professional caring systems. The family's adaptive capacities and their general strategies for coping with crisis will obviously be tested. It is at this stage that the psychosocial tasks of adjusting

to the illness and possibly altering life plans, because of the changed life expectancy, will begin to present themselves. The counselling task involves facilitating the expression and discussion of issues and feelings involved in facing these psychosocial tasks. It is, however, important at this stage not to overload the family, whose members are in a state of crisis. Information counselling, advocacy, practical and emotional support are likely to be the major roles demanded of the primary care counsellor, though it may be helpful for some individuals to know that the opportunity of more personal counselling is available, should they wish it. Attention should be given to the creation of a relationship with the family which may be long term, requiring different roles, skills, and levels of involvement at different times.

3. *The chronic phase*—In general terms, this is the phase between diagnosis and (where relevant) terminal care, in which the ability of the family to maintain a semblance of normal life in the 'abnormal' presence of chronic illness is the key task. It is at this stage that the family may need to be helped to tease out the tasks which the illness creates from those of ordinary family life. One cannot afford to dominate at the expense of the other. When a condition leads to disfigurement or is degenerative, the family will have to deal with the issues that arise repeatedly from this throughout this stage. A feeling of inadequacy, in the face of the tasks of chronic care, is often experienced by carers and counsellors alike and is indeed the universal human response to the plight of chronic illness. This feeling does not indicate the counsellor's inadequacy for the role. It does, however, provide the counsellor with a useful insight and the empathy necessary to stick with these families through what is often a long and arduous phase. The demands of this type of relationship often do not fit comfortably into a traditional counselling role. It is, however, a vital component of the continuing care of the chronically ill. Counselling is regularly about the struggle with chronicity. Whilst the counselling may not need to be continuous and intense, it does need to be available as part of a system which supports continuing care. Promotion of coping and stress management strategies can be an important component of counselling at this stage. It is necessary to talk explicitly with patients about the nature and length of the specific involvement, which should be linked to the continuing care of the team. This will help to ensure that the patient does not feel abandoned, and is facilitated in a continuation of support from the ongoing care system.

4. *The terminal phase*—Here the issues surrounding separation, death and grief, future life and consideration of the past predominate. These are covered elsewhere (see Chapter 12) and there are a number of excellent, practical texts available (Worden 1982).

Between each phase of the condition itself there will be transition episodes, which in themselves mark the movement of an illness from one phase to another. These episodes themselves may or may not be of crisis proportion, but families will need to undertake major re-evaluations of how they have organized and dealt with matters in the past, to decide how they need to change in order to meet future demands and tasks. Problems can emerge during these period of transition, when unfinished business from a previous phase prevents movement into a new phase and families become stuck into a way of relating that was helpful at one time, but has now outlived its usefulness. The counsellor, aware of the process of transition, can assist in the adaptation process necessary. For example, it may become apparent that home care can no longer be maintained and the sick person needs to enter hospital. During this transition the family have to change from those tasks required in caring for someone at home, to those concerned with having a family member in hospital. Emotional themes of relief, disappointment, loss of function, and loss of an intimate relationship will accompany the structural changes that need to be made in this particular situation.

Using this conceptualization, the initial detection of symptoms and the diagnosis of multiple sclerosis in a young married woman will precipitate a crisis phase in adjusting to the diagnosis and prognosis. In the chronic phase, the family's attempts to maintain normal life will become gradually harder and will be disrupted by periods of relapse/exacerbations, when there is rapid deterioration. The progressive nature of multiple sclerosis will require repeated adaptation and redistribution of roles within the family and there will be many transitions which have the potential to trigger a crisis, for example loss of driving licence, becoming wheelchair-bound. Transition into the terminal phase may be perceived differently by families and medical staff. It is important that counsellors are sensitive to the patient's understanding, which is often idiosyncratic, as it is this that determines the psychosocial themes and tasks. It may be, for example, in the case of multiple sclerosis, that the family have always held a belief that loss of sight is the worst and last symptom and it is this that triggers anticipation of death.

The notion of linear, progressive phases of illness can be misleading, in that different illnesses and different families will have their crises at very different times. There may also be repeated crises within the chronic phase as the condition of the patient changes. This simple categorization does, however, point to the principal psychosocial foci that occur within the condition overall, and provides a generalized map which the counsellor can use to anticipate the type of role and input required.

The family life cycle

The family life cycle perspective (Carter and McGoldrick 1989; and see Street 1994) suggests that, whatever the nature of the illness or its time-phases, it is important to place this within the context of the different developmental stages that individuals, marriages, and families encounter.

The requirements of the medical regime, and particularly the level of dependence of the identified patient, will require renegotiation of current and expected roles within a family. Examples of this potential conflict include the adolescent relying on his mother for physical care, or the business man who has to adapt to managing care of the home and his wife, as her multiple sclerosis progresses. These role changes not only require considerable personal adaptation and consequent changes in relationship patterns, but they may deviate from the expected developmental task for that individual. For example, adolescents expect to become increasingly independent and a middle-aged man, at the height of his occupational power, does not expect to face an increase in dependency at home. A range of feelings and development concerns are thus created which will influence the way in which the tasks of the illness and of care are met.

One can, therefore, relate specific disease issues to the tasks and transitions that are facing the family in terms of their normal development. For example, when considering a young 16-year-old man with muscular dystrophy, his current, normative developmental task would be in relation to his developing sexual identity and differentiation from his parents. Simultaneously, the parenting task would be the acceptance of an intense mixture of childlike and adult behaviour and of the impending adulthood of their offspring. At the same time the parents, in mid-life and as their children grow up, will be facing their own developmental tasks, including creating new roles for themselves,—other than work,—as well as beginning to accept their own mortality. These normative developmental tasks will underlie the tasks of the illness, which in this case will focus on the increasing dependency of the young man and the imminence of his death. The specific requirements of the illness as previously discussed are superimposed on to the ongoing process of balancing all the individual developmental needs in the family. Awareness that these divergent trends need to be balanced will constitute the content of the counselling process. The counsellor needs to be aware of the three elements (1) individual developmental tasks, which contribute to the (2) family's developmental tasks, and (3) the current and future tasks of the illness, in order to help the family arrive at some balancing of needs. The tendency for the tasks of the illness to take precedence in a family is strong, but counselling can promote a more even balancing of needs, in a way that will minimize future problems for the whole family and maximize developmental potential.

THE COUNSELLING PROCESS

It may be helpful at this stage to summarize the general implications of this conceptual model for the counselling process. The model can be used to inform sufferers and carers of the process that they are going through.

This can reduce anxiety, by normalizing many of their experiences, and facilitate open exploration of their associated feelings, many of which will be uncomfortably ambivalent and focus on helplessness. It is not uncommon for feelings associated with the existence of a chronic illness to generalize to other areas of a family's life and, therefore, their elucidation can be beneficial. The conceptualization of normal development within this model can be used helpfully to delineate problems for which solutions can be found, from those which require adaptations to be made. This approach provides a completely different reference point to the 'he/she/they haven't accepted the illness—counselling for this please'. It allows for the maintenance of the family's own history, whilst they make the necessary changes to their developing family story as the illness or disability takes its course.

The conceptualization of chronic illness in terms of a continuing process which presents different tasks at different times, in the context of a developing family with its own gamut of needs and relational adjustments, helps to visualize the counselling itself as a process running alongside and requiring adapting roles of itself. It can be helpful to perceive the counselling role in this way and to monitor its progression and correlation with the presenting tasks and needs of the family. At its core, the concept of counselling being applied here is one that emphasizes it as being an essential part of care rather than a separate discrete treatment.

Some of the specific tasks of counselling in chronic illness that we have identified include:

- providing information;
- assisting in decision making by exploration and clarification of the options available;
- communicating empathy;
- ensuring open communication;
- ensuring a balancing of needs of the individuals involved;
- ensuring continuity of care, and long-term monitoring;
- identifying and assisting at times of transition;
- a supportive/advocate role in obtaining required practical assistance;
- identifying a need to refer on for more specialized help;
- maintaining a developmental perspective in looking at family changes and crises.

Case history 1

These specific tasks can be seen in the following example of Mr M., who at the age of 47 suffered a stroke which left him with a severe mobility problem, necessitating the use of a wheelchair, and cognitive changes which resulted in him not being able to continue work. The stroke occurred when his children were still in full-time education: the eldest (a boy) was away from home, the other (a girl) had a similar plan in mind. Mrs M. was in full-time work and she had a busy social diary. In the initial crisis phase of the illness, Mr and Mrs M. required much information as the prognosis for the condition became apparent; this information had to be provided very sensitively as Mr M. experienced great sadness and disappointment at the limitations he now bore.

Four sessions were conducted with him and his wife, with the focus on the need for him to cope with the disabilities, in order that he could take an active part in the process of helping his wife to help him. This was particularly important, as the usual decision-making process they had as a couple needed to change, with Mrs M. taking more of a lead. At that time Mrs M. also received three sessions of an individual nature, so that she could explore and express her feelings about the changes that she was having to make to her life plans, as well as the loss of reciprocity she was experiencing in her relationship with her husband. The family dealt adequately with the initial phase and made use of most of the offers of practical help. Mrs M. took the opportunity to meet with a specialist counsellor to discuss the different sexual relationship she had with her husband, but she declined joint sessions on this theme.

The next transition the family faced was not so much related to the disability as to the developmental changes; the girl was about to enter higher education, her mother had persuaded her to study away, but her father became angry about her leaving 'all the work for Mum'. At this time Mr M. had refused to continue his attendance at the Day Centre and Mrs M. presented to the GP with some feelings of depression and distress about the family atmosphere. Again, counselling sessions were organized for Mr and Mrs M., one of which the girl also attended. The focus of these sessions were a discussion of what is known as the 'empty nest syndrome' that faces all parents when children leave home. The girl herself appropriately made a decision to study in another town and the counsellor agreed with Mr and Mrs M. that they would be seen shortly after the girl had left, to see how things were progressing.

This case will continue for some time and one can predict the future transitions the family have to face—Mrs M. retiring from work, Mr M.'s increasing dependency and Mrs M.'s age not allowing her to meet all those needs, the question of whether one of the children will then provide care in the family which, given the history and our social traditions, is likely to be the girl. Of course all this is predicated on the assumption that Mr M. does not become more disabled through illness, or indeed that he does not suffer another CVA which could end his life. It can be seen that the process of counselling will run alongside the development of the family history itself and will, therefore, be integral to it.

COUNSELLING, CHRONICITY, AND PRIMARY CARE

It can be seen, when counselling individuals and families coping with chronic physical illness and disability, that the counselling process does not indicate an intensive period of one-to-one work, but rather it is variable over an extended period of time. Indeed, given the family nature of the problem, it can be argued that the most appropriate location in which to dispense psychological assistance of this focus and quality is in primary care. The primary care team is very well placed to have knowledge, at least, of the degree to which 'pre-morbid' family relationships were satisfactory and then to monitor the progress of the care, in terms of the development of the family itself through its own life cycle. Whilst continuity of care is important, it would be a fallacy to believe that all the elements of the 'counselling' or psychological care package can or should be supplied by the same person. Division of labour can readily be organized into:

(1) ongoing medical care of the condition and providing information on its development;
(2) assessing and responding to the practical tasks that emanate from the care of the condition;
(3) providing the same space to consider the emotional responses to the development of the illness;
(4) placing these in the context of decision making and the adoption of coping mechanisms in the family.

Clearly such a process will involve a number of different individuals undertaking different tasks at different times, all of whom need to be part of an integrated and supportive primary care system. It would be inappropriate to consider that 'counselling' only involves the empathic listening to the emotional response. In this context, counselling involves all aspects of care and it is important to ensure that a well co-ordinated caring system is able to operate, which picks up each and every aspect of individual and family need. Within the primary care setting, therefore, resources must be available to meet these varying demands, with sufficient flexibility to ensure that roles can be taken on in different ways in different circumstances. Similarly, in any one case flexibility of response is important, so that whatever the stage of the illness or the family's life cycle, the need can be met appropriately. When a caring system is able to indicate to its customers that it knows exactly what response is required to a crisis, this can reduce stress enormously. Similarly, individuals feel more reassured when they know that local services can deal with them directly, rather than automatically needing to refer to a specialist.

AUDIT, EVALUATION, AND EFFECTIVENESS

The elucidation of a model for understanding physical disease within a family life cycle context readily allows for the creation of appropriate criteria and standards of practice when assessing the effectiveness of a counselling service. The predictable transitions and crises of the illness itself and of the family life cycle allow the practitioner to specify when identifiable care events should and can happen. Similarly, the predictability of some events enable adequate time to be given to family and patient for information, education, and preparation. This means that standards of practice can be set for differing conditions at differing periods of their history, such that it can be ascertained generally and specifically whether services are addressing the need adequately and at the right time.

The relational/interactive framework that has been presented here also indicates that efforts at evaluation need to address the presentation of the whole family, rather than evaluate discrete events of counselling or the impact on any one individual. 'Counselling' in this context is the central and pivotal element of a package of psychological care to a number of individuals. Evaluation of this approach to care, therefore, needs to adopt a systematic approach, by considering the general health of everyone, as the best indices of adaptability to a very difficult family situation. Indeed, once evaluation becomes more sophisticated in the understanding of family processes, it should become possible within an audit framework to distinguish between those features that would have occurred in that family regardless of the illness, those features resulting from that family dealing with a specific illness in its usual way, and those features emanating from the family's inability to cope with the illness. In this sense, therefore, there are strong arguments for the use of family diagnostic categories in the evaluation of this type of work (Fredman and Sherman 1987). In terms of developing effectiveness, not only do counsellors need to be familiar with the tasks set by particular illnesses, they also require some general background knowledge of families and their processes. Knowledge of the tasks faced by individual members of the family can help the counsellor to empathize with each individual. As well as skills for counselling individuals, counsellors also need to be skilled in interviewing and counselling couples and family groups. Last, but not least, such counsellors require an ability to work flexibly as part of a multidisciplinary team.

The change of emphasis towards teamwork and from an individual to a family focus is very necessary, given the philosophy of community care, combined with the economics of diminishing resources. Families coping with the tragedies of chronic illness and disability need our very best attention and help. We trust this small contribution will add something to that process.

REFERENCES

Bunn, T. A. and Clarke, A. M. (1979). Crisis intervention: An experimental study of the effects of a brief period of counselling on the anxiety of relatives of seriously injured or ill hospital patients. *British Journal of Medical Psychology*, **52**, 1991–5.

Carter, B. and McGoldrick, M. (1989). *The changing family lifecycle—a framework for family therapy* (2nd edn). Allyn and Bacon, Boston.

Fredman, N. and Sherman, R. (1987). *Handbook of measurements for marriage and family therapy*. Brunner/Mazel Inc., New York.

Hart, M. (1990). *Press and public relations*. Crossroads care. Caring for carers—a nationwide survey. Sunday Observer, 18 March 1990.

Hasler, J. and Schofield, T. (1990). *Continuing care: the management of chronic disease* (2nd edn). Oxford University Press, Oxford.

King's Fund (1989). *Carers needs—a 10 point plan for carers*. King's Fund, London.

Nichols, K. (1991). Counselling and renal failure. In *Counselling and communication in health care* (ed. H. Davis and L. Fallowfield), pp. 85–9. Wiley, Chichester.

Nichols, K. and Springford, V. (1984). The psychosocial stressors associated with survival by dialysis. *Behaviour Research and Therapy*, **22**, 563–74.

Rolland, J. S. (1984). Towards a psychosocial typology of chronic and life threatening illness. *Family Systems Medicine*, **2**, 245–62.

Spiegel, D., Kraemer, H. C., Bloom, J. R., and Gottheil, E. (1989). Effect of psychosocial treatment on survival of patients with metastic breast cancer. *The Lancet*, October 14, 888–91.

Street, E. S. (1994). *Counselling family problems*. Sage Publications Ltd., London.

Tyler, A., Harper, P. S., Davies, and Newcombe, (1983). Family breakdown and stress in Huntington's Chorea. *Journal of Biosocial Science*, **15**, 127–38.

Wai, L., Richmond, J., Burton, H., and Lindsay, R. M. (1981). Influences of psychosocial factors on survival of home dialysis patients. *The Lancet*, November, 21, 1155–6.

Welsh Office NHS Directorate: Welsh Health Planning Forum (1991). *Protocol for investment in health gain—physical disability and discomfort: physical and sensory disability*. Welsh Office, Cardiff.

Worden, J. W. (1991). *Grief counselling and grief therapy*. Routledge, London.

12 Terminal illness

Dorothy Poingdestre

INTRODUCTION

In this chapter I discuss the range of issues and of feelings that are likely to be important in relation to care for those with a terminal illness (see also Spilling 1986), in an attempt to demonstrate the contribution which counselling can make to that care. Much of what I say is relevant to terminal illness at any stage of life, but particular attention is paid to those who are seen as dying 'before their time', as it is often in these circumstances that the most difficult issues arise and specialist counselling can be of most evident help.

In my view, counselling is the act of helping people to look comprehensively at their situation and empowering them to make their own decisions for their own future. Working with the terminally ill requires of the counsellor the ability to stand where they are standing, on the threshold of death.

Death is the only unavoidable event that confronts us all. The aim of counselling is to enable patients to face death as a reality and to lead them forwards positively, comfortably, and peacefully; enabling them to do what needs to be done, both emotionally and practically, before death.

Time is the most precious gift that can be offered to the dying. Through time spent in counselling, dying patients are enabled to see their worth as people in their own right. Dame Cicely Saunders has said, 'You learn the care of the dying from the dying themselves.' Most people are afraid of dying. Talking about death and working with the dying faces counsellors with fundamental questions about life and death, and their own limited lifespan. This requires a certain maturity, which only comes from experience of life. Only then can empathy be shown to patients, families, and friends.

Counsellors have to take a serious look at their own attitude towards death and dying before they can sit quietly and without anxiety next to terminally ill people; letting them know by their words and actions that they are not going to run away if dying is mentioned. Counsellors need to have the ability to maintain an attitude of concern, acceptance, and tolerance; to enable patients and carers to express their inner feelings and to feel safe doing so.

RESPONDING TO LOSS

When people realize that something valuable is about to be lost, there is a sense of shock and the usual activities of life are disrupted. Severe trauma produces a protective emotional numbness, which, together with denial, allows time to adjust to the new situation. Once the truth is faced, questions come: 'Why me?', 'What have I done to deserve this?', or 'I've lived a long life, I suppose I've got to die of something.' Anger may come if others can be blamed, even to the point of reacting violently against them. If patients think if is their own fault, guilt or a feeling of retribution for past deeds may be felt, as well as grief and sadness; a longing to turn back the clock; self-blame and regret followed by a sense of emptiness and despair.

Dr Elisabeth Kubler-Ross, one of the pioneers of the 'dignity in death' movement in the United States of America has listed five stages faced by terminally ill patients (Kubler-Ross 1969):

1. Denial and isolation, when patients select the facts they want to accept.
2. Anger, often directed to those nearest to the patient, who find such a response confusing.
3. Bargaining, when patients attempt to prolong their lives by promising to be better people if only God will let them live a while longer.
4. Depression, when patients may turn their face to the wall, not wanting to communicate their feelings, and are difficult to help.
5. Acceptance, when patients admit the truth of what is happening to them.

Patients rarely pass through stages 1–5 in that order, but these can serve as guidelines. Counsellors need to discover what the loss of function, loss of independence, and loss of life mean to each terminally ill patient.

THE DYING PATIENT: TO TELL OR NOT TO TELL

All people who know they have a terminal illness will go through, at their own pace, some of the emotions explained above. If depression or communication difficulties are inhibiting their functioning, counselling intervention may be helpful.

If patients want to know the truth, they will ask someone they trust. If they are not answered truthfully, trust disappears. Patients are the counsellor's best guide regarding how and when to tell. Never collude with fantasy. First, discover how much is known already. What is understood from what the individual knows? Would he/she like any further explanation? Is he/she asking to be told? If the answer to any of these questions is met with hesitation, the truth must not be forced, but an opportunity must remain open to learn more when he/she is ready. Confronting reluctant patients with the truth will be unhelpful and may seriously damage the counselling relationship. Attentive listening, once the function of neighbours and church, may be sufficient to allay feelings of distress and isolation.

Unlike sufferers from a fatal heart attack, patients with a progressive illness have time to realize what is happening to them, and to prepare for death. Not all patients think this is such a bonus! Many experience a feeling of helplessness or of events taking over. It is hard to be assertive when one's life is in the hands of a hospital team. Counsellors can rebuild the patients' confidence and help them regain the control they may have lost.

SHOCK AND DENIAL

Patients and carers are numbed with shock when first told there is no more that can be done. They need space and time to accept the news. Counsellors can help by going over their reactions with them. Tears may not have been shed yet. Encourage them to cry, as tears are part of the healing process. Talk about their plans for the future which may not now be fulfilled. Most people need help to express suppressed anger and fears. There is nothing wrong in being worried about what is happening to them; we would all be upset and anxious in their situation.

Some fears, however, are unrealistic, and can disappear after discussion. Most people are not so much afraid of death as of dying and what it will be like, for example 'Will I be in pain?' or 'Will I go into a coma?'. Counsellors can be sounding boards for such fears and provide a trustworthy and safe environment for the open exploration of feelings, which helps to relieve anxiety.

ANGER

Displaced anger can cause problems. We all believe we should live into old age, and find the concept of dying before then unbelievable. Once permitted to do so, dying patients are likely to express a flood of hurt feelings, together with past feelings which re-emerge with force. They may be angry with the world in general, or with the general practitioner who did not send them to the hospital early enough, or with themselves for ignoring the first signs of illness.

Some are resentful at having to leave a loving family, which they have worked so hard to achieve. They may feel cheated, angry, and bitter at having to die. Counsellors can allow patients to express such feelings, without saying too much at this time. Being able to tolerate such remarks, while showing that it is natural for patients to have such strong negative feelings is sufficient at this stage. Counsellors understand where the anger is coming from and where it needs to be directed. Once patients realize their anger is against the disease itself, they can be at peace with those around them.

Counsellors can explain that it is difficult for carers to tolerate anger because they themselves are worried, feeling vulnerable, and concerned to say the 'right thing'. Nobody knows instinctively how the patient feels. Everyone deals with trauma differently. They are the one who is dying. Counsellors represent what patients are losing—health, emotional and physical strength, control, confidence, the ability to fulfil a role in society and plan for the future. While patients want to talk to people who are sufficiently sure of their own identity not to be overwhelmed, these very characteristics reflect their own forthcoming losses.

GRIEF

In his Foreword to Elisabeth Kubler-Ross's book *On death and dying*, Colin Murray Parkes writes: 'Whatever we believe is to come after death, the loss of so many of the things that we prize must be painful, and since our own death gives grief to others it is natural that we feel sad on their behalf.' (Kubler-Ross 1969.)

Grief takes us through varying emotions: confusion, turmoil, sadness. At this time patients may well wish to review what has happened during their lives: the lost opportunities or the things they regret having done, but cannot change. These can be relatively small incidents which seemed unimportant at the time, but which assume significance in the face of terminal illness. In stressful situations, the negative aspects of life are dwelt on. By careful listening, the counsellor can confirm the individual's value as a person and help them remember the positive experiences, relationships, and achievements which may be lost amid the regrets, assuring them that everyone's life is a mixture of success and failure. With a counsellor, they can be sad without being told to stop being morbid, or made to feel that their sadness is upsetting everyone else. A conflict of emotions may be experienced—the hope that carers will not be distressed by their death, but also the fear that they have not made a lasting impact on the carers' lives and will soon be forgotten.

RESIGNATION AND ACCEPTANCE

Not all patients want to accept that they are dying. Seeing their distress and fight against death right up until the end is painful to watch. It is always easier to see someone slip away peacefully. Some patients only reach a stage of resignation; they seem hopeless and give up, turn their face to the wall, withdraw from life, and wait for death. Some go a little further, into a more positive attitude, determining to live as much as possible in the time they have left or to rethink their priorities. As the illness progresses, reassurance is sometimes needed that acceptance of care is not a failure, but is a yielding to the love of others who want to make their last days as easy as possible.

Dying patients who are depressed or anxious are not usually suffering from a depressive illness or an anxiety state in the psychiatric sense. They are likely to be facing difficulties in coming to terms with their own mortality, in communication with professionals and carers, in coping with the effects of the disease or treatment, or in adjustments in their role as the illness progresses.

Patients may become despondent when, having accepted their impending death, they do not die as quickly as they would wish. 'It's like a death sentence, without knowing the date it's going to happen', one said. Some patients scan the newspapers for news of any breakthrough treatment for their illness. They would rather be a guinea-pig in testing, than lie back and accept their fate. Counsellors need to recognize what stage patients have reached in adapting to their illness. Are they facing and accepting the reality of their own death? Are they giving up the hard work of staying alive? Has social interaction become less important? They may not want to joke or take responsibility for maintaining social exchanges. Withdrawal is understandable. It is distressing for patients who are tired and who have had enough, to be reminded that they have in some way a duty to keep fighting; not to let down their family and to be chivvied back into a social world which they are ready to give up.

COMMUNICATION

Counsellors aim to answer any questions from patients and carers with honesty and to deal with the issues such honesty produces. Some patients do not know much about their diagnosis and prognosis. This can be because they have not asked, or they have not been offered the information, or they have not heard what they have been told. They are sometimes dissatisfied with the information given by medical staff either because it was insufficient, or they did not understand the terminology, or they were confused and felt too diffident to seek further clarification. There is also the fear of taking up too much of the doctor's valuable time. Counsellors need to ensure that there is effective communication about what they know, the proposed action, and the likely outcome.

Different patients react differently to the news of having a terminal illness, depending on their personality and past coping strategy. People who use denial as their main defence will use denial more extensively now. People who faced past stressful situations with open confrontation similarly will do so in their present stressful situation. They may not want to discuss their terminal illness, but may want reassurance that counsellors are available should they want to do so later. Counsellors need to let patients know that they are ready and willing to share their concerns, however painful they may be. By stating: 'This is a difficult time for you', counsellors are expressing their willingness to see things from the patient's point of view. Alternatively, they may just wish to talk about their feelings of anger, confusion, and fear. They may be concerned about upsetting carers; causing embarrassment; worrying about protecting their carers from distressing experiences, and feeling socially and emotionally isolated. There should be no false attempts at cheerfulness, though humour can be found in most situations. They should be allowed the relief of being sad without being alone. The opportunity of simply expressing themselves to someone who is perceived as being reliable and trustworthy is often a great relief in itself.

Some carers insist that the patients are not told their diagnosis, but this can leave them thinking their condition is even worse than it is. Terminally ill patients have special needs, which can be fulfilled if time is taken to sit and listen to what they are for that patient. In the hospice movement, highly trained doctors, nurses, and social workers are there to acknowledge the forthcoming death; concentrate on easing physical pain and give true emotional support to patients and carers. This enables patients to come through the shadow of death and be calm, up to the moment when they simply and acceptingly cease to live. The skilled application of common sense, human sympathy, and honesty helps to ease physical, emotional, and spiritual pain. Once such pain has been conquered, patients are freed to be themselves again to live until they die.

DYING PATIENTS AND THEIR CARERS

Most dying patients have a suspicion of how ill they are. The carers have their own suspicions, but neither side is able to be open for fear of upsetting the other. This makes for tension when they meet, with everyone avoiding that which is uppermost in their minds; questions such as how long the patient has to live. There is the conflict between the wish to confide and be comforted and the wish to protect each other from the distress of the truth. Children and elderly parents, though vulnerable, still need time to talk and be prepared for a death in the family, giving them the opportunity to say those special things that are not often put into words. Counsellors can help people understand what is happening to them; arranging to see carers on their own, with a partner or within the whole family group to facilitate open discussion.

Relationships can change under the stress of dying. A fiancé may break off the engagement, or a divorced spouse may return to be the carer. Difficulties can arise when one partner is naturally outgoing and open about problems and feelings, while the other likes to keep thoughts and feelings bottled up. Patients are likely to feel trapped and frustrated as they become more housebound. This personal pain may lead to social isolation and further relationship breakdown. Counsellors can enable each to express these feelings by acknowledging that they exist; making direct statements about patients and carers looking tense, angry, sad; saying that many people feel like this in these situations and that it is natural both to have such feelings and to talk about them together. Counsellors can provide an element of safety and control for such talking to happen. Counsellors may feel ruffled, but need to be perceived as calm, reliable, tolerant, concerned, and unshockable in threatening situations.

Counsellors must be able to act in a way which cannot be expected of friends or family, and to provide some continuity and stability which is missing from life at that time.

Overwhelming tiredness can make some patients withdraw from family life. Even visits from friends can seem too tiring. Patients living alone may wish to die at home alone. Some dying patients in a close relationship may wish to marry before they die. The registrar will conduct the wedding ceremony at the bedside or at home. Some carers try to protect patients from the daily problems they are facing in their own lives, but being left out of ordinary discussions only makes patients feel worse—as though they may as well be dead already. Counsellors need to show that their carers are not trying to deprive them of their role, but trying to protect them, and in some sense themselves, from having to make the changes which are required.

Some carers want to know what to expect at the end. Many will never have seen a dead person. Counsellors can give practical advice as to who to contact when death occurs—the general practitioner, the ambulance, the hospice home care team, etc. Carers often experience helplessness, watching the patient die. It can be some comfort to be informed about the process of dying. There is a time in a patient's life when the mind slips off into a dreamless state; when the need for food becomes minimal, and the awareness of the environment all but disappears into darkness. Carers who have the strength and the compassion to sit with a dying patient in the silence will know that this moment is neither frightening nor painful, but a peaceful cessation of life.

Carers do learn to cope and gain much in return. Counsellors can help partners and other carers explore their feelings about having to give up work to look after the patient, as well as the regrets associated, for example, with death happening on the threshold of retirement, just when time could have been spent together. Some carers turn away from the truth, and do not want to discuss a future without their partner. It would be cruel to make them face the truth, if they are not ready to do so.

Various issues need to be addressed, for example, have the roles changed within the relationship? Who paid the bills and wrote the cheques and shopped and cooked? The remaining partner may not be equipped with the knowledge and resources to take on these tasks. The terminally ill partner may be well enough to instruct the other while there is time. Some carers cannot cope with toileting, medication, or washing, and may need support in finding appropriate help in these tasks. Having a lower threshold of coping does not make a person less of a human being or less caring.

Counsellors need to gain a general overview of possible problem areas and assess at what stage carers are in relation to their own grief prior to the death. Often carers cannot understand that someone can stop fighting to stay alive and may interpret their readiness to die as personal abandonment. Counsellors can explain that this is a common reaction and not a personal rejection.

Common patient/carer problems are:

1. Coping with patients' illness at home; fear of causing unnecessary suffering; fear of finding them dead.
2. How to answer patients' questions about deterioration; wanting to protect them from the truth.
3. What to tell children and other family members.
4. How to live with anticipated loss; the disruption of life and the struggle to see meaning in what is happening.

Carers and patients sometimes need to shelve their anticipation of loss in order to keep on living. It is hard for most people to be expected always to talk of their death in a deep, meaningful way. Sometimes they need encouragement to enjoy the time they have left. It does not have to be doom and gloom. However, difficulties can arise as time goes on. The caring can become quite a strain; the patient is on the carer's mind all day long. Carers may become physically tired. Counsellors may have to help the carers sort out what they can realistically expect of themselves and of the patient during this terminal stage, thus helping to alleviate any feelings of guilt, frustration, and helplessness.

PROBLEMS RELATED TO THE DISEASE AND TREATMENT

Patients often fear that, as their disease progresses and they change their physical appearance in some way, they will become less acceptable to their carers. Many issues need to be explored—body image: feeling infected, mutilated, unclean; becoming emaciated or being bloated; coping with a colostomy or hair loss; becoming housebound; loss of interest in sex; the effects of the various treatments; the lack of a cure and the disappointment at hearing there are no more treatments to try. Do they feel loved, cherished, and cared for? Is having to depend on others difficult after a lifetime of independence? Are they worrying that their previous life style has contributed to this illness? Do they understand what is and is not contagious?

Some treatments aimed at cure may have severe side effects. The time may come when a decision has to be made about whether such treatment should continue. Perhaps it is no longer effective, or the distress it causes outweighs the possible benefits. Some patients find it difficult to discuss this with their physician. A few may want to give up prematurely, because they have become tired of the struggle to live. Others, perhaps because they are so afraid of death, or of accepting defeat, may want to persist with treatment when it is clear that they would be better off with palliative treatment, giving a few weeks of comfort and tranquility with their carers before death. Counsellors are not in charge of treatment, so they may be in a good position to explore these issues with patients and help them make the best decision for themselves. If they work closely with the doctors and nurses, for example, as members of a primary health care team, then they can make themselves well informed with regard to the value or otherwise of persisting with treatment.

PROBLEMS IN ROLE ADJUSTMENT

Terminal illness brings with it a series of role changes, from, for instance, on active, care-giving, wage-earning parent to a weak, helpless dependent patient. Counsellors can help patients and their carers to adjust appropriately to these changes. Some patients give up too soon, or are pushed into the sick role by over-anxious carers when there is much they can still do. For many hours, patients have to be in bed, or sitting in a chair, with time on their hands to think about their illness. They then become bored and upset because they feel useless and a burden. They are less in control of their lives than before: less in control of their timetables; less in control physically and financially; less in control of the ordinary activities of daily living—washing, cooking, cleaning.

Some patients give their carers undue distress because they are unable to accept the care they really need. They exhaust themselves trying to prove that the illness is not that serious. They find it hard to watch someone else take over jobs around the house that they once did. Resentment and jealousy about this can turn relationships sour at the time when they need to be a source of strength. Some patients and carers become 'out of step' in the adjustments they each have to make. The patient may feel ready to stop fighting and rest, while the carer cannot bear to see this happen, encouraging them to get up when they are too weak to do so. Many carers want to see the patient eat when they are no longer hungry. Counsellors can help carers see that in trying to keep their loved one with them a few days more, they are making those days even harder for them.

RELIGIOUS BELIEFS OR LACK OF THEM

Counsellors seeking to help dying patients should be aware of their own prejudices concerning the role of religion and their attitude towards ministers of religion as sources of help. Some patients find comfort in religion, or may have become more aware of a need for religion in their lives since becoming terminally ill. Awareness of the spiritual aspects of dying may produce questions about what will happen following death. Ministers may well provide a source of reassurance, clarification, and spiritual comfort which some counsellors may find difficult to convey. Counselling which takes religious problems seriously, and which is informed by the counsellors' concern for ultimate value and meaning is religion in its widest sense.

It is important to find words which patients would use to discover where they stand concerning their faith. Most people have a faith or a philosophy of life, even if they would not call themselves religious. Do they think life has a meaning? People who have had a near-death experience state that they are more accepting of death the next time. Some patients turn to healers and find comfort and strength. Dying need not be the dread experience most of us imagine it to be. One patient, not a churchgoer, was realistic about her death, although she still did not want to leave her loved ones. She was convinced she would meet her mother and her first child again. During a church service, she felt all her worries slip away and was at peace for the first time in years. Her newly-formed belief in an afterlife brought her comfort. While on holiday, she bought a painting of an open doorway, leading into a distant garden, which symbolized for her what would happen to her in death. She was glad her family would have that painting to see after her death. When nearer to death, she found novels too shallow, finding comfort in the Bible instead.

It is important to discover if patients' beliefs have changed since becoming ill. Is their faith still important to them? Are they still practising their faith? Would a visit by their chaplain be helpful? In what way has their faith been challenged by this illness? Do they believe their illness is God's will? They may need help in looking at their fear that God is punishing them through this illness. They may be guilt-ridden about some real or imagined 'sins' and may be greatly relieved when offered an opportunity to share these thoughts. All human beings are vulnerable and make mistakes. They sometimes lose touch with God and need to know that God has never lost touch with them. Patients' anxieties can then be relieved, allowing them to die without a struggle.

CHILDREN OF DYING PARENTS

When a parent is dying, the child needs to know that the parent loves him; that the death is not his responsibility. One parent was able to share all that was happening to her with her children, but did find difficulty acknowledging their anxiety about her illness. Some parents find it difficult to tell their children that a family member is dying, and are confused about how and what to say. Some of the concern is the fear of coping with the children's reaction to such news. Who is there to listen to the children in a family when each is concerned with their own grief and fear? Counsellors can see children on their own, or assist relatives to tell the children. If parents have been ill for a while, the children will understand that they are not getting better. Older children often tell younger siblings, but all may still need emotional support from carers and/or counsellors.

Any emotional problem at home can cause major behavioural problems at school. One boy, playing up at school, did not want to be there, but with his dying parent at home. Teachers should be kept informed of such major life-crises in the homes of their pupils. Children are imaginative creatures and it is better to tell them the truth gently than to let them imagine what is happening for themselves.

Children are also startlingly frank with their questions, which may upset carers. On being told, 'Mummy is very ill', a child is likely to ask, 'Will she die?' This can be answered truthfully by saying that the doctors are doing all they can for her, but they may not be able to make her better. Children can become fearful that the remaining parent might die and leave them. 'Who would look after me then?' As with other close relatives, children might imagine they have symptoms similar to the dying parent. Counsellors can prepare carers with possible dialogues before they speak to the children. Parents can only be advised to tell the children. If they are adamantly opposed to this, there is nothing else to be done, except to be available, if needed.

CONCLUSIONS

Not all counsellors have the temperament to stay alongside the dying, sharing the feeling of helplessness felt in the face of death. Poignant counselling situations are those where the dying patient is the age of one's spouse, child, parent, or friend. It is a reminder of how precious are one's own relationships; how no one knows when death will come; how every day must be lived fully as if the last. Counsellors have to travel along a tightrope of avoiding not only over-involvement, but also cold detachment, for to see a patient only as a sickness and not as a person who happens to be sick is dehumanizing. People never lose the need for warmth and affection, the need to care about others and be cared about. As in all counselling, some patients may feel better able to face what is happening to them after a short counselling intervention, others may need more support, right up until the moment of death. Experience will show the counsellor what is right in each circumstance, but much will depend on the strength of the patient's own support system.

Even though death is seen by many to be a sad subject, giving cause for wonder at how anyone could work with the dying all day, every day, it has much to give counsellors. It is a privilege to be entrusted with patients' inner feelings, fears, and hopes, and to be allowed to offer guidance and support at this time; helping them maintain some sense of their own value and individuality. This reinforces that they are valued for themselves and for their unique contribution to the life they have made for themselves and for those connected with them.

REFERENCES

W. Dryden, D. Charles-Edwards, and R. Woolfe (ed.) (1989). *Handbook of counselling in Britain*. Tavistock/Routledge, London.

E. Kubler-Ross (1969). *On death and dying*. Tavistock Publications, London.

C. R. Smith (1990). *Social work with the dying and bereaved*. Macmillam Education Limited, London.

R. Spilling (ed.) (1986). *Terminal care at home*. Oxford University Press, Oxford.

13 Bereavement

Sheila Thompson

A hazard rather than an illness, bereavement comes to us all. Caplan, following Lindemann, (Caplan 1964) first brought bereavement within the area of primary preventative care, including it among the crises which come to disrupt established coping mechanisms and force change not only in outer circumstances but throughout the inner worlds of the people involved.

Although it is difficult to demonstrate a clear and direct link between an illness or disturbance and any one precipitating factor, considerable evidence has now been accumulated about the risks that bereavement brings to mental and physical health.

Unresolved bereavement has been shown to lead to psychiatric illness (Bowlby 1980) and also to impaired physical health (Parkes *et al.* 1969), and, at every age, to higher mortality and suicide rates. (Smith 1978.)

There is also some evidence, despite the difficulty of precise measurement, that skilled bereavement counselling can significantly improve the outcome, in particular if introduced early and promptly for individuals considered at high risk (see Parkes 1981 for a comprehensive review and also Parkes 1988; Raphael 1984).

More specifically, it has been found that widows receiving counselling showed a significantly lower incidence of sleeplessness, back pain, panic, poor appetite, excessive tiredness, weight loss, and visits to the doctor, as well as less smoking, drinking, tablet taking, and depression. (Raphael 1977)

With different professions and different services now becoming interested in this field, there are important questions to be considered, relating to what is involved in bereavement counselling, who needs it and who should deliver it? These questions need to be placed within the framework of an understanding of the process of loss.

LOSS AND ATTACHMENT

In the development of attachment theory and the study of the formation of close interpersonal bonds, equal attention has come to be paid to loss and the survival of loss. Bowlby (1967, 1980) drawing widely upon animal ethology as well as upon a range of studies of human development, has shown that as strong attachments between mother and infant and between mating couples have been necessary for the evolution and preservation of human and more evolved animal life, so threats to these bonds produce intense anxiety, and their severance strong and painful reactions.

However, parents and offspring eventually have to separate and in almost every attached couple one survivor is left. As we have the capacity, vital to our survival, to make attachments, so we have the capacity to survive when they come to an end.

THE PROCESS OF LOSS

Bereavement can be looked upon as a period of transition, and mourning as a process of recovery from loss.

Process implies progression, and this progression can for our convenience be divided into stages. Following Worden (1983), four developmental phases or stages can be identified, with each bringing a specific task for the bereaved person which has to be mastered and completed, in an approximate sequence, before the mourning is finished.

This gives a framework to help us to enter into the process, with tasks of the bereaved indicating the tasks of the bereavement counsellor. But the framework has to be used with caution. It is a simplification of a complex and confused experience. We should, as Feifel (1988) has warned, 'beware of promulgating a coercive orthodoxy of how to mourn'.

The first stage

This comes in the immediate aftermath of the loss. The task at this stage is the realization of what has happened.

There may first of all be a feeling of numbness, disorganization, and helplessness, and then of disbelief and denial. Even with an expected death, the reality of the dead person's presence can be felt so strongly that it overrides the knowledge of the death.

There may be an apparent searching for the lost person, as a mother searches for a youngster who has become detached and as migrant birds are known to search for a lost mate. This activity appears to be an involuntary biological response, necessary on the assumption that losses are retrievable.

What is happening at this stage can also be understood as an attempt to make the unmanageable manageable, to force a postponement of the full realization. It is a delaying tactic, a managing tactic, a brake that some survivors need to apply in order to slow down the process and bring it within the individual's capacity to absorb shock and change.

Stage two

Stage two begins with full realization of the loss and its permanence. X is dead and will never return. The depressed feelings that are a feature throughout the mourning process are at their most acute now. This can be a period of intense despair and pining. The survivor may withdraw his or her energy from daily life and devote it to the contemplation of the loss. There may be a persistent preoccupation with memories of the dead person and with the details of their life together, in which each segment of this life has to be retrieved and recollected.

This process cannot be cut short. The grief has a purpose. It is only through this activity that the bereaved person can achieve sufficient mastery of what has happened to make it possible to let the acute grief go and regain personal autonomy and independence. Before this can happen, the internal mental image of the dead person, and of their relationship, has to be re-formed to include the fact that he or she has died.

With the pining come other complex feelings, anger, guilt, anxiety, fear, and self-reproach. These feelings may be less acceptable than grief and difficult to express and share with others. Anger may be the response to feeling abandoned by the dead person, and may be directed elsewhere, at the medical services for instance, or at the self. The irrational components of these feelings need to be recognized and abandoned as more accurate perceptions of reality return.

The grief may never be given up altogether, sadness may continue, but there comes a time when it no longer dominates, when the establishment of a new equilibrium, or a return to something like a former state, becomes possible.

How long does this stage take? One answer is 'as long as it takes', and it is important that the bereaved person is allowed the time required. It may be a month or two, it may be a year or more. But all the same there comes a point where this stage needs to be brought to an end.

Stage three

This is the stage of new adjustment, the acceptance of a life of which the dead person is no longer a part, the start of an attempt to fill the gap left in practical activities, to find the new resources needed, to reach out to a new life, and perhaps a new identity.

Even though some sadness may remain, the emotional energy that has been absorbed in dealing with the grief now needs to be released to tackle the more practical tasks of readjustment. The woman who has been X's wife now has to establish her new position as X's widow. She has a new role and a different place in society and in her family, with new tasks to undertake.

The bereaved person may have been permitted or encouraged to regress during the period of intense grieving, but now it is necessary to move on.

Stage four

Now comes the stage when the emotion that has been invested in the dead person is available to be reinvested in other activities and other relationships. Patterns of sleep, appetite, and energy, should have been restored. Sexual feelings, if lost, return. This stage may open up the possibility of a remarriage for someone who has lost a spouse; for others it may be characterized more by the ability to take up hobbies, join clubs, and have a social life again. When the bereaved person can reach out to new relationships, take up former interests, or develop new ones, the bereavement tasks have been completed.

ASSESSING THE RISK

Many people come through bereavement safely with no wish or need for help. Some of the factors that help or hinder in this can be identified through the following questions which draw attention to those who are likely to be at greater risk and who may be helped by counselling.

1. What social support network is available?

Are there close family ties, family members near at hand, and supportive friends and neighbours? The dispersal and geographical separation of the extended family can leave many people isolated.

The support a family provides may be insufficient. People grieve at different rates and, even if there is a family presence, the slow mourner may find that other family members who are through their mourning become impatient. Social networks can also fail to respond; friends and neighbours may withdraw from the bereaved, or even stay to hinder the grief work because of their own incompletely resolved losses.

2. *Was the death timely and generationally appropriate?*

Deaths of old people are anticipated and adult children expect to have to mourn their parents. Problems are compounded when the death seems untimely, if a young marriage partner dies, if parents are left to mourn their children.

3. *Was the death expected, providing opportunity to prepare for it?*

If death is anticipated, and the survivors can prepare themselves, much of the grief work can be done in advance. Deaths that are sudden, violent, or unanticipated can leave behind an additional legacy of fear, blaming, regrets, and greater existential insecurity, a stronger feeling of one's own vulnerability, and the fragility of all life.

4. *What was the nature of the relationship with the dead person?*

An unequal relationship with exceptional dependence on one side, or an ambivalent relationship, are among the pointers to a difficult bereavement. The more mature and better founded the relationship and the fewer regrets about unfinished business that remain, the easier it is to let go.

5. *How open was communication at the end?*

Experience in terminal care teams has shown that if the family members are able to share with the dying person the knowledge that the situation is serious and that death is a likely or inevitable outcome, they will find it easier to let him or her go after death. The fears and fantasies about death itself, about what the dying person may have been experiencing or concealing, any guilt at being the survivor, seem to be reduced. Counselling can, with advantage, begin at this stage (see Chapter 12).

6. *What losses has the bereaved person sustained in the past, and how were they resolved?*
Poorly resolved losses from the past will be recalled to add their load on top of the grief of the present and interfere with its expression. Losses encountered early in life, losses that brought deprivation, losses that were inadequately mourned, can make people less resilient and less able to trust in the help that others can offer.

7. *Is there any history of depressive episodes?*
Depression is an expected feature of bereavement, but a feature that is expected to pass. It may become intractable if it is loaded on to a more chronic depression from the past.

8. *Are there any concurrent stresses?*
Illness, another recent bereavement, financial worries perhaps caused by the death of the breadwinner, or any other concurrent circumstances leading to stress, can further deplete reduced resources, divert attention from the loss itself, and delay the completion of the mourning.

9. *Is this a death by suicide?*
These need separate mention and special attention. The stigma and taboo of suicide can cut off survivors from the usual sources of help and leave them particularly isolated and at risk. Also to be borne in mind, when there is a death by suicide, is the likelihood of a pre-existing family disturbance needing more specialist treatment than can be provided by bereavement counselling alone.

Bringing together many of the above pointers, Parkes (1972) has identified, as being at particular risk, the young widow with dependent children and without other relatives nearby, now financially insecure and ill-equipped to manage on her own, with a strained marital relationship in the past, difficulty in expressing feelings, and a past history of depressive episodes.

Skynner (1976) quotes research into so-called 'exceptionally healthy families' characterized by open communication and flexible relationships, showing that such families have an enhanced ability to cope with change and loss of all kinds, including losses brought about by the death of close family members.

COUNSELLING THE BEREAVED

Another dimension now needs to be added to the description of the process of loss. Though humankind may have become required and equipped, during the course of our evolutionary development, to allow for the severance of interpersonal ties, the way in which grief is experienced, expressed, and resolved depends upon the social context.

Mourning is shaped by cultural and social expectations, and the process is promoted or hindered by the feedback and reactions received. With bereavement counselling, we enter the social context in order to influence and augment it, and introduce feedback and reactions that are skilled, deliberate, and focused.

Care needs to be taken to ensure that this intervention is not allowed to replace or discourage other existing relationships. The risk of this was brought home by the comment of one family member—'We are so glad the bereavement counsellor has taken on Mother now. The family were finding it a strain to have to do so much visiting themselves.'

Bereavement counselling requires an understanding of the circumstances of the loss, of the nature of the relationship that has been lost, and of the sources of the survivor's response.

It includes the following factors: the provision of a safe relationship; the concept of normality; the facilitation of the mourning process; and the monitoring of the progress.

The safe relationship is a relationship with someone not personally caught up in the grief, who will not withdraw or criticize or try to cut short the mourning process, with whom all the overwhelming, conflicting, and perhaps seemingly unacceptable feelings can find expression and be safely contained.

It is a relationship with someone familiar with the grief process who accepts its normality among the apparent abnormality and who under-stands that mourning is a process of recovery. Like adolescence, another time when bonds are being severed, different, apparently abnormal pat-terns of behaviour can be accepted as transient phenomena within this framework.

Facilitation supports and eases the bereaved person through the tasks and difficulties of each stage of mourning. Monitoring identifies any aspects that are not being resolved, any stages at which the bereaved person risks becoming completely or partially fixated and where more intensive help may be needed.

The first stage

Returning to Worden's developmental phases, in the first stage the task of the counsellor is to support and help the bereaved person through the process of becoming aware of the loss. In doing this, it may be necessary to represent the reality and to discourage evasion, but always keeping within the survivor's current capacity.

This involves talking about what has happened. The counsellor may need to ask specific and detailed questions about the death and the funeral, using words like death and dead, avoiding euphemisms, helping the survivor to recall and understand that the dead person has gone and will never return,

Occasionally, the survivor may find it hard to accept the fact that the loss has occurred at all, particularly in the case of a violent death where no body has been recovered and so there has been no opportunity to view the body and dispose of it with funeral rituals. Alternatively, it may be the finality and irreversibility that are hard to accept.

During this time the presence of two contradictory ideas competing in the survivor's mind, that X is dead and that X cannot be dead, can bring instability and a fear of madness. The counsellor may have to provide reassurance that the bereaved person is not going mad.

Bereaved people, particularly if they perceive themselves abandoned and unsupported, may try to remain at this stage, resisting the realization of what has happened and its consequences for fear of a full understanding of the loss from which there can be no going back.

The second stage

In the second stage, the task of the counsellor is to help the survivor to experience and work through all the pain of grief, as he or she relives the lost relationship in order to be able to abandon it.

Problems at this stage include not only the prolongation of this period of intense grief, but also the misdirection of anger, the persistence of guilt and self-blame, the denial of negative feelings, and the idealization of the dead person.

There can also be denial of the significance of the loss and the importance of the lost relationship: and there can be a failure to mourn with an apparent rapid return to normality. 'Sooner or later, some of those who avoid all conscious grieving break down—usually with some form of depression' (Bowlby 1980).

Where the identification has been close, and much has been shared, the survivor may struggle to preserve the continuing presence of the dead person within. This may lead to attempts to replicate outward characteristics, sometimes even symptoms of the last illness. What is feared is the extinction of the parts of the self that were invested in the dead person. The survivor may need help to go over the past and identify all the aims and ideals that were shared, so that they can now be freed from any exclusive attachment to the dead person and retained to become part of the life ahead.

All the feelings involved in the lost relationship need to be identified as accurately and completely as is possible. Sadness and grief may be intermingled with more complex feelings such as anger, guilt, self-reproach, and fear. If these feelings are not expressed they are likely to persevere to delay the mourning process and go on to interfere with and distort relationships in the future.

Anger appears to be felt by a majority of bereaved people, sometimes in intense outbursts, sometimes as a more prolonged bitterness. Anger felt towards the deceased may be too painful to experience directly, and so may be turned into anger towards others, towards medical staff for example. It can be also be directed against the self and be experienced as self-blaming, bringing lowered self-esteem, depression, even suicidal thoughts.

Acute anxiety and fear may also be felt. A major component of personal safety and security may have been lost, bringing a heightened awareness of personal mortality and fears for other members of the family. Memories of being lost and unsupported as a child may be revived. If bereaved people can now find access to the sources of these feelings, they may be able to reduce their impact through talking them over with the counsellor.

Guilt is also a feature of mourning. Even being the survivor can be a source of guilt. Reproaches, with the memory of things said and done, or not said and not done, are left as a residue even when relationships have been happy. A long illness, the burden of caring, may have brought a wish that it could soon be over. The counsellor may need to emphasize the inevitability of such wishes, representing reality and bringing back reminders of the care that was given and the efforts made.

The counsellor may need to help acknowledge the fact that all relationships have their ambivalence with positive and negative feelings coexisting, that not everything that has been lost will be missed, aware that after a death the negative feelings may come to be suppressed in idealization of the deceased.

Some counsellors may encourage their patients to say or write all the things that they wished they could have said to the dead person, if it seems that the pressure of unfinished business is making it hard to leave the relationship. However, it is important to avoid ending such activities on a new negative note, to maintain a balance, and to emphasize the way in which good and bad feelings are a part of all relationships.

If feelings of guilt and depression remain at an intense level, the counsellor may need to ask if the survivor has ever had thoughts of harming him or herself, enquiring about thoughts rather than intention. When such thoughts can be shared and accepted they lose some of their force, and the sense of isolation is reduced.

The third stage

In the third stage, the task of the counsellor is to help the survivor to return to daily living. The loss may have depleted existing resources, and now help may be needed in regaining confidence, negotiating a new reality, acquiring new skills, and taking on new responsibilities.

Now the counsellor may focus the counselling more on practical tasks and their significance. There may have to be a reallocation of roles and responsibilities within the family. Now may be the time to explore how needs that are no longer being met can be satisfied in other ways. The spouse who has gone may have been companion, sexual partner, tennis partner, dancing partner, chauffeur, housekeeper, gardener, cook, family disciplinarian, etc., and adjustments will have to be made to fill some of the gap. Where grieving is seen as a duty to the dead, the counsellor may need to support the idea that the duty has been completed.

Difficulties at this stage appear in a failure to adjust to the new circumstances, and in the prolongation of helplessness and dependency after the period of acute grief has ended.

The fourth stage

In the fourth stage, the task of the counsellor is to help the survivor to invest energy in new relationships and activities.

Some bereaved people may be held back at this stage by a fear of being disloyal, or of being thought disloyal. They may carry in their mind conflicting models from the past, or within their culture, in which unions are for life and mourning is perpetual. They may be looking for confirmation that the time has come when it is acceptable to take up active life again, and to find enjoyment and fulfillment in relationships and activities that the dead person never knew.

FAMILY COUNSELLING

Most discussions of bereavement counselling focus upon the needs of one individual. The elderly widow, or less commonly widower, is the most frequent subject of research and treated as the typical recipient of bereavement counselling.

However, bereavement is a family event and often plays an important part in family development. Even when bereavement counselling is sought for one family member, there may well be other family members at risk who are not brought forward. The bereavement counsellor needs to have an awareness of the family as a system in which the different members interact and in which the loss of one of them influences each other individual through its impact upon the system as a whole.

Who has gone? What gap has been left within the family? How are the family members communicating with each other about the loss?

Different family members grieve and recover at different speeds. There may be frustration with the ones behind who threaten the recovery of the whole. There may be anxiety about the health of other family members, as security in well-being has been shaken and personal vulnerabilities have increased.

Families appear to deal best with crises if there is an open pattern of communication and flexible boundaries, if members can move towards each other and change and adapt their roles within the family. Families, like individuals, that are more rigid, that struggle to remain unchanged, tend to deny the loss and fail to grieve adequately. An attempt to preserve those qualities of the dead person that were important to the family may bring unrealistic and burdensome expectations of others; a junior family member, for example, may be expected to show some of the characteristics of a dead parent or sibling; a surviving parent may impose unrealistic tasks on him or herself, or have them imposed by others.

The counsellor who is seeing one family member needs to make a point of enquiring about the others, noting who is, or who is not, being mentioned, and looking to see if there is need and opportunity to bring them together and facilitate a discussion in which they can share their feelings about the loss.

Children

Children need special consideration. Studies of the effects of bereavements in childhood have been summarized by Black (1978).

Bereavement counsellors are frequently asked for advice by a parent wondering what to do about the children. What should the children be told, may be asked, and when and how should this be done?

All the considerations that apply to helping the adult bereaved apply with equal force to children. Children also need to comprehend what has happened and to have opportunities to express all the complex feelings involved, even though their intellectual understanding of death and finality may not be complete.

There are added considerations. With less maturity and ego strength, children have less capacity to bear concentrated pain, and the younger they are the longer it will take for them to absorb what has happened and to realize that it is irreversible. This process may not be completed for many years, perhaps not until they are grown up themselves. Adults responsible for children can help by keeping memories and feelings alive and accessible, so that the children can continue to work on them as and when they are able to. This does not always happen. The bereavement may be complicated by secrecy as adults strive to protect the children, or to protect themselves from exposure to the children's grief, by concealment or evasion. It is in these circumstances that adults will sometimes report that children do not seem to have been very affected, even by the loss of a parent or sibling.

On one such occasion a counsellor, told by the adults that the children were unaffected, and going to check this out, found the children repetitiously playing funerals. When this was pointed out to the parents, they began to talk to the children for the first time about the death of their baby. Through this they were able to start expressing their own feelings, which had been blocked by the efforts they had been making to shield the children from awareness of their grief.

There is a possibility that children will come to make links between a death in the family and some previous unsatisfactory behaviour of their own, particularly if there is secrecy and the order of events has not been made clear. A feeling of responsibility for what has happened may then persist and become permanent.

It seems desirable for the adults to be as open and frank with the children as they can manage to be, not excluding the children from family discussions and explanations, offering them, with appropriate preparation, an opportunity to go to the funeral. Children too need to say goodbye.

Secrets in the family are considered to do more harm than the truth can ever do; and when children are supported by adults whom they trust they are better able to deal with reality, however upsetting, than with the misunderstandings and misconceptions that may otherwise remain (Pincus and Dare 1978)

Help for children should come, if possible, from those adults who are closest to them rather than from a stranger. The role of the counsellor, therefore, is likely to be focused upon helping the adults to help the children. The adults, involved in their own grief, may have difficulty in finding the words to use. As when helping parents to discuss sexual matters with their children, it may be helpful to talk about the event with them in the simple words that will give them a vocabulary they can then use in communications with their children.

Teenagers

Teenagers may also need special consideration. The death of a parent may come at a time of great ambivalence when the teenagers are beginning to pull away from the family.

One 15-year-old boy avoided his mother's sick room because he found the details of her last illness intolerable, and took little part in her care. After her death he was blamed for being uncaring and his isolation from the rest of the family intensified. Only after the counsellor had made a prolonged and ultimately successful effort to include him in the discussions with the rest of the family was he able to reveal and share his grief.

How long should bereavement counselling last?

Concentrated work may be needed for a few weeks or a few months. Less concentrated involvement may then need to continue, with the contact being kept open.

There are identifiable landmarks—the first Christmas, the anniversary of the death, birthdays, and important family events, when vulnerability may temporarily increase and it may be necessary to counsel in advance that these can be difficult times.

OTHER SIGNIFICANT LOSSES

Bereavement does not always involve loss by death. The process of loss is the same process whether the loss is of a spouse or child, a dog or cat, a breast or a limb, a loss of status or a loss of abilities and valued functions, or any other difficult life experience that impinges upon the security of the person and the conception of the self.

The intensity and duration, the significance and impact, of these events may vary greatly, but the process still passes from loss through recognizable stages to recovery. The amputee has to realize what has happened and then identify and grieve for what has been lost, experiencing a complicated range of feelings before he or she can find the resources to adjust to what has happened and build a life again. Any counsellor involved will have to bear in mind all the considerations we have already discussed.

There are also the losses where accident or illness drastically alters a relationship although the loved one survives physically. The family of a head-injured victim, for example, also need to 'know and name and express the pain' (Raphael 1984). To do this they have to separate out what has been lost from what still survives, so that they can mourn those aspects of the relationship and of their future hopes that have been taken away while they continue to hold on to what remains.

GRIEF THAT FAILS TO RESOLVE

If a survivor is not responding to bereavement counselling, then the counsellor will need to identify the stage at which he or she remains fixed, and focus more narrowly and more intently. It is possible that the problem lies in specific unresolved elements in the relationship with the dead person, such as business left unfinished, conversations not completed, or feelings not identified, that are making it impossible to let go.

If the grieving still persists, the counsellor will need to consider whether the problem may extend beyond the immediate circumstances of the bereavement. Bereavement is a receptacle for disturbances of all kinds, and other difficulties may have become attached to it. Caplan (1964) noted that during crises old problems in some way linked to the present problem are reactivated to constitute an additional burden if they were not satisfactorily dealt with in the past. Other problems in existing relationships may be intensified.

Case history 1

Mrs A. was still in black two years after her husband's death, weeping frequently, and making a three-hour bus journey every week to visit the grave. Enquiry revealed that Mr A. had been an only child, and that his mother was still actively grieving too. It gradually became clear in counselling that the two women had always competed for Mr A.'s attention and that now neither was prepared to relinquish the role of principal mourner. After they were seen together, and the counselling focus shifted to the relationship between the two of them, the older woman was able to take the lead in moving on.

Case history 2

Mrs C. was overwhelmed with anxiety after her husband's death and some months later was still unable to leave her flat on her own. In counselling she recalled the mysterious disappearance and death of her twin sister in early childhood, never explained, and the panic attacks she had herself suffered from in adolescence. These symptoms had receded during her marriage, but now returned. In this case, bereavement counselling was not considered sufficient to address the deep-seated problem that the bereavement had brought back into the open and she was referred for psychiatric help.

Case history 3

Mrs F. came for help more than a year after the death of her mother complaining of restlessness, inability to concentrate, and pains in her hands and wrists. It transpired that she had had an acute grief reaction to the death of her father 12 years earlier and her family had arranged for her to see a psychiatrist at that time. Prescribed tranquillizers by the psychiatrist, she subsequently had a difficult time weaning herself from them, and she considered that they had done her a lot of harm. After her mother's death she was afraid to express her grief directly for fear that her family would once more treat her as mad. In counselling it was necessary to go back through the mourning process for both her parents, but it was equally important to work through her anger with her family for the way she felt they had treated her, and her fears of madness or of being perceived as mad. After eight one-hour sessions she reported that the immediate symptoms were much reduced and family relationships had improved. The way was left open for her to return if she needed to.

WHO PROVIDES BEREAVEMENT COUNSELLING?

Bereavement counselling is now offered by specialist hospice and terminal care teams, and by some hospitals, for the families of their patients, as well as by community-based bereavement services. There are specialist services, for example for homosexuals (Gay Bereavement) or for parents who have

lost children through cot deaths (SA'NDS). The counsellors may be specialist bereavement counsellors or trained volunteers. Increasingly bereavement counselling is being provided by the traditional caring professions who
have extended their work to include this area.

The primary health care services

The question for the family doctor and the practice team is not whether or
not to become involved in bereavement care (as they already are), but how
far the involvement should go. Should formal bereavement counselling be
included within the work of the team, and at what stage should there be a
hand over to specialist services?

The case for keeping bereavement counselling within the traditional
professions, for not treating it as a pathology requiring a specialist service,
has been argued by Reilly (1978) and endorsed by Worden (1983).

If the first need of the bereaved is for a supportive network, including
a broadly based facilitating response, then the caring professions have a
responsibility, not only to respond to particular bereavements themselves,
but also to promote this response in the community at large. They are the
pace setters. The message given when bereavement is passed over to others
by the primary health care services could be seen as a counterpart to the
message given by the neighbour who crosses the road to avoid talking to
someone recently bereaved.

Bereavement is a time when consistency, familiarity, and continuity of
past, present, and future life, is important, when people may be ill-equipped
and often reluctant to encounter a stranger, when a known and trusted
source of help is preferred to unknown specialist services.

The counselling should be readily accessible and available at any point
during a bereavement process which may be of long duration, which is
difficult to fit within a time frame, and in which symptoms may appear
or reappear after an interval, or be activated or reactivated by subsequent events.

Bereavement is a time when general health may deteriorate and when
more frequent visits tend to be made to doctors' surgeries. The symptoms
identified in the studies of Parkes and Raphael as responding to bereavement counselling, were largely physical symptoms. The ability to eliminate
specific disease, or access to those who can, may be important.

The counselling should take place in a context which makes it possible
to include other family members where this seems appropriate.

If counselling is to be offered within the general practitioner services,
the question of who should provide it remains.

There are several possibilities. A specialist counsellor may be recruited
to join the team and work within its shared experience and authority. Alternatively, or in addition, an existing member of the team could be designated

to provide counselling as a primary function, or one or more members could undertake it as an extension of existing practice. Alternatively, counselling could be a shared responsibility of the team as a whole, with a specialist counsellor available for consultation.

Additional training may be needed. Bereavement counselling has its own knowledge and skills and brings us into an area in which we are required to make use of the self in a disciplined way, dismantling or reducing the defences that we all (professionals and non-professionals alike) use to protect ourselves against the misery of others. Training sessions in bereavement counselling habitually have a large experiential content in which the participants are given the opportunity to explore personal attitudes to loss.

Some of the implications of extending the practice of counselling had to be considered by a home care team attached to a hospice. Bereavement counselling was at first undertaken by social workers who had had specific training. This was then extended at the team's request to include the nurses and doctors as well, so that bereavement counselling could be seen as an extension of the terminal care in which all were involved, continuity could be preserved, and opportunities for professional and team development increased. Consultation with colleagues was always available, and resources shared, with time set aside for this, and all bereavement cases were regularly reviewed at meetings of the whole team.

The change brought the question of professional boundaries to the fore. Some knowledge is specific to a particular profession, but, in addition, each professional worker also draws upon a wide area of knowledge that is shared with others, but in which some other profession may have primacy.

To carry work deliberately into this shared area, and to learn from colleagues of other disciplines, requires a confidence from each worker in his or her own professional identity and area of exclusive knowledge or primacy. It is only when one is secure within one's own traditional boundaries, and secure in the knowledge that colleagues of other disciplines understand and respect these boundaries, that one can take the risk of 'crossing the frontiers of professional practice' (Thompson and Kahn 1988).

Such developments within and between disciplines, including the growth of multidisciplinary teams, can be related to the adoption of open systems concepts in the place of the static closed systems thinking of the past. Formerly, as Skynner (1976) has described, a training was considered to have been completed when 'enough' knowledge had been acquired, after which the worker would remain within his boundaries and try to protect them from disturbing change. However, we now think in terms of more open systems, and of more permeable boundaries that permit the constant intrusion of information from outside. The task now is to make selective use of what comes in without being swamped by it, and to preserve stability in conditions of confrontation, challenge, and feedback unknown in the past

Supervision

This leads on to the final point, the need for ongoing supervision. (Consultation may be a preferred term for a process which need carry no hierarchical implication and which is largely concerned with the pooling of resources and the sharing of knowledge and skills.) Bereavement counselling shares an area of professional work with psychotherapy and social work, in which such supervision is considered a necessary and valuable resource and protection.

There are a number of models. There could be supervision with a specialist superviser, with a senior colleague in the same discipline, or with a member of another discipline who happens to have more experience in this particular area. With a different area of concern, the roles might be reversed. It could be group supervision, or peer group supervision in which some may have more experience that others, and with or without the presence of a group facilitator.

Supervision/consultation recognizes that the observer often sees more of the game, and that it is possible to become lost in the counselling maze. As bereaved people use their counsellor not only to help them through the mourning process but also to act as a reference point outside it, so too the counsellors themselves gain through an opportunity to discuss the problems encountered with someone who can also provide an outside reference point.

CONCLUSIONS

We have discussed the task and process of bereavement counselling within the context of primary health care. It can be argued that this is where it most appropriately belongs. It is to the general practitioner and the primary health care team that patients in need come, and it is here that many patients find their first and only resource.

This is despite the fact that in many ways it is hard to place the consequences of bereavement within the traditional medical model. We are dealing with the destabilization of interpersonal relationships with potential long-term consequences, and with the search for a new stability that can only be facilitated through interaction with others. Outcome is hard to evaluate beyond the short-term relief of symptoms.

So whatever model a primary health care team may choose to follow, whether or not the work is extended to include formal counselling for some, the members of the team will continue to confront the consequences of bereavement and loss in their daily work. The need for an informed recognition and response from all workers remains.

This response is likely to be facilitated in teams which give bereavement a higher profile through the addition of structured bereavement counselling and the availability of a trained counsellor. The additional facility for patients can also be a resource for the whole team.

But equally counselling is only as good as its context, and is most effective when it comes as a development and natural addition to the work that is already taking place.

REFERENCES

Black, D. (1978). The bereaved child. *Journal of child psychology and psychiatry*, **19**, 287–92.

Bowlby, J. (1967). *Attachment and loss. 1. Attachment*. Hogarth Press, London.

Bowlby, J. (1980). *Attachment and loss. 3. Sadness and depression*. Hogarth Press, London.

Caplan, G. (1964). *Principles of preventive psychiatry*. Tavistock, London.

Feifel, H. (1988). Grief and bereavement: overview and perspective. In *Grief and bereavement in contemporary society*, Vol. 1, (ed. E. Chigier), p. 5. Freund Publishing House Ltd, London.

Parkes, C. M. (1981). Evaluation of a bereavement service. *Journal of Preventive Psychiatry*, **2**, 197–188.

Parkes, C. M. (1988). Can we predict outcome after bereavement? In *Grief and bereavement in contemporary society*, Vol. 1 (ed. E. Chigier), pp 125–33. Freund Publishing House Ltd, London.

Parkes, C. M., Benjamin, B., and Fitzgerald, R. G., (1969). Broken hearts, a statistical study of increased mortality among widowers. *British Medical Journal*, **1**, 240–3.

Pincus, L. and Dare, C. (1978). *Secrets in the family*. Faber & Faber, London.

Raphael, B. (1977). Preventive intervention with the bereaved. *Archives of General Psychiatry*, **34**, 1450–4.

Raphael, B. (1984). *The anatomy of bereavement*. Hutchinson, London.

Reilly, D. (1978). Death propensity, dying and bereavement: a family systems perspective. *Family therapy*, **5**, 35–55.

Skynner, A. C. R. (1976). *One flesh: separate persons*. Constable, London.

Smith, K. (1978). *Help for the bereaved*. Duckworth, London.

Smith, K. (1978). *Help for the bereaved*. Duckworth, London.

Thompson, S. and Kahn, J. (1988). *The group process and family therapy*, pp. 19–29. Pergamon Press, London.

Worden, J. W. (1983). *Grief counselling and grief therapy*. Routledge, London.

Part III

Perspectives on counselling

14　The counsellor's perspective

Margaret Graham

AN INTRODUCTORY EXAMPLE

I've just seen my GP and he suggests that it might be a good idea for me to see a psychiatrist.

This was Ann's second session with the counsellor, Valerie, in a large, progressive general practice. Ann, a woman in her late twenties, sat on the edge of her chair in the counsellor's room, slightly hunched, fiddling in a desultory way with her car keys. She glanced up at Valerie to see her reaction to the statement, conveying in her expression her own mixed feelings about the GP's suggestion.

Both the GP and Valerie were familiar with Ann's family background and current difficulties. Ann had had counselling with Valerie three years before when she had found herself in crisis, her inability to cope with her work as a research chemist accompanied by feelings of worthlessness and inadequacy, but also much anger. Ann had struggled with her belief that she 'ought' to be able to cope and constantly berated herself for 'being so pathetic'.

In counselling, Valerie had heard about the death of Ann's mother aged 50, when Ann was entering adolescence, and her father's subsequent inability to cope with her either practically or emotionally. As the only child of her parents' marriage, Ann was sent to live with her mother's much younger sister. She had formed a good relationship with this aunt. At the time of the first series of sessions it was the first anniversary of the death of her aunt at almost exactly the same age as her mother. Both had died of breast cancer.

The second series of counselling sessions marked a return of some of Ann's feelings of hopelessness, following an outburst one evening after work while out with her boyfriend. Ann described how, as if from nowhere, she became overwhelmed with feelings of rage and violence. 'It was like an explosion and all this stuff I've kept inside me for years just began to pour out. I felt I had no control over it. It was very scary.' Since then she had been unable to face her work because of her fear that she might have another outburst, with her negative feelings about her job coming out in a destructive way.

On hearing the GP's suggestion Valerie was taken aback. She had assumed the GP was aware that Ann was having counselling since he himself had suggested it, and was surprised that he had not discussed the possibility of a psychiatric referral with her.

It emerged that when Ann had gone to her GP after the outburst of rage some five weeks earlier, saying she felt unable to cope, he had put her on a course of antidepressants and suggested she might try counselling again. Ann had reluctantly accepted both these 'treatments' but felt, 'I ought to be able to sort this out for myself'.

She had made her own appointment with Valerie, as was the practice in this surgery, but Valerie was unable to see her until almost four weeks later because of her own holidays. Meantime Ann had had another two GP appointments. The second of these was with a trainee GP and happened to be on the same day as her first appointment with Valerie, which meant that Valerie did not have access to the medical notes and had, therefore, not written anything in them. The trainee was thus unaware that counselling was starting and felt concerned that the practice might not be offering Ann sufficient 'holding', particularly since she was talking openly of having little to live for. At this point the trainee suggested a psychiatric referral, but asked Ann to discuss the idea with her own GP first.

Ann saw her own GP the next week, just before this second counselling session. There was still nothing in the notes to say that counselling had begun. Ann and the GP discussed the trainee's suggestion and Ann eventually agreed.

In Valerie's room that morning, Ann brought a great deal of ambivalence. She began to express some of her confused feelings:

Maybe at last someone [the idealized expert—the psychiatrist] is going to help me get rid of these terrible feelings: they [the doctors] must think I really am crazy— maybe I am. No I'm not! Anyway. I know that seeing the psychiatrist will only label me for the rest of my life. You don't seem to think I'm mad or that I need to see the psychiatrist. Who do I believe? Who can I trust?

At the same time as Valerie was trying to attend to Ann's needs she was also wrestling with her own feelings and questions. She was aware of how Ann must be experiencing this present situation much as she had her earlier personal struggle. She might be experiencing the GP's implied inability to cope with her by sending her to the psychiatrist in the same way as she had experienced her father not coping with her after her mother's death. The psychiatrist might turn out to be someone 'good' to take the pain away, or he might fail her, as her aunt had done by dying. Valerie felt it was important for her as a woman, and possibly as a mother-figure to Ann, to be willing to explore even her most difficult feelings and not to abandon or give up on her too.

Valerie's own feelings were as ambivalent as Ann's:

I should have gone to greater lengths to retrieve those notes to make sure I mentioned that counselling had started. Why didn't either Ann or the GP mention counselling during her consultation? What sort of messages does this communication failure give Ann about the safety of this setting? What is this saying about the GP's perception of my experience in the management of emotional disturbance? I don't think Ann will gain anything by seeing a psychiatrist: what she is experiencing at the moment are the delayed, previously denied feelings associated with her experience of loss as well as the realistic fear that she may also develop breast cancer. I'd like to work with Ann, without antidepressants, for as long as it takes but I only have a limited number of sessions here.

This anecdote gives a flavour of some of the issues with which many counsellors in general practice will be familiar.

The appointment of a specialist counsellor to work as part of the primary health care team (PHCT) is both exciting and challenging. Most recent accounts of such appointments are enthusiastic and positive from both the GP's and the counsellor's perspective (Grimwade 1989; Hoag 1992; Marsh 1992; Martin and Mitchell 1983; McLeod 1992; Sabin 1992). However, the integration of someone from a different professional background into a team of professionals, whose expertise and methods of working are already well established, can raise issues for everyone involved. If counsellors, GPs, and other PHCT members are to work together as effectively as possible in the interests of their patients, it is important that these issues should be acknowledged and discussed.

In this example I have identified five dilemmas which are common to all counsellors in general practice and which distinguish working in this setting from counselling in personal private practice, working for a counselling agency, or providing a counselling service for an industrial or educational establishment.

Working in a team

The first dilemma which Valerie faces is that she is probably the only non-medically trained person among the clinical staff of the PHCT. She shares with Ann's GP the goal of wanting to alleviate Ann's distress and to help her function more fully in the world. However, Valerie has a different perception of the nature of that distress and different skills for achieving that goal. The GP uses the long-established, trusted, and accepted medical model to deal with psychological disturbance. Ann, as a patient, is familiar with how it works and respects it; the GP has diagnostic skills and experience in the use of medication for people with a wide variety of problems, most of which have a physical manifestation, but may not be physical in origin. He can also call on the additional skill of the specialist consultant in the relevant area; in Ann's case psychiatry.

Valerie has skills for working with emotional disturbance, which rely on creating an environment, over time, in which it is possible for Ann to explore, in relative safety, her feelings associated with the distress she is experiencing. The GP's focus is on symptom removal, the counsellor's on helping her client discover what role the symptoms are performing and what they are saying about the true essence of the disturbance.

Thus the challenge for the counsellor is to find a way of becoming integrated into the PHCT, given the shared goal yet using different methods for achieving that goal, in such a way as to honour her own expertise while still acknowledging the medical method of dealing with the same person. From this example, it looks as if Valerie and the GP are working in isolation from each other rather than in collaboration.

Psychotropic drugs

Valerie's second dilemma concerns the medication prescribed for Ann at her first consultation with the GP. Ann probably expected to be offered some tablets and part of her undoubtedly wanted them, although another voice was telling her that she was being pathetic and should pull herself together. The GP wants to relieve Ann's suffering and he knows that antidepressants, although they take time to work, may take the edge off Ann's symptoms. They will not be addictive and they are likely to be tolerated well enough without side effects. Above all, they will probably help her to sleep better and to be calmer. If they don't work, no real harm will be done.

Valerie, meantime, is able to provide another possibility which involves neither symptom removal with drugs, nor advice to Ann 'to pull yourself together'. Based on her previous knowledge of Ann's situation, she believes that her current distress has meaning and needs to be fully experienced if anything is going to change in Ann's life. In order to 'get better' Ann needs to discover that her feelings can be understood and are survivable, eventually without medication. Valerie also believes that the benefits of counselling are likely to be greater in the long term than those from medication alone.

If Valerie is to retain her credibility she needs to be able to debate with her medical colleagues when to use antidepressants, in an informed, confident, and flexible manner. Some people quite clearly are not able to tolerate their emotional pain without psychotropic drugs, but nevertheless benefit from a more supportive style of counselling. Ann is perceived by Valerie as being well able to work at a psychological level, therefore Valerie would prefer it if Ann was not taking any drugs. This connects with Valerie's third dilemma.

The counsellor's availability

One of the considerations the GP must have had in mind when he prescribed antidepressants was that he knew Valerie was unlikely to be able to see Ann immediately. By giving Ann something tangible at her initial consultation, he was seen by her to be taking her symptoms seriously and to be responding quickly, both important ingredients in any treatment.

Much as Valerie might like to offer an instant service, she is only available for 10 hours a week, the maximum which the practice has been able to negotiate with the FHSA.

Ann has come to expect reasonably instant access to her GP, perhaps having to wait a few days for a non-urgent appointment, but being able to see a GP on the same day for an emergency. It is confusing for her that the counsellor, although working in the same team, does not operate a system of such prompt access.

The counselling system becomes jammed because, after an initial assessment, Valerie can work for a maximum of eight sessions with any one client. Valerie's 10 hours in the surgery can thus easily be filled. The waiting time for a counselling appointment in general practice may not be as long as it would be in a counselling agency in the community, or for a psychiatric out-patient appointment. It is, nevertheless, one of the things which a GP must take into account when making a counselling referral. In general practice the primary treatment is delivered by doctors, and counselling is one of several treatment options. The dilemma for GPs and counsellors is thus to establish which patients are to be offered this scarce resource and what is to be done if there is a gap between the referral for counselling and the first appointment.

Working in the short-term

Some counsellors choose to work in the short term; others like to be able to decide how they will work according to the individual needs of their clients. In general practice there is a major constraint on time, and short-term work is seen as the most appropriate method of counselling by many GPs and counsellors. In recent years there has been much development of models of working in the short term (Hawkins 1992; Ryle 1991) which can be seen not as second best, but as a valuable way of working in their own right.

In the example, Valerie has to decide what Ann can hope to achieve in a limited number of sessions. She needs to check if she has a 'genuine customer', or if Ann is simply being a 'good patient' by doing what the doctor has suggested. Compliance does not necessarily mean that the counsellor cannot work with the client, but the nature of this compliance must be addressed at an early stage. Valerie needs to know what other appropriate resources are available once the eight sessions are finished. She needs to have a clear appreciation of the dangers of encouraging Ann to uncover a lot of difficult material, without having the expertise within the limited time available to bring Ann to the point where she can finish her counselling sessions satisfactorily. With any new client, a counsellor needs to be able to recognize those situations where the client is unlikely to respond to the type of counselling offered—the deeply-damaged client with years of dysfunction behind her, the borderline or psychotic person who may have slipped past the GP without the psychosis becoming obvious, the client who may be unable to make use of a 'talking treatment', or one whose problems might respond better to a very different approach such as might be offered by a community psychiatric nurse (Chapter 6), a psychiatric day hospital, a clinical psychologist, or a self-help group. In Valerie's situation, she must think carefully, using her knowledge of the local psychiatric services and the availability of other longer-term ways of working which might be acceptable to Ann, before deciding how to resolve this dilemma with Ann's GP.

Communication of information about a client

Valerie has developed a system of recording in the medical notes when she sees her clients. She knows that Ann legally has access to her medical records and that she has a contract of confidentiality with her, as with all her clients. Valerie will have had to decide how to manage the boundaries of confidentiality, alongside the need to communicate with the referring GP.

In our example, Valerie, for various practical reasons, does not manage to retrieve the medical notes in order to record her initial contact with Ann. She neither finds the time to talk to the GP directly after the first session, nor to write a formal letter as would a hospital consultant immediately after seeing a newly referred patient.

This highlights another of the differences between counselling in general practice and counselling elsewhere: who carries ultimate responsibility for the patient? There is no doubt that GPs are deemed to hold that responsibility. If Ann did commit suicide, as was the trainee GP's fear, how would that be viewed by the outside world? What are Valerie's responsibilities to the GPs, to Ann and to herself?

GROUND RULES TO HELP ESTABLISH
A COUNSELLING SERVICE

This section will examine some of the decisions which need to be taken and the processes which need to be put in place, in order to be able to deal with the key dilemmas highlighted above. Here I draw primarily on my own experience as a counsellor in general practice for the last 16 years. I also have a private psychotherapy practice, which allows for a certain amount of cross-referencing of ideas and expertise. The development of my practice counselling role has been based on the belief that GPs and counsellors, when working sensitively and co-operatively together, have a great deal to offer their patients. This role has evolved through learning by trial and error, through being supervised and supervising others, through discussion with peers, and through reading and further training. It continues to evolve even as I write.

For a counsellor to be able to work to his/her full potential, it is important that he/she feels valued and accepted by the team. This is of course a two-way process, requiring a willingness by the established team and by the counsellor to acknowledge each other's skills and expertise, to learn from each other, and to be prepared to confront each other honestly about their differences in an atmosphere of mutual trust.

Contract with the practice

The contract between the counsellor and the practice plays an important part in helping the counsellor establish a sense of being part of the team. Hoag (1992) suggests that it was important early on in her contract with the GPs to negotiate a salary commensurate with the expertise she knew she was bringing to the team. The method and amount of payment of the counsellor can influence how valued and autonomous the counsellor feels, and can also spill over into the counselling relationship. Research shows that there are wide variations in the method of payment for counselling (Curtis-Jenkins 1992; McLeod 1988). These can range from a private arrangement with the GP, or between the client and the counsellor in which the counsellor negotiates a fee directly with the client and the surgery provides the clients and the room, to a much more rigid contract in which the counsellor is required to see a certain number of clients in a specified, often limited, time.

In the practice in which I work, one of the partners had the imagination 16 years ago to see a role for someone with counselling skills in the PHCT. The then FPC had the vision to support the idea, by agreeing to my employment under the regulations of the day for the employment of ancillary staff, thus making me an established part of the team. Since those early days, my salary has been increased to take account of my experience, further training, and BAC accreditation. It has also been important to negotiate payment for administration and communication time, as well as supervision expenses. The practice now has two counsellors, able to see, between us, 12 clients a week. Time to meet my colleague is built into the contract, so that we can offer each other support and continue to improve the quality of the service we provide.

The establishment for the counsellor of a clear and appropriate contract means that if, for example, a client fails to turn up for a session, the counsellor is able to work with the client's process (that is with the less-conscious reasons why the client did not keep the appointment) rather than having to worry about failing to reach the quota of clients for that month. A similar dynamic is at work regarding supervision. The practice's acknowledgement of the need for supervision, by paying for it, lessens the likelihood of resentment creeping into the work with a particularly challenging or overwhelming client.

Another aspect of the practice contract concerns the types of referral the counsellor is expected to accept and their source. For example, there is sometimes an expectation that the counsellor will automatically see people with certain presenting problems, such as all women requesting a termination of pregnancy or anyone who has recently been bereaved. Other counsellors are expected to see all comers, at least for an assessment. Some practices with a long-established counsellor will find that they have a lot of self-referrals, because the word has spread from other satisfied patients. Other practices expect the GPs only to make referrals. Whichever is the chosen system, it needs to be clear to the counsellor and the rest of the team.

Recently appointed counsellors may sometimes feel themselves to be set up to fail, by being asked to see people who are unmotivated or unable to make appropriate use of counselling. Inappropriate referrals often arise because GPs have to account to their FHSA for the use of the counsellor's time. Certain practices, for example, only receive funding for a counsellor by spelling out the sort of 'problems' which they expect their counsellor to handle. In this scheme, selection for referral may be based on symptoms or immediate presenting problems, such as 'abnormal grief reaction' or 'stress', without taking into account the patient's suitability or preparedness for this type of treatment.

Some writers, in giving a flavour of the potential for counselling in general practice, have outlined the main presenting problems in a specific way: depression, anxiety states, phobias, bereavement, loss, stress-related physical symptoms, relationship problems, sexual dysfunction, post-trauma difficulties, addiction, eating disorders, and so on (Cocksedge 1992; Hatswell 1992; McLeod 1988.) The difficulty with categorizing 'problems' in this way is that it diminishes the importance of the client's own feelings and ignores the interrelatedness of many of these categories. For example, the development of an eating disorder may be the only way for a client to cope with the overwhelming feelings associated with sexual abuse in childhood, or a relationship problem may be the tip of an iceberg, covering up unworked through feelings about growing up in a family where one parent is an alcoholic or manic depressive.

It is important, therefore, that the counsellor and the GP discuss the nature of referrals and any expectations of the outcomes of counselling.

The frame for the client

One of the tenets of counselling is that the outcome is likely to be more successful if the client has had the experience of feeling contained and held in a safe therapeutic relationship with the counsellor. The counsellor in general practice needs to be aware of how some routine procedures and systems in the surgery may make it more difficult to create a secure frame for the client. Langs talks about how the 'deviant frame' of general practice can adversely affect the outcome of therapy (quoted in Hoag 1992). It is particularly important, therefore, that the counsellor establishes a clear and secure frame for his/her clients.

We have evolved processes to achieve this secure frame. The GP, having made his/her own assessment that the patient might benefit from counselling, usually discusses the implications fully with the patient. The patient is then given a short leaflet, which outlines what counselling involves, followed by details of how we work and how to make an appointment. The leaflet invites the patient to phone one of us at specified times to arrange to come for an initial assessment. We explain that the session will last for 50 minutes, that it will take place in our own room in the surgery where there will be no interruptions, and that it will be entirely confidential, unless we choose together to share information with the GP. We also say that, after the initial assessment, a decision will be made whether to offer a series of sessions, at weekly or more widely-spaced intervals, or to suggest some more appropriate intervention.

The benefit of this approach is that it empowers clients to decide for themselves whether or not they wish to take up the suggestion of counselling, by making their own appointment directly with the counsellor. In a setting where compliance with the doctor's authority is more usual, the requirement for clients actually to ask for what they want can be the first step in taking themselves and their situation seriously. The advantage to the counsellor is that some sort of assessment of the situation can begin to be made over the phone and appointments are better able to be planned.

Having an upper limit to the total number of sessions and to the length of each individual session, can serve to offset clients' frequently expressed feelings of being 'undeserving' or of 'taking up so much of your time'. In general practice, where doctors are quite visibly very short of time and are unashamedly relieved when there is a cancellation, it is important to emphasize that counselling works differently. The counsellor and client decide together whether to contract for a particular number of sessions, with the understanding that they will not be limitless. Our experience is that we have very few cancellations, largely as a result of the careful consideration given to setting up the counselling.

It may be seen as a disadvantage of this system that it does not cater easily for counselling emergencies. We believe, however, that (with the possible exception of somebody considering a termination of pregnancy, when counselling needs to be carried out quickly) most situations can be contained by speaking to the client on the telephone, or by talking with the referring GP about the client's distress as soon as possible. It is usually possible to demonstrate that we have heard the client's difficulty and acknowledge how hard it is to cope: this can often be enough to hold the client until one of us has a vacancy. My colleague also keeps one emergency session a week for any client whom the GP considers must be seen within the week.

The ability to maintain a secure frame in this way may demonstrate to others in the team that anxiety can often be alleviated if it is acknowledged and taken seriously, without having to respond with an immediate appointment.

A final aspect of the development of a secure frame lies in making clear the boundaries of confidentiality at the initial assessment interview. If the client has been referred by a GP, we receive a card on which is outlined the problem as presented to the GP. It is explained to the client that the counsellor records, in a client's medical notes, the date and number of any counselling sessions. The content of the counselling remains entirely confidential. However, we are currently exploring ways of sharing with the GPs some of the issues looked at in counselling, in an effort to treat the client as holistically as possible. At all times the emphasis is on giving power to the client to decide how much information is included in the medical notes.

An example of how the counsellor's procedures differ from those of the rest of the team lies in the way we communicate confidences to the GPs even when permission to do so has been freely given by the client. It is standard procedure, for example, for a practice nurse or midwife to discuss patient care, during a coffee break, with other members of staff in the room. While this works well for some team members, it is important for counsellors to adhere to their own model of confidentiality which does not allow for the disclosure of any identifiable information about a client to anyone other than the named GP, or other specified member of the clinical team who shares the care of the client. If, at times, this seems unnecessarily fussy, it soon falls into perspective when faced in a session with a client who says, 'I've never told anyone this before', or 'This is very difficult for me to say, but I feel I can trust you'. It is the privacy and safety of the counselling situation which is essential for its effectiveness.

The only exceptions to these boundaries of confidentiality are those delineated in the BAC code of ethics (BAC 1992), for example, when the counsellor believes that the client may cause serious harm to others or to themselves, or when the client is in danger. In the case of overt suicidal thoughts and intent, the clients are always encouraged to share their feelings with the GP. The counsellor must always ensure that the client knows the boundary of confidentiality and must discuss with the client any reason for wanting to change that boundary.

Supervision and support

One of the requirements of the BAC code of ethics and that of accredited counselling training organizations is that counsellors must have adequate supervision and support. The professional isolation which many counsellors feel in the setting of general practice is well documented (McLeod 1988). It is, therefore, essential to achieve a good balance between supervision on individual client material, issues to do with working in a team, and peer support from those working in a similar setting.

It can sometimes be difficult to arrange the necessary quality and frequency of supervision because of the prevailing ethos, in many doctors' surgeries, that all supervision and support can be taken care of within the practice. This relies on the operation of the hierarchy to attend to the needs of team members, but does not allow the GPs at the top of the hierarchy to give themselves the quality of attention and support which they must also need. Some counsellors find it hard to persuade GPs of the essential nature of supervision from another counsellor or trainer outside the surgery with expertise not only of counselling issues, but of the setting itself.

Hawkins and Shohet (1989) suggest that a counsellor or other helping professional can survive the negative attacks of clients through the strength of being held within and by the supervisory relationship. This notion is not one particularly espoused in medical training or practice, perhaps to their detriment, since both alcoholism and suicide rates are significantly higher among doctors than among other professionals.

Integration into the PHCT

The challenge here is for the counsellor to find a way of becoming integrated into the team which acknowledges the validity of a different working method, and at the same time to find a balance between holding his/her own authority and acknowledging the expertise and training of colleagues.

One potential difficulty in such integration is connected with the different emphasis attached to a medical as opposed to a counselling model. This difference is vividly demonstrated by the 'Defeat Depression' drive of the Royal College of Psychiatry. The notion of 'defeating' depression is a very medical one and ignores the possibility, for example, of 'depression' being the means by which people can let themselves know that they need to rebalance their lives, or of it marking the reappearance of something unfinished, such as bereavement. Medical training places great emphasis on the classification of illness and the need to develop good diagnostic skills, in order to be able to put an appropriate treatment plan into operation. Doctors often see their role in a compassionate way, as one of finding the quickest and most effective method of removing painful symptoms. The counsellor, on the other hand, may take the view that since body and emotion are inextricably bound together, it may not always be in the patient's best interests to attempt to remove the symptoms immediately. Most GPs are all too aware of the patients who bring recurring, though different, physical complaints week after week. Although the dysfunction of some of these 'somatizers', as they are frequently labelled, may be too deeply entrenched for counselling to have any effect, there are many who might be prevented from becoming the frequent attenders of the future, if their symptoms are regarded in a more holistic manner earlier in their consultations.

Jones (1986) suggests that for the integration of someone from a different discipline into the PHCT, the structure needs to be one which 'reinforces professional independence and responsibility while encouraging maximum contact'. However, many of us have difficulty in arranging this contact despite its significance in determining the success or failure of a counselling scheme. McLeod (1988) suggests a number of reasons, including the ambivalence which some GPs feel about the work of counsellors, their very different use of time, and the possibility that many doctors are more used to directing and acting than to consulting on a peer level. Perhaps there is an unconscious resistance to substantive contact between GPs and counsellors, on the GPs' part, because they may not regard counsellors as their peers, and on the counsellors' part because they find it easier simply to get on with their work with the clients.

One group of GPs and counsellors have recently made what sounds like a highly effective start towards building up good communication between them (Draper 1992). The group of three GPs and three counsellors met regularly over 18 months, with the purpose of exploring issues of common interest. The members were able to share some more personal issues within the safety of a small group, including the fantasies each profession had of the other, the envy and the prejudices, as well as more patient-centred issues.

They noted the high incidence of suicide and depression among GPs and the difficulty they have in asking for help, believing that attention to one's psyche is only considered legitimate if disguised as 'training'. Counsellors on the other hand are clear that their own personal growth is important in order to help clients. The group provided its members with the opportunity to develop a mutual respect for and confidence in each other's role. Among different perspectives explored were the doctors' feelings that on occasions they need to take active responsibility for their patients, whereas the essence of a counselling relationship lies in the counsellor's encouragement of the client to take control.

Out of their report comes the very clear message that a good working alliance must be of benefit to the patients, both directly and indirectly. If, for example, GP and counsellor in collaboration can create a feeling of containment and safety in which the patient's feelings of anger, grief, fear, or low self-esteem can be truly heard and found to be survivable, preferably without recourse to medication, the patient will have discovered something of life-long value. This working alliance can only develop if the need to communicate effectively within the PHCT is taken seriously. There is no doubt that this takes time and energy and a will to confront and challenge existing methods.

The focus of this section has been primarily on the integration of the counsellor with the GP. Although GPs make the majority of referrals to counsellors, other team members, for example health visitors and practice nurses, can make referrals to the counsellors. These referrals can often be particularly appropriate and fruitful because the health visitor or nurse is frequently in a good position to pick up people's difficulties. The less pressured environment of the home visit, the baby clinic, the family planning session, the insurance medical, and so on can provide an opportunity for people to indicate that all is not well. This demonstrates the importance of the counsellor being available for referrals from all members of the PHCT.

Impact of the counsellor on the PHCT

The presence of a counsellor in a general practice has an impact at different levels. At the client/patient level, the impressionistic evidence from my surgery suggests that the availability of a counsellor to attend to some of the more overt emotional difficulties among patients helps the practice provide a more comprehensive and readily acceptable service. One GP has frequently said that the impact of the counsellors goes beyond their direct work with patients. The very fact that the GP can offer a patient a counselling service indicates to the patient that the GP is not thinking solely in medical terms about the patient's well-being, and has helped many patients move forward without actually seeing a counsellor.

At present, our surgery has no formal audit of the number and nature of referrals to the counsellors, nor is there any assessment of the outcome of counselling as perceived by the client. We are currently considering inviting clients to return some months after their counselling sessions have finished, to hear if any benefit from the sessions has been maintained.

At the level of the counsellor's impact on other team members, there has been a raising of consciousness about emotional distress, not just in the patients, but amongst each other. Most counsellors become familiar with casual remarks from other staff such as: 'If you've got a spare slot I could do with a bit of counselling myself'. It is important for counsellors to be clear about the boundaries of their role in relation to staff. He/she often becomes the person to whom staff turn when they have a problem in the workplace, but is not in a position to offer specific counselling to a colleague, particularly if that person is an employee of the GPs. Perhaps the role here is to show the colleague how to take the problem to a more appropriate person, such as one of the GPs or, if necessary, to an outside counsellor.

Some general practices encourage their counsellor to increase his/her impact on the team by asking that presentations on aspects of the work are given to other team members. Other practices have regular team meetings to discuss patient material. This can be a useful forum for counsellors to share their perspective on the different situations, discussed in a general way, without breaking the boundaries of confidentiality regarding specific clients. Any such meetings can only serve to strengthen the counsellor's position within the PHCT.

CONCLUSIONS

In conclusion, I will return to my case study example. Ann continued to explore with Valerie her confused feelings about whether or not she wanted a psychiatric referral. Valerie suggested that Ann might like to prepare her own referral letter as a way of retaining control over her own situation, but although Ann liked this idea she eventually thought that she preferred not to see the psychiatrist at all. Valerie consulted with both the GP and the trainee, who were happy with this decision and glad that Ann was to continue in counselling, even though it would only be for a few more sessions. However, having considered the case with her supervisor, Valerie realized the importance of the GP's original suggestion being seen to be followed through, in line with the GP's perception of Ann's psychiatric state and his understanding of the most appropriate choice of treatment. At the next session Valerie discussed further the implications of a psychiatric referral. Ann wrote a draft referral letter asking for a psychiatric assessment and this experience in itself turned out to be very useful, for both herself and Valerie, as part of the counselling process. At her psychiatric appointment two weeks later, Ann saw a junior member of the department who did not suggest any alteration of Ann's medication, but recommended further counselling by one of the staff at the psychiatric day hospital. Since Valerie and Ann already had a good working relationship, Ann decided, with the full knowledge of her GP, to finish the remaining sessions and to set a goal of transition from short-term work with Valerie to private open-ended counselling outside the surgery.

This case has highlighted many of the facets of my role as a counsellor in general practice, including the overlap of professional expertise between GP, psychiatrist, and counsellor. Its ultimate resolution has shown the need to address those key dilemmas discussed earlier within the framework outlined for the successful operation of a counsellor as an integral part of the PHCT.

REFERENCES

BAC (1992). *Code of ethics and practice for counsellors*. British Association for Counselling, Rugby.

Cocksedge, S. (1992). Counselling in general practice: a brief review of the literature. *CMS News* (British Association for Counselling), **32**, 8–11.

Curtis-Jenkins, G. (1992). *Counselling in primary care*. Counselling in Primary Care Trust, Staines.

Draper, J. (1992). *A study of a group of counsellors and general practitioners working in general practice*. Unpublished paper.

Grimwade, K. (1989). *Counselling within primary care: results of a survey of GPs in Lewisham and North Southwark Health Districts*. Lewisham and North Southwark Community Health Council Publication.

Hatswell, V. (1992). Counselling in general practice. *CMS News*. (British Association for Counselling), **32**, 6–8.

Hawkins, P. (1992). A humanistic, integrative and psychodynamic model for short-term counselling and psychotherapy. Unpublished paper.

Hawkins, P. and Shohet, R. (1989). *Supervision in the helping professions*. Open University Press, Milton Keynes.

Hoag, L. (1992). Psychotherapy in the general practice surgery: considerations of the frame. *British Journal of Psychotherapy*, **8**, 417–29.

Jones, D. (1986). General Practitioner attachments and the multidisciplinary team. *British Journal of Psychotherapy*, **2**, 196–200.

Marsh, G. (1992). The counsellor as part of the general practice team. In *Counselling in general practice* (ed. R. Corney and R. Jenkins), pp. 67–74. Tavistock Routledge, London.

Martin, E. and Mitchell H. (1983). A counsellor in general practice; a one year survey. *Journal of the Royal College of General Practitioners*, **33**, 366–7.

McLeod, J. (1988). *The work of counsellors in general practice*. Occasional Paper, No. 37. The Royal College of General Practitioners, London.

McLeod, J. (1992). Counselling in primary health care: the GP's perspective. In *Counselling in general practice*, (ed. M. Sheldon), pp. 8–14. RCGP Enterprises, London.

Ryle, A. (1991). *Cognitive-analytic therapy: active participation in change*. John Wiley, Chichester.

Sabin, J. (1992). The therapeutic alliance in managed care. *Mental Health Practice Journal of Psychotherapy Practice and Research*, **1**, 31–7.

15   The GP as counsellor

Marie Campkin

Whilst ideally all GPs should have some counselling skills, can the GP be regarded as a counsellor in his/her own right? If counselling is narrowly defined as a process involving fixed sessions, at regular intervals, for a contracted period, and between a person with specific counselling training and a client with whom the relationship is exclusively of that nature, it would appear to have little in common with general practice.

For the general practitioner undertakes to be available to his/her patients at short notice, year in, year out, on an unlimited number of occasions, for appointments of variable, but usually brief duration, and with an agenda open to matters physical, psychological, and social, and often extending to include the legal, the bureaucratic, the financial, and the rest.

Yet, since the words consult and counsel share a common origin, it is not surprising that the general practice consultation should include a counselling component. In the widest sense, a counsellor can be defined as an adviser, a source of information, a person to be consulted. Further definitions, obsolete in the UK but still current in the United States, include advocate, representative or defender. Most GPs would readily identify themselves as carrying out many of these functions, even if they prefer to regard themselves primarily as clinicians.

At the same time, many GPs value those aspects of their work which enable them to practise the more specifically therapeutic arts of counselling: listening without judging, sharing rather than pre-empting the patient's struggles towards self-understanding, and avoiding the use of reassurance, good advice, and 'doctor's orders' as a substitute for acknowledging the patient's anxiety and autonomy.

Tension between the roles of counsellor and clinician may be a cause of discord if the doctor and patient have conflicting expectations. If the doctor sees him/herself only as a clinician, when the patient feels in need of a counsellor, both may be frustrated; the doctor because the patient fails to provide appropriate symptoms and signs for a clinical diagnosis; the patient because the doctor ignores his/her tentative offers about real anxieties and problems.

Conversely, if a patient convinced that an ailment is purely physical meets a doctor intent on counselling, that patient may resent what he/she regards as an intrusive and irrelevant interest in his/her personal background, particularly if the patient feels that complaints are not being taken seriously at the clinical level.

Within this setting, therefore, counselling is not something doctors should sometimes 'do to' patients. Rather it is a way of 'being with' patients; not so much a process, more a state of mind. For the doctor with this attitude, and aptitude, it is not an optional extra, but as integral to the consultation as history taking, diagnosis, and treatment, and may play a part in all these activities.

This is not a new role for general practitioners; it is as old as medicine. In past generations, the relative absence of effective treatment for most serious illnesses rendered the doctor's empathy as crucial to his/her reputation as clinical acumen and therapeutic skill. With scientific progress, the conquest of many of the old killer infections and the ever-widening scope of surgical and pharmacological intervention, this aspect of the doctor's role might have been expected to diminish. Instead it seems that our society is ever more reliant on the family physician to perform functions ranging from those of the priest to those of the grandparent. Consultations requiring counselling as well as clinical skills continue to increase.

Inevitably there is considerable variation in doctors' innate ability and inclination to appreciate the psychological aspects of their patients' presentation. Practitioners' estimates of the proportion of surgery attenders suffering from mental illness have varied widely in different studies. Goldberg and Huxley (1980), having quoted ranges of 15 to 64 per cent and 0 to 85 per cent, comment that the difference between the doctors giving high and low estimates 'resides not in their patients, but in their concepts of psychiatric disorder and the threshold they adopt for case identification.'

Nonetheless, to some extent the individual doctor's 'bias' may be self-fulfilling, on three counts. Patients usually know whether to trouble their particular doctor with problems or whether that GP prefers them to bring physical symptoms. Those patients unaware of the possible relationship between overt physical symptoms and underlying emotional distress are unlikely to make the connection if the doctor fails to recognize it. Finally, those doctors known to be sympathetic to patients with emotional problems tend to acquire more and more of them.

Given the evidence that around half of all patients suffering from depression in general practice go unrecognized, current initiatives to 'defeat depression' by increasing awareness and improving training are timely (Paykel and Priest 1992). However, the present climate in general practice is not conducive to an enhancement of doctors' sensitivity to patients' emotional needs.

The agenda for the brief average surgery consultation suffers increasing encroachment by matters not determined by the patient. The objectives are worthy, but the activities time-consuming: preventive—let me just check your blood pressure; health promotional—not still smoking are you?; and opportunistic/financial—just three more smears needed for the target, and here is one of them. This not only pre-empts some of the consultation time, but also establishes a doctor-centred environment which influences its style.

After these matters have been addressed there may be little time, and less space, for the doctor to hear what the patient has to say, still less to listen for what may remain unspoken. No wonder our patients appreciate the undivided attention they obtain from the 'alternative' practitioner, whose listening ear may be more potent than the treatment, just as, in the words of Balint (1968) the drug 'the doctor' is the general practitioner's most valuable therapeutic agent.

There needs to be flexibility for the doctor to devote a longer time to a particular patient when necessary, without the stress of knowing that this is resulting in an ever-increasing wait for others. The compensatory 'short consultation' seems to be disappearing, for the reasons suggested above, and despite a general move towards longer appointment times— ten minutes rather than six—the problem remains.

Meanwhile it is all the more important for the doctor to remain receptive to the patient's communication whilst engaged in 'routine' activities. The concept of opportunism need not be confined to the purely physical.

THE INFLUENCE OF BALINT

It is inevitable and proper that the name of Michael Balint should arise in any consideration of the doctor's counselling role. From the 1950s onwards he, with his wife Enid and their GP colleagues, explored and defined the doctor–patient relationship and its use in the processes of diagnosis and treatment. He devised a form of training to enable general practitioners to apply this in their everyday work, and as a method for further research (Balint 1968).

A relatively small number of doctors undertook this training, but Balint's influence pervaded general practice thought and education for a generation, through the eminence of Balint-trained doctors within the Royal College of General Practitioners, the academic departments of general practice, and the developing establishment of vocational training. As a result many of his ideas are now taken for granted, though not necessarily put into practice.

The most effective way for doctors to acquire the counselling attitude remains this method of discussing cases in a group with a Balint-trained analyst or GP leader. Some vocational training schemes offer this experience during the trainee year. There are also weekend events and ongoing groups for established practitioners, but few doctors undertake the ideal programme of at least two years of weekly seminars. (Some GPs do undergo similar training in seminars run by the Institute of Psychosexual Medicine. Though this work has a precise focus, the doctor's general consulting and counselling skills are bound to be comparably enhanced.)

The advantage these have over a more standard form of counselling training is that the work is grounded in general practice experience. When the participating doctor presents one of his/her difficult and puzzling cases, the GP and the group examine encounters with the patient and their relationship for clues both to the patient's problems and to the doctor's 'blind spots', which may have interfered with his/her ability to understand them.

Exploring their own and each others' cases encourages the members to engage what Enid Balint described as their 'hunches, fantasies and feelings' (in Elder and Samuel 1987) in a manner quite remote from anything in their previous medical experience. This broadens the clinical diagnosis to take account of the psychodynamic factors revealed by the discussion, and allows predictions to be made and tested. The doctor learns to monitor personal feelings and to use imagination in the consulting room as well as in the group.

The improved understanding which the doctor acquires enables the patient to be treated more effectively, and as he/she reports continuing work the group and its leader provide support, criticism, and a degree of supervision. Eventually, as with other forms of psychological training, the doctor develops his/her own 'internal supervisor' to refine new personal skills.

Conventional supervision is not a practical proposition for the average GP, though forms of peer review and audit are gaining ground on the clinical side. However, those GPs who wish to extend their interpersonal skills may seek further individual training and supervision of their casework.

The caricature of the 'Balint doctor' is of someone earnestly enquiring into the sex life of a patient who came in with an ingrowing toenail. The reality is more to do with the development of a particular curiosity: an interest in why people behave as they do: why they present with this symptom at this time; why they engender in the doctor a feeling of anger, confusion, or despair: and how to be more useful to them.

This is not greatly different, perhaps, from the attitude of the professional counsellor, except that when a client sees a counsellor he or she has already determined that there is a problem for which counselling may be an appropriate strategy, whereas the doctor has to discern, from amongst the many attenders at the surgery sessions with their diverse complaints and requests, which one or two may also have hidden problems to which his/her antennae should particularly be tuned.

THE NEED FOR TRAINING

Michael Balint himself acknowledged that his form of training was only suitable for a minority of doctors. Vocational course organizers with a Balint-style group in their halfday release course expect all trainees to participate, but recognize the wide variation in their response to the process. Nonetheless, even the most sceptical may eventually gain much from the experience.

If Balint training remains an ideal, but is accessible or acceptable to relatively few doctors, what other forms of training could help doctors acquire 'the counselling attitude' for the benefit of themselves and their patients?

Most undergraduate departments in medical school now devote some time to teaching 'communication skills', while GP vocational training schemes focus on 'the consultation' in a variety of ways. Much of this work is behavioural in style and concerns body language, styles of questioning, an agenda for the conduct of the proceedings, and the elimination of bad habits, as revealed by the video camera (Pendleton *et al.* 1984).

Studies with a behavioural emphasis tend not to address what is going on inside the doctor's head, or what might be deduced about what is in the patient's head. One may observe the patient's tears or anger, but not know the doctor's internal response to them. If the consultation is confused and dysfunctional, this will usually be considered more in terms of how the doctor might have managed it better rather than what it may be saying about the patient's state of mind or way of life.

Goldberg and Huxley (1992) describe research studies aimed more specifically at determining which are the desirable characteristics in doctors' interviewing techniques which correlate with the accurate diagnosis of emotional distress. In one study Goldberg and his colleagues had been able to show that:

A brief set of videotaped feedback sessions succeeded in modifying the doctors' interview behaviour over the next six months, and this in turn caused them to be more sensitive in detecting emotional distress in their patients.

(Goldberg *et al.* 1980)

Another approach would be through the use of counselling skills training. Here there may be less emphasis on the doctor's conduct of the event, but more on the art of listening with full attention and the suspension of judgment; clarifying the patient's presentation rather than organizing it; asking for feelings rather than facts; and regarding the listener's response as an aspect of the patient's communication.

Sessions along these lines are occasionally offered in vocational training, but the majority of doctors in practice have not been exposed to them. For interested GPs such courses could be of great value, provided the training takes account of the particular circumstances of general practice.

Brief intensive courses could cover much of the groundwork of basic counselling skills training, with some theoretical background, the provision of practical experience as counsellor, client, and observer, and consideration of the scope for applying the skills within the normal consultation.

Ideally this would be a standard ingredient of undergraduate and vocational training. Its value does not lie merely in giving the doctor an additional resource; the nature of the training also enables the GP to experience being the client, and looking, however briefly, at his/her own human needs. This is indeed a rare experience in medical education at any level, but one which might, if more widely practised, profoundly alter the attitudes of doctors towards their patients, themselves, and each other.

Ultimately the place for further counselling training could be within general practice itself, using the practice-based counsellor as a resource. With increasing involvement of all the members of the primary care team in direct patient contact and care, they too could benefit by taking part in ways relevant to their own work. This is not in order to turn them all into counsellors, but to enable the counselling attitude to prevail throughout the practice.

THE PROMOTION OF HEALTH

Such an attitude should surely feature in the interrelated areas of health promotion, disease prevention, and patient education. Yet the procedures involved here have tended to be ruled by protocols and delegated to ancillary staff, and the criteria have been largely determined by bureaucratic rather than clinical, let alone psychological, considerations.

Freeling and Tylee (1992) comment:

> The emphasis on proactive care with practice nurses providing preventive care for defined conditions may affect their ability to recognise underlying depression unless suitably trained.

This is not a criticism of practice nurses, many of whom, like many doctors, health visitors, and others, show great sensitivity and empathy in their everyday interactions with patients.

However, the carrying out of specific protocols and procedures, particularly in the environment of the 'health promotion clinic' in its recent heyday, may militate against the ability of the health care worker to discern and respond to the patient's personal concerns, in a setting more geared to the collective than to the individual.

Advice and education on diet, exercise, smoking, and alcohol can all too easily be dealt with by a nurse or a doctor at autopilot level, whilst possibly being experienced by the patient as bullying, patronizing, or irrelevant.

The psychologically secure may take it or leave it; for the emotionally vulnerable it could damage their health. Many are already preoccupied with ill-informed fears about the risks and dangers of everyday life, from cholesterol and AIDS to 'mad cow disease'. Propaganda may increase their anxiety without beneficially altering their behaviour.

Yet opportunities do exist to intervene helpfully, perhaps by exploring factors underlying the 'unhealthy' behaviour before deciding how it should be changed. If all the staff involved in clinics are trained and encouraged to consider the psychological aspects, the whole enterprise may become more effective as well as more patient-friendly.

For example, one can safely assume that most people who are seriously overweight are seriously unhappy about it. The last thing they may be needing is yet another lecture on calories and exercise from another slim nurse, doctor, or dietitian. Some sympathetic fellow-feeling and a chance to talk about their distress might not make them lose weight, but could make a small dent in their vicious circle of diet, frustration, misery, and comfort eating.

Similarly, for some smokers their habit is one factor in maintaining the fragile balance of a difficult life. A 30-year-old woman with a cough agreed with the doctor that she should stop smoking, but feared gaining weight. She was sent to the nurse for advice, but later returned to ask the doctor about relaxation, because she kept shaking.

This time, encouraged to talk, she described her early life as the youngest of seven children, whose mother was ill after her birth and died before she was two. She spent long periods in hospital with skin trouble, sent back whenever the family could not cope with her. She used to cry and scream a lot, until one day she 'stopped crying'. At twenty she escaped into a disastrous and violent marriage, which finally broke up two years ago. She took to drink for a while, but overcame this problem by herself. She sincerely wanted to give up smoking, but with the overwhelming tension in her life as evidenced by her shaking, this seemed quite the wrong time to attempt it.

This story illustrates several points. In automatic 'health promotion' mode, both doctor and nurse initially failed to recognize the distressed person behind this 20-a-day smoker. Once she had been 'seen', the priorities changed. Promotion of her mental health may now determine that she should continue smoking for a while if she needs to, whilst action is taken to address her emotional state—surely a place here for the counsellor.

An important factor was that though this patient had been with the practice for some time, her past history was not known. Nowadays, like most practices, we have an initial registration procedure which includes the obligatory physical check-up and the recording of family and personal medical history.

Had this been available, this patient's distress could have come to light earlier, given the obvious pointers in her history of bereavement and childhood illness to the emotional deprivation which is still taking its toll.

This first contact with the patient offers an unparalleled opportunity to anticipate problems in both the physical and psychological spheres. The family history may reveal adoption, early bereavement, separation, divorce, and the acquisition of step-parents and siblings. These facts—and family deaths from alcoholic liver disease, accident, or suicide—are just as important as predictors of psychological vulnerability as family members with diabetes or heart disease are of a hereditary predisposition to physical illness.

Other significant events in the personal medical history may include teenage drug problems or eating disorders, previous emotional illness, accidents, illnesses, and operations. Asking a woman specifically about pregnancies may often reveal one or more 'forgotten' terminations.

It may be easier for the patient to give sensitive information in this matter-of-fact way than to be asked for it later, perhaps when discussing an associated problem. For example, with a woman anxious about her fertility, it is important to know about previous pregnancies; yet one might not want at that moment to remind her of a past abortion. The doctor who already knows can use his judgement about bringing the subject up.

Just as a patient's bad family history of heart disease may alert the doctor to take especial note of his blood pressure and serum cholesterol, so a woman's history of several terminations of pregnancy might lead the doctor to consider the possibility that she may have suffered sexual abuse. This does not mean rushing in with a direct question; simply being aware of it may allow for an opening when the time is right.

From the counselling viewpoint, these initial encounters, as well as other routine activities such as baby and family planning clinics, create many openings for health promotion in its broadest sense, provided those carrying them out are trained and alert to the possibilities. Likewise, the concept of preventive care can extend beyond that of physical disease to encompass keeping watch on children in dysfunctional families, recognizing the anniversaries of traumatic events, and maintaining contact with bereaved families or spouses.

Patient education, too, is not just about telling patients what is good for them; it may include interpreting for them links between present events and past unfinished business; suggesting ways of understanding the behaviour of those around them; recognizing the symbolic value of certain symptoms; and so helping them to care better for their own psychological as well as physical well-being.

For the patient described, this could mean exploring the possible connection between her years of unshed tears and her shaking hands, and seeking a means of dealing with both.

The foregoing story illustrates the ease with which depression in a patient presenting with other complaints initially went unrecognized. A greater use of counselling skills by GPs could improve their management of depression, currently recognized as seriously under-diagnosed and inadequately treated (Freeling and Tylee 1992; Paykel and Priest 1992) (see also Chapter 6).

The need for the doctor's counselling skills does not end with the diagnosis; the whole matter of negotiating and reviewing treatment and encouraging perseverance remains. This is only the start of a process which may require many more consultations, over many months. But it may be the culmination of years during which the patient has been struggling under the burden of his/her own history. The investment of time by doctor and patient will be amply rewarded.

A COUNSELLOR IN THE PRACTICE

Should those doctors with both interest and some skill in counselling have less need of a counsellor in their practice than those without? In one sense the opposite may be the case. The more psychologically minded the doctor, the greater the number of patients whose need for counselling will be recognized. Paradoxically, therefore, the doctor with the counselling attitude will be more likely to appreciate having a counsellor in the practice and will find more work, both in volume and suitability, for that person to do.

Each week the doctor may discover one or two people who would benefit from formal counselling, as well as others whom the GP will continue to manage personally within the framework of a series of ordinary consultations.

Assessment can then be made by the practice counsellor who may decide to offer some sessions or to place the patient elsewhere, whether privately, or with a training organization, or an agency like Cruse or Relate.

A doctor with little psychological interest may be glad of a counsellor to whom to refer the 'heartsink patients', or those who specifically present with their emotional problems, but is unlikely to discern the needs of those who do not. His/her patients, however, may well appreciate the availability of a counsellor, especially if they have direct access to the counsellor's services rather than depending on the doctor for referral.

In either case the relationship between counsellor and doctor or partners is of crucial importance. If each tries to understand the way the other works and they can share and compare their views about patients, there is great scope for mutual education and stimulation, to the ultimate benefit of the whole practice. If, on the other hand, there is no meeting of minds, referrals are unlikely to be appropriate, and the consequent failures will lead to mutual recriminations.

Our own experience of having a counsellor/psychotherapist in our practice has been extremely rewarding. Apart from taking referrals from the five partners for assessment, her most valuable contribution is to facilitate a fortnightly doctors' meeting, in which we may talk about patients whom we are managing ourselves, share feedback about those we have referred, deal with 'hot' issues in the practice (such as relationships between ourselves or with members of the staff), and discuss any other problems of the moment.

THE GP AS COUNSELLOR?

I have described some of the ways in which a GP who is so inclined can use the many opportunities that daily work affords to engage with patients in a counselling mode. This may result in a single, spontaneous, prolonged consultation, a series of planned appointments of brief duration, or random encounters of varying length and at irregular intervals, where some piecemeal progress is made.

For some patients it will be simply the provision of support without much expectation of change, often over many years—a common enough situation in practice, whatever the doctor's attitude to it may be. But perhaps the doctor with a psychological bent may find it easier to avoid getting caught up with the patient who is a therapeutic 'black hole', to tolerate the frustration of the ones who refuse to get better, and to capitalize on the unexpected 'moments of change' which sometimes occur to enliven even the most intractably static relationship. (Elder and Samuel 1981).

Is there any place for the general practitioner to take on the task personally of providing counselling in a more formal sense; to offer a number of long sessions outside normal consulting hours, using standard counselling techniques and without recourse to prescriptions, certificates, or referral?

It is worth noting that in the early days of Michael Balint's work with general practitioners, there was considerable use of the 'long interview'. The doctor would see the patient for an hour at a time, maybe on several occasions, initially to take an exhaustive history to establish and clarify the diagnosis, and then to practise a kind of psychotherapy to try to help the patient achieve some resolution of the problems. (Balint and Balint 1961)

Later on however, the emphasis shifted towards trying to apply the understanding and insight which had been developed through this earlier form of work within the constraints of the ordinary surgery consultation, so that these skills might be used with any patient at any time rather than lavished on a few who had been singled out for special attention.

It was felt that the long interview was a 'foreign body' in general practice, and the 'detective inspector' model was relinquished in favour of a more intuitive and concentrated attitude of receptive listening and seeking to tune in to the patient's distress (E. Balint and Norell 1973).

In this way the doctor is aware of his/her own feelings and the effect that the patient has on them and observes what changes take place whilst the patient is allowed to dictate the pace, decide when to attend, and how to use the relationship (Elder and Samuel 1981). This remains the basis of the counselling attitude I have been describing.

Nonetheless, some Balint-trained doctors may feel disposed to carry out more intensive work with individual patients, as may other GPs who have undertaken formal training in counselling, group or family therapy, or one of the other psychotherapy disciplines.

If such work is carried on privately with patients who have a separate GP then the doctor's situation is little different from that of any other therapist in private practice. However, a number of difficulties can arise when the GP undertakes therapy with patients within his/her own practice or partnership.

First, it is virtually impossible to maintain rigid boundaries between the doctor's responsibilities as a therapist and as a GP. Even if the patient is registered with a partner, the doctor may sometimes have to provide general medical services at the surgery or at home. The physical surroundings of the consulting room emphasize this ambiguity, unless the practice is fortunate enough to have a separate room available, furnished for therapy rather than clinical activity.

Secondly, the GP may have considerable knowledge of the patient's spouse or other family members. This could create dilemmas about confidentiality and possible conflicts of loyalty, either in reality or in the patient's fantasy.

Thirdly, however experienced a therapist the doctor may be, some patients may find it difficult to accept this alternative guise, or to understand the different ground rules which apply. These include a rigid commitment to times and appointments rather than the more casual view which may prevail in the surgery setting, where patients often miss appointments, and doctors may be poor timekeepers.

The doctor also shares with the practice-employed counsellor the likely constraint that no charge may be made to the patient for therapy. This may make it more likely that the patient may miss appointments, or 'drop out' if the going gets tough. (The apparent paradox arises, of course, because of the normal contract in private practice that missed sessions have still to be paid for.)

Finally it is unlikely that a doctor in full-time practice will be able to undertake many hours of counselling within the working week, and the GP's availability may be affected by practice emergencies or a partner's illness.

Given all these problems, what is there to be said in favour of the proposition that the GP might personally do some counselling?

The principal advantages lie in his/her availability and continuity. In a crisis, especially if there is no counsellor in the practice, the GP may be best placed to offer some time without the patient having to go through a process of referral, assessment, and being put on a waiting list.

In a long-established relationship, where the doctor has already done a good deal of groundwork over months or years, an opportunity may arise to make better progress with some more intensive sessions. Afterwards there will be a return to the normal situation.

Yet another patient might be frightened of the idea of counselling therapy, but could be given an introduction to the process to prepare the way for a referral elsewhere.

The doctor's acquaintance with a patient's family can be a source of strength, provided the role of 'honest broker' is established, listening to all without betraying confidences. Where a marital or family difficulty is central to the patient's problems, the doctor may work with the couple or family, either alone or jointly with a practice counsellor if available.

There is considerable flexibility in the structure of general practice, which allows for a greater variety of possible arrangements as to the number, frequency, and duration of sessions to be offered than would be available anywhere else.

Many of the hazards for the general practitioner counsellor can be negotiated by careful selection of patients, adequate explanation, and agreement of a contract before starting out. Like other therapists, the doctor will need to be aware of personal limitations, and to seek advice and supervision, preferably from someone who understands the peculiar difficulties of the healer who wears two hats.

A PERSONAL REPORT

I have written this from my perspective as a doctor with experience of four years' Balint group training in the early 1970s, many subsequent years of leading groups, mostly for vocational trainees, and participation in a Balint research group. Both my bias in favour of Balint training and my account of the pros and cons of the GP as counsellor in the practice arise from my personal experience.

With this longstanding interest in the psychological aspects of general practice I eventually decided to undertake training in psychodynamic psychotherapy. Subsequently, I began to see patients within the practice for therapy sessions, under weekly supervision and whilst continuing in personal therapy.

I recently reviewed the work done in the first year of my dual existence, to consider the relative merits of my two forms of consulting. Inevitably, the long-session patients formed a fairly insignificant proportion of the whole.

Of 3670 consultations, 486 were for psychological problems which arose during normal surgery appointments. Of these, nearly one-third become 'long consultations' lasting 20–45 minutes. Some of these would occur where a problem came to light for the first time; others might take place in the course of treatment of a depressive illness, or following a bereavement, or during a marital crisis. Although it is disruptive to the appointment system I feel there are occasions when important work needs to be done immediately. You cannot tell a patient in tears to come back tomorrow, or cut short someone who has just found the courage to disclose a painful secret. Once this crucial matter has been dealt with, more orderly follow-up can be arranged.

During the same period I had 59 50-minute psychotherapy sessions with 11 patients, ranging from 1 to 21 sessions each. These 50-minute sessions were intended to be for patients who would be seen long term. In fact, while the system was getting into gear there were sometimes vacant slots which I used for single assessment sessions or for brief therapy. Some patients who I thought would be long term dropped out after a few sessions—one by mutual agreement, one without notice or explanation, and one to my considerable relief.

I experienced the pitfalls of trying to play two roles, and the problems of insecure boundaries and have concluded that for me the difficulties of doing therapy and practice side by side outweigh the benefits. It would be preferable to see these patients, at another time and place.

What I have found particularly valuable is to have a couple of weekly slots available for assessments or brief therapy. For the doctor with an interest in counselling this could be seen as equivalent to the partner who does a minor surgery session or an asthma clinic, enabling the doctor to pursue his/her interest and to offer an additional service to the patients without distorting his/her general contribution to the work of the practice.

REFERENCES

Balint, M. (1968). *The doctor, his patient and the illness* (revised 2nd edn). Pitman Paperbacks, London.

Balint, M. and Balint, E. (1961). *Psychotherapeutic techniques in medicine.* Tavistock Publications, London.

Balint, E. and Norell, J. (ed) (1973). *Six minutes for the patient.* Tavistock Publications, London.

Elder, A. and Samuel, O. (ed.) (1981). *While I'm here, doctor.* Tavistock Routledge, London

Freeling, P. and Tylee, A. (1992). Depression missed or mismanaged. In *Long-term treatment of depressions* (ed. S. Montgomery and F. Rouillon). John Wiley, London.

Goldberg, D. and Huxley, P. (1980). *Mental illness in the community.* Tavistock Publications, London.

Goldberg, D. and Huxley, P. (1992). *Common mental disorders.* Tavistock Routledge, London.

Goldberg D., Steele, J., Smith C., and Spivey, L. (1980). Training family doctors to recognise psychiatric illness with increased accuracy. *Lancet,* **ii**, pp. 521–3.

Paykel, E. and Priest, R. (1992). Recognition and management of depression in general practice: consensus statement. *British Medical Journal*, **305**, pp. 1198–9.
Pendleton, D., Schofield, T., Tate, P., and Havelock, P., (1984). *The consultation: and approach to learning and teaching.* Oxford University Press, Oxford.

RECOMMENDED FURTHER READING

Freeling, P. and Harris, C. (1984). *The doctor–patient relationship.* (revised 3rd edn). Churchill Livingstone, Edinburgh.
Salinsky J. (1993). *The last appointment.* The Book Guild, Sussex.

16 The client's perspective

Jane Keithley and a client

This chapter considers counselling in primary health care from the perspective of those who use the service—the clients. It will explore what is known about their views of counselling and counsellors; about the ways in which they perceive that they are helped (or not helped) by counselling; and about their perceptions of 'outcomes'. In addition, it looks at the evidence, from the clients' point of view, on the advantages and disadvantages of a counselling service being provided in a primary health care setting and on how far counselling in this setting is likely to be 'different'.

The chapter is divided into two parts. The first draws on the published literature as well as some unpublished research on the client's perspective. The second is a personal viewpoint, written by a client, from her own experience of receiving counselling on two separate occasions.

STUDYING CLIENT VIEWS

Introduction

It is still true that relatively few studies have explored the experience and views of the users of counselling services, whether these are provided by psychologists, community psychiatric nurses, counsellors in private practice or working for a voluntary organisation such as Relate, or any other professional. However, over the last 15 years or so, there has been more interest in and acceptance of the value of such information (Llewelyn 1988). For example, the National Marriage Guidance Council (now called Relate) supported a follow-up study of clients in the early 1980s (Hunt 1985). Increasing emphasis on the need for and value of user views in planning and auditing health and social care services, reflected in policy documents such as *Working for patients* (HMSO 1989) and *Caring for people* (HMSO 1989) strengthen the case for paying more attention to the voices of counselling clients.

The relative paucity of such work seems to reflect a number of concerns. First, there is seen to be an ethical dilemma in following-up counselled clients, associated with a strict ethos of confidentiality:

It seemed like an invasion of privacy, a breach of confidentiality, and was seen as contrary to the principles of counselling which include respecting a person and not using him or her.

(Hunt 1985)

The opposite case can, of course, be put. Is it ethical **not** to take account of client views, in the context of a service which places so much emphasis on being 'client centred'? However, there are undoubtedly sensitive issues for researchers and practitioners to consider when seeking out and questioning individuals about what could well have been a very painful time for them, about a service which involved them in discussion of very personal matters and which they may not have admitted to others that they have approached.

Secondly, there has been some scepticism about the reliability and validity of client reports. Marsh and Kaim-Caudle discussed this in relation to patient satisfaction in general practice:

A dissatisfied patient of one doctor may have received better care than the satisfied patient of the same or another doctor.

(Marsh and Kaim-Caudle)

Clients (like researchers!) are likely to have difficulty in assessing the contribution of counselling to their improved or worsened state of health, well-being, or circumstances, compared to the contribution of all the other things that are likely to have happened to them over the same time. Their memory is likely to be selective and subsequent experiences can lead them to re-formulate the past in ways which 'make sense' in the light of their present circumstances. (Gurman 1973; Hunt 1985).

Thirdly, it has been argued that counsellors themselves are reluctant to engage in studies of the 'outcomes' of their work, including those which seek client views, on the grounds that it is impossible to develop measurable criteria of the effectiveness of counselling and even that to attempt this would conflict with the model of counselling as a non-directive activity, where the aims are unique to the client and to be decided by her/him (Keithley 1982; Timms and Blampied 1980).

The uniqueness of counselling may make generalizable analysis difficult, but strengthens the case for seeking client views. This is even more so, given that there is some evidence that the perspectives of clients and counsellors on the process and the outcomes of counselling can differ (Keithley 1982; Llewelyn 1988).

To sum up, client views are an important element in assessing the success or otherwise of a service which aims to enhance the individual's understanding, personal growth, and capacity for self-determination. In addition, publicly provided health care services are increasingly expected to justify and provide evidence of their effectiveness through auditing of process and outcomes which includes user views. If counselling is to be an accepted part of those services, it needs to participate fully in these activities.

Clients and counselling in primary health care

This section considers the client's perspective on the inclusion of counselling among the range of services provided within a primary health care team. It draws heavily, though not exclusively, on research carried out by the author on a service provided by National Marriage Guidance Council (now Relate) trained counsellors in a general practice in Norton, Stockton-on-Tees in the late 1970s. Despite the age of the data, it still reflects the questions that are being asked about the attitudes of clients to counselling in this setting. The major changes since that time are the expansion in the number and diversity of counsellors practising in this setting (Sibbald *et al.* 1993 found 31 per cent of their sample of 1542 practices in England and Wales had a counsellor) and the increased awareness of GPs and others in the NHS of costs and of the need to justify service provision in cost-effectiveness terms.

From the client's point of view, there are obvious reasons for locating counsellors in the primary health care team. Many people already 'medical-ize' (perhaps inappropriately) their emotional and relationship problems. It is estimated that between 10 per cent and 30 per cent of consulting patients have mainly emotional problems (Gray 1988). Thomas (1993) found that over half of a sample of people coming to see their GP said they had felt the need to talk to an 'independent' counsellor about a problem at some time during the previous three years. Most people who experience marital breakdown consult their GP at some time (Chester 1971; Hart 1976). Open, free, and non-stigmatized access, the high respect in which GPs are held and cultural expectations about how best to tackle such problems all contribute to people being more likely to approach their doctor than any other professional. Similar arguments apply in respect of other members of the primary health care team. The almost universal coverage of the population and the broad-ranging services involved in the continuing care of a practice population mean they are likely to be aware of many of the problems and life changes of individual patients. Having a counsellor as part of the team can also sensitize other members to the emotional problems which may lie behind some patients' somatic symptoms.

Elsewhere in this book (Chapters 3 and 16) it is suggested that even if GPs have the expertise, it may be preferable to encourage patients to seek specialist help from someone else. Most evidently, the 'ten-minute consultation' offers little scope for the exploration of complex circum-stances and feelings, compared with the hour-long appointments usually offered by a counsellor. It may also be difficult for 'patients' to become 'clients', presenting medical issues (which the GP as 'expert' is expected to investigate, diagnose, and treat) and emotional difficulties (for which a very different counselling response is appropriate) to the same person in the same context (Cocksedge 1989).

Other advantages can accrue if the specialist counsellor is clearly a member of the primary health care team. Clients may be more confident that different aspects of their care are fully co-ordinated. It may be easier for individuals to seek counselling help once a trusted nurse or GP has explained something of what is involved and has made a definite recommendation or referral. Locating the counsellor on practice premises means that counselling takes place in surroundings which are familiar to those referred to him/her. These premises are also likely to be fairly geographically convenient and to house a wide range of services. They are not clearly labelled as specifically for those with relationship or emotional problems, so avoiding any possible stigma or embarassment.

Of the 82 clients interviewed for the Norton study, 78 supported the provision of a counselling service in general practice, including quite a number who had not personally found it helpful. By far the most frequently mentioned advantage was the link between GP and counsellor, which was seen by most clients as both relevant and of value. They also talked about the convenience and reassurance of receiving counselling in the familiar, accessible, and pleasant surroundings of the practice (a factor which may not, of course, apply to the same extent in all practice premises). About one-quarter also spontaneously mentioned the anonymity and lack of stigma in attending counselling at the surgery (Keithley 1982). Another advantage sometimes mentioned (for example Thomas 1993) is that the service is free, whereas there is often a charge for counselling in other settings. However, this is not always the case, as funding of the service depends on local arrangements. Charging for counselling in the context of an NHS service which is largely 'free' can raise issues for the counsellor, the PHCT, and the clients.

However, the Norton clients also voiced some of the reservations which have been expressed about counselling in this setting. These are, in some respects, an alternative interpretation of the features which are seen as advantages. For instance, referral to a known and trusted counsellor is also likely to mean a restriction of choice for the prospective client. A general practice may offer anonymity in the sense of not being identified solely with one service, but in other ways, the proximity to the clients' homes and the increased likelihood of meeting people they know threaten anonymity. Opportunities for professionals to collaborate and co-operate in caring for people could be seen by individuals as a threat to the confidentiality of the information they impart, or as meaning that a breakdown in their relationship with one professional makes it difficult for them to make a 'fresh start' with another. In the Norton study, however, it is important to note that it was doctors and counsellors who were most concerned about confidentiality. Clients were much more likely to view the sharing of information between GP and counsellor as a matter of course and as a positive benefit. Only one of those interviewed mentioned confidentiality and even he said that it was not something which had personally worried him (Keithley 1982).

It has been suggested that if clients come to counselling because it is 'prescribed' by their doctor or another primary health care team member, they may lack motivation or even feel resentful at being 'passed on' (Heisler 1979). All the GPs interviewed in the Norton study admitted to engaging in some fairly active persuasion of initially reluctant clients. On the other hand, of the clients interviewed, only four or five indicated that they felt 'fobbed-off' by their GP. However, a much larger number (26 out of the 67 referred by a GP) reacted negatively to the idea of counselling, mostly because they were pessimistic about what might be achieved, and 22 had mixed feelings. These are all people who did eventually agree to see the counsellor (Keithley 1982). A particularly pertinent question for GPs and other team members is how far it is worthwhile persuading initially reluctant individuals to seek counselling. The answer appears to be that it is. There was some indication of a relationship between initial reactions and how helpful the individual eventually found counselling to be. However, nearly half of the 'reluctant' clients reported substantial and lasting help, and approaching three-quarters reported deriving some benefit (Keithley 1982).

It is unlikely that many of these would have approached a counsellor outside the surgery setting. This and other studies have suggested that many clients of counsellors in general practices would not have sought counselling elsewhere (Waydenfeld 1980) or known how and where to find a good counsellor.

It has also been suggested that having a counsellor as part of the practice team can enable GPs and other team members to act as a filter: to ensure referrals are appropriate and to prepare individuals for their initial encounter with counselling by ensuring that they have realistic and accurate expectations (Marsh and Barr 1975; Waydenfeld 1978). However, the accounts by the Norton clients of their referrals did not suggest that the GPs in that practice, with the possible exception of one, were performing a particularly active filtering function. There seemed to have been a widespread lack of explanation of who the counsellor was, or what he/she may be able to do (Keithley 1982).

Clients on counselling: process and outcomes

There are a number of studies which have asked clients to describe their experience of counselling in a general setting, their satisfaction with the service, and their assessment of the outcomes.

In general, reported levels of satisfaction and helpfulness are very high. Waydenfeld and Waydenfeld (1980) in their study of counselling in nine general practices, found that almost all of the 47 clients who returned questionnaires had found counselling to be at least of some help to them, would seek counselling in this setting again, and would recommend it to others. Similar responses were reported by Anderson and Hasler (1979) and Martin and Mitchell (1983).

Hunt (1985) asked the clients of counsellors working in Marriage Guidance Council centres about their views on the counselling they had received. Her respondents seemed a little less enthusiastic. Nearly half of the 51 clients said they were satisfied with the service, one-quarter had mixed feelings, and one-quarter were dissatisfied. Nearly half reported that they had derived some benefits from the counselling.

There is also some evidence of higher levels of client satisfaction with counselling services than with alternative ways of responding to problems brought to the GP. The Edinburgh primary care depression study found that counselling was evaluated more positively by patients, in terms of meeting needs and helping with problems, than drug therapy prescribed by a psychiatrist, cognitive behaviour therapy from a clinical psychologist, or routine care by a GP. It was also the only form of treatment which more than a small minority of patients would definitely want again should they become depressed in the future. However, it should be noted that this counselling costs about four times as much as routine GP care and the study found no evidence of greater clinical efficacy (Scott *et al.* 1992). In addition, care must be taken in reading too much into the varying, but often high levels of satisfaction found in many studies. Different studies are likely to ask questions which produce rather different patterns of responses. In addition, most such studies have a response rate well below 100 per cent and it could well be that non-respondents would have different accounts of their experiences.

The Norton study was no different. Of 149 people approached, 83 were eventually interviewed. However, this group was very diverse, including men and women, people of different ages and marital status, from a range of social class backgrounds, and whose contact with the counsellor ranged from one interview to more than twenty (Keithley 1982). The research looked in detail at client views of their counselling and uncovered a complex picture.

When clients were asked the question: 'Did counselling help you at all?', just over half (55 per cent) gave an unequivocally positive response, about one-quarter expressed mixed feelings, and one-fifth said that it had not (Keithley 1982). However, when they were asked to expand on this initial response, it was found that clients expressed a complex mixture of feelings, which was very inadequately conveyed, if at all, by a unilinear concept of helpfulness—unhelpfulness. Most expressed some reservations and most described some positive aspects. In some cases, the initial response was actually misleading. This suggests that practitioners who wish to seek the views of individual service users in order to make the services offered more sensitive to their expressed needs and preferences, or to make it clearer to potential users what they can or cannot expect the service to provide, would do well to adopt an in-depth, qualitative approach rather than rely on simple answers to simple questions.

The principal sources of clients' dissatisfaction with counselling were that it failed to have any impact on their problems, or that it was an inadequate or inappropriate type of help. Some of the clients found it difficult to see how 'just talking' could help them and were disappointed at the lack of 'expert advice' or 'practical help'. Others reported that any benefits there were tended to wear off over time. It may be that some of these felt a need for periodic 'booster' counselling sessions; an option which, it should be made clear to such clients, is of course open to them (Keithley 1982).

The principal sources of satisfaction were firstly that counselling offered a chance to talk to someone, who was impartial, an outsider, with professional expertise and personal qualities which were admired and who could offer a guaranteed and substantial period of uninterrupted time. In common with other studies, it was clear that personal liking for the counsellor is important, though not sufficient for 'successful' counselling as perceived by clients. Indeed, Hunt suggests that the most significant factor in determining the effectiveness of counselling, whether clients felt satisfied and whether they felt helped, was how both counsellor and client felt they had 'got on' together and the degree of rapport, understanding, trust, respect, and goodwill they had for each other (Hunt 1985).

The other reasons for finding counselling most helpful cited by the Norton clients included that it increased their understanding of themselves, of other people, and of their problems; it improved their marital and other relationships; and it helped them as individuals.

Of the 83 clients interviewed, 45 also specified improvements in their health, although some expressed this improvement in very general statements such as, 'it made me feel better'. All of these talked about improvements in their mental health: they felt less depressed, less tense, more relaxed and at ease, or less anxious about their health (Keithley 1982). The value and validity of these comments should not be in doubt. However, those who look to them as evidence of potential savings to the health services should beware. The Norton study, despite the fact that the GPs had the impression that the counselling service reduced the consultation and medication rates of many of those who were referred, found little concrete evidence to support this when the medical casenotes of the 33 clients referred by one of the GPs were examined. In nearly three-quarters of cases, there was no apparent impact on either consultation or prescription rates and, in some of these, the rates actually rose following referral (Keithley 1982). Other studies have been more optimistic (for example, Waydenfeld 1980), but a recent editorial in the *British Medical Journal* drew fairly pessimistic conclusions from a summary of the evidence (Pringle and Laverty 1993). Other chapters in this book address the complexities of evaluation and the assessment of 'value for money' in this field (Chapters 3 and 17).

In the Norton study, counsellors and GPs were also asked to assess the helpfulness of counselling to individual clients. Their responses were less detailed than those of the clients. Nonetheless, overall, the proportions who rated the counselling as helpful, who expressed mixed feelings, or who rated it unhelpful, were quite similar. However, this apparently high level of agreement broke down when responses relating to individual clients were considered. In the case of 44 (nearly three-fifths) of the 74 clients for whom comparison was possible, there was some disparity, and in the case of 17 this disparity was marked. There did not seem to be any pattern, in the sense that one group was more or less likely to rate the counselling favourably, or that disparities were particularly associated with a particular type of client (Keithley 1982).

In addition, disparities also emerged in a comparison of the reasons that counsellors and clients gave for describing counselling as helpful or not helpful. Where counselling was not felt to be helpful, perhaps unsurprisingly, clients tended to point to the inadequacies of counselling in relation to their situation, whereas counsellors concentrated on the inappropriate expectations of clients and their inability to 'use' counselling. Many clients seemed to value highly a kind of help that would be seen by the counsellors as something less than 'real' counselling. The benefits most frequently mentioned by clients were 'someone to talk to' and 'feeling better'. Counsellors, on the other had, mentioned these relatively infrequently, instead emphasizing 'increased understanding' and 'helping the client as an individual' (Keithley 1982). This tendency for clients to specify more simple forms of help, perhaps requiring less professional expertise, than do counsellors has been found in other studies, and Llewellyn (1988), in a study of psychological therapy, argues cogently that this reflects a 'real' difference in the degree of importance and relevance for clients and therapists of different aspects of the therapeutic process, rather than different ways of talking about the same aspects.

This, as well as the disparities in perceived helpfulness, strengthens the arguments for ensuring that client views are represented in assessments of counselling services. Of course, these disparities also raise complex issues about how to interpret them and whether the views of professionals and 'experts' are to be considered as more valid than those of service-users, or vice-versa, especially if the aim is to draw implications for policy developments.

A PERSONAL ACCOUNT

As a Community Development Worker, I am very aware of the need for counselling services. The subject has been an issue of concern for many years as the lack of such services, free at the point of delivery, generates a number of difficulties, not only for community development staff, but for a wide range of people employed in areas of disadvantage. The gap between provision and demand results in many such workers taking on a quasi-counselling role in relation to the people with whom they come into contact on a daily basis. This often creates anxiety for workers who feel they do not have the appropriate skills and training, yet the demand exists and the provision does not—there are few places to which people in need can be referred. The concept of developing counselling services within GP practices is welcome as a means of going some way towards meeting that need.

However, it is as a recipient of counselling that I now share my experiences. These experiences do not, perhaps, fit neatly into the overall context of this book, as in one instance I was referred by my GP to a counselling service separate from his practice and in the other I referred myself to a counsellor based within a practice of which I was not a patient. These two experiences took place within a time span of eighteen years, for different reasons and in different circumstances.

The first was in 1974 when I was in the final year of a degree course at a polytechnic a hundred miles from home. Within the space of six months, three members of my family (all in their own ways very important to me) had died and a long-term relationship had ended. The black clouds of depression gathered over my head and I would find myself, for no apparent reason, washed by feelings of misery and hopelessness. My concentration went, my work was suffering, I was overwhelmed by feelings of anxiety about my parents—I was convinced that they too would die and rang them every day just to make sure they were still alive. I didn't seem to be able to **do** anything and there seemed little point in continuing my own existence when I couldn't work and everyone I cared about was leaving me. Physically, I felt permanently 'unwell'—I had one cold after another and even my bones felt tired.

I decided to visit the students' doctor, there had to be something he could give me to stop me feeling so ill! I recounted my physical symptoms and somehow (I don't remember how) ended up telling him of the recent events in my life and how I was feeling. He suggested that the two things were related and instead of giving me the antibiotics I had expected, he prescribed a one-month supply of antidepressants, telling me to come back when I had finished the bottle. He told me that they would 'calm me down' and enable me to get on with my work. He didn't, mention any side effects but he did stress that it was only a month's supply so I needn't worry about taking them.

The primary effect of the drug was to make me sleep, which I did with complete disregard for where I was (I even fell asleep in a nightclub once!). With hindsight, I can recognize the beneficial effects of so much sleep and I certainly felt distanced from my anxieties, but my concentration was worse, not better, and I still could not work. By the end of the month I still felt tired and ill and I did not feel any more able to cope with completing my degree.

On my return visit to the doctor, he spent slightly longer listening to how I felt and said that he would not give me another prescription but that I should go and see the students' counsellor and talk to her. He did not offer to make the appointment for me, but told me how to go about doing it. I had very mixed feelings about his response. Whilst I was unimpressed by the effect of the antidepressants and unsure about taking any other drugs (I knew about addiction), I was also wary of going to see a counsellor. Other students, who were known to be seeing the counsellor, were felt by 'the rest of us' to be the inadequate ones, the ones who couldn't cope, the ones who had 'cracked up'. These were not labels I would readily apply to myself, however accurate they might be. I feel that the need to be seen to be 'coping' is particularly relevant within an academic environment where there is an underlying atmosphere of competition and the 'fear of failure' abounds.

Needless to say, I did not rush off and make an appointment with the counselling service. I dithered and pondered and felt myself lapsing into the state of high anxiety which had taken me to the doctor in the first place. Eventually, in desperation, I made the appointment via the student union office. This in itself was a difficult task as I felt that everyone would know what I was doing, a feeling which was reinforced by the location of the counsellor's office. It was situated in a corridor nowhere near the medical centre, the door was clearly labelled, there was nowhere to hide—if you were in that area, the chances were that you were seeing the counsellor. By now, I felt too ill and desperate to care.

Given the anxiety surrounding the process, visiting the counsellor was in reality a very positive experience. I saw the counsellor over a period of about three months for an hour a week. We talked through the issues which confront anyone who has suffered a bereavement and she helped me to find ways of getting back to work. It felt good to be able to unload my problems on to someone who clearly understood how I felt and who didn't seem to mind when I spent a large part of some sessions in floods of tears. Physically, I felt much better—less prone to coughs, colds, headaches, and cold sores and much less 'weary'. Mentally, I gradually began to feel much more capable of dealing with things myself and developed a much more positive perspective on life . . . and death.

It was several months before I felt really well, in fact it was not until after I had left the polytechnic and had started a job. However, I feel that this episode of counselling was definitely beneficial in the long term. For example, a couple of years later there were two more deaths in the family—I felt much more able to deal with that situation and although I grieved, this was a positive process not a disabling one. I also felt more confident about making relationships with people—I had a much more philosophical outlook, valuing what I had rather than fearing loss. The experience was also valuable when I later became a community development worker as I could use the insights I had gained through counselling in my work with people in disadvantaged communities.

My second experience of counselling again took place whilst I was a student in higher education. It is tempting to suggest that education seems to be bad for my health, but death does not acknowledge term dates and, on the second occasion, being a student was the least of my problems. These were a result of a combination of several factors including an accumulation of stress built up during my previous employment, the grieving process associated with leaving that work behind, and relationship difficulties rooted in childhood experiences. Other than severely disrupted sleep patterns, I had no obvious physical symptoms to focus on this time around. Instead I was beset by feelings of guilt, failure, and confusion.

Probably the key difference in my approach to this situation was that I clearly recognized that my problems could not be solved by the medical profession directly. My reluctance to take drugs had increased over the years and my own experience (both at work and personally) told me that what I needed was counselling. Whilst being reluctant to admit that I could not 'be my own counsellor' (at least on this occasion), I was also aware that it might be difficult to get access to appropriate sources of help. My own GP practice does not offer a counselling service and I was, in any case, very wary of 'entrusting my psyche' to just anyone.

There is a free counselling service available to students at the academic institution I was attending and, having found out a little about it, I attempted to make an appointment. The process of trying to do so proved to be a very negative experience and I 'retired hurt', reflecting that had I been a young undergraduate, I might have felt even worse. Fortunately, a friend and former colleague is a counsellor and I sought her advice as to where I could find a reliable source of help. She suggested that I contact a counsellor that she knew and trusted, who worked in a medical centre in a nearby town. I was rather anxious about the ethics of using a service intended for other people but she reassured me, pointing out that as I was not registered with the practice, I would have to pay for each session. As an impecunious student this could have caused some problems, but I had support from a number of sources which enabled me to pay my way.

Making the appointment was straightforward and my first visit to the practice felt very comfortable even though I was on unfamiliar territory. I reported to the desk just like any other 'patient', sat with everyone else in the waiting room and was collected by the counsellor after a short wait. It all felt very simple—there was no feeling of being particularly identifiable and the atmosphere in the medical centre was very relaxed.

For the first five weeks I saw the counsellor for one hour a week, then five sessions at fortnightly intervals over a period of three months. This was followed by a gap of one month as, at the time of writing, we are in the process of tying up loose ends. I would envisage that only one or two more sessions will be necessary to complete the process.

I have found this process extremely useful, as the issues which came up were of a much more overtly 'psychological' nature and required a different approach from myself and the counsellor. For most people, bereavement tends to occur in adulthood and to be a relatively isolated event. The issues this time around were the result of repeated events spread over a number of years. My own levels of knowledge and self-awareness had developed a great deal in the preceding eighteen years but I did acquire new insights that I feel will be of long-term benefit. It is difficult to evaluate precisely what those benefits are at this stage. However, even in the short term, I have shifted from a situation where I was incapacitated by my mental state, to one where I can face the future not only with equanimity but with a reasonable degree of confidence.

In comparing the two experiences, it is important to acknowledge the differences in my age, experience, outlook, and the different nature of the problems I experienced. The most difficult step to take in approaching a counsellor is the first one, that is making an appointment. Back in 1974, it was that process, and the location of the counselling service, that deterred me from making an appointment until I was desperate. In 1992, that process deterred me from making use of the free service available to students altogether. The location of the counselling service within the medical centre made the process much easier—it felt no more difficult than making an appointment to see a doctor or nurse. I believe that it is essential to create an atmosphere which makes it feel easy for people to make an appointment to see a counsellor. The medical centre felt welcoming, comfortable, anonymous, and safe.

As an extremely infrequent user of primary health care services, it was not the familiarity of visiting my own doctor that eased the process. It was rather that going to the doctor is, in itself, an acceptable thing to do—no one expects to be told why you are there and, in a busy medical centre, there are lots of people that you could be there to see.

A second potential barrier to access is finance. In the first instance, the counselling service was free to students of the polytechnic and finance was not, therefore, a consideration. In the second instance, I was deterred from using the free service available to me as a student by the poor experience that I had in trying to make an appointment. It is possible that if I had been unable to identify an alternative, I would have been forced by need (as I had been in the past) to overcome my reluctance and use that service. I was fortunate in being able to draw on support from other people to avoid that necessity. Had I been a patient of the practice concerned or had my own practice offered a counselling service, then this potential barrier would probably not have existed.

A third potential barrier to access is information. I know that my own GP practice does not offer such a service, not by being a patient, but by being a community worker who is required to be familiar with the services available to local residents. As previously mentioned, I visit my GP extremely infrequently and I would not necessarily know whether counselling services were available. My awareness of my own mental state enabled me to identify what service I felt I needed and an approach to the medical profession was not an obvious choice. Other people who do not visit their doctors regularly may be unaware of precisely what services are provided at their practice. It is important that the availability of a counselling service, including a brief explanation of how it can help, is widely publicized. Many practices now produce brochures that tell patients what is available, but unless such information is mailed out it will still only be available to people who go to the surgery. However, with the recent rise in preventative primary health care and, especially, well-person clinics, a larger proportion of the practice population should become familiar with their GPs surgery.

To sum up, from the perspective of being a service user and as a community development worker, I feel there are certain key issues which should be taken into account when considering the provision of counselling services:

1. People in need require assistance and support in recognizing the source of their problems and in overcoming any prejudices they may have about the counselling process.
2. Making an appointment with a counsellor should be as 'matter of fact' as making any other appointment.
3. Counselling services should be free at the point of use, particularly for people in disadvantaged communities. Those of us who are fortunate enough to be able to pay are likely to have fewer difficulties in gaining access to the services we need.
4. People must be given information about the availability of counselling services—it cannot be assumed that every patient of every practice knows what is available.
5. The attitudes and behaviour of all the staff concerned in the provision of counselling services are paramount in making the service accessible.

REFERENCES

Anderson, S. and Hasler, J. (1979). Counselling in general practice, *Journal of the Royal College of General Practitioners*, **29**, 352–6.
Cocksedge, S. (1989). GPs should not counsel long-term. *Journal of the Royal College of General Practitioners*, **39**, 347.

Chester, R. (1971). Health and marriage breakdown: experience of a sample of divorced women, *British Journal of Preventive and Social Medicine*, **25**, 231–5.

Gray, P. (1988). Counsellors in general practice. *Journal of the Royal College of General Practitioners*, **38**, 50–1.

Gurman, A. (1973). The effects and effectiveness of marital therapy: a review of outcome research. *Family Process*, **22**, 145–70.

Hart, N. (1976). *When marriage ends*. Tavistock, London.

Heisler, J. (1979). Marriage counsellors in medical settings, *Marriage Guidance*, March, 153–62.

Hunt, P. (1985). *Clients' responses to marriage counselling*, Research Report No.3, National Marriage Guidance Council, Rugby.

Keithley, J. (1982). *Marriage counselling in general practice* PhD thesis (unpublished), University of Durham.

Llewelyn, S. (1988). Psychological therapy as viewed by clients and therapists, *British Journal of Clinical Psychology*, **27**, 233–7.

Marsh, G. and Barr, J. (1975). Marriage guidance counselling at a group practice centre. *Journal of the Royal College of General Practitioners*, **25**, 73–5.

Marsh, G. and Kaim-Caudle, P. (1976). *Team care in general practice*. Croom Helm, London.

Martin, E. and Mitchell, H. (1983). A counsellor in general practice: a one-year survey. *Journey of the Royal College of General Practitioners*, **33**, 366–7.

Pringle, M. and Laverty, J. (1993). A counsellor in every practive? *British Medical Journal*, **306**, 2–3.

Scott, A. and Freeman, C. (1992). Edinburgh Primary Care Depression Study: treatment outcome, patient satisfaction, and cost after 16 weeks. *British Medical Journal*, **304**, 883–7.

Sibbald, B., Addington-Hall, J., Brenneman, D., and Freeling, P. (1993). Counsellors in English and Welsh general practices: their nature and distribution. *British Medical Journal*, **3306**, 29–33.

Secretaries of State for Health (1989*a*) *Working for patients*. HMSO, London.

Secretaries of State for Health (1989*b*) *Caring for people*. HMSO, London.

Thomas, P. (1993). An exploration of patients' perceptions of counselling with particular reference to counselling within general practice. *Counselling*, February, 24–30.

Timms, N. and Blampied, A. (1980). *Formal friendship: an exploratory study of marital counselling clients and their counsellors*. University of Newcastle, Department of Social Work Studies.

Waydenfeld, D. and Waydenfeld, S. (1978). *Counselling in the general practice setting*. North London Marriage Guidance Council.

Waydenfeld, D. and Waydenfeld, S. (1980). Counselling in general practice. *Journal of the Royal College of General Practitioners*, **30**, 671–7.

17 The researcher's perspective

Roslyn Corney

INTRODUCTION

In a time of limited resources, it is important that the addition of any member to the primary care team is carefully assessed and evaluated. Counsellors in general practice may find that their work is particularly under scrutiny as there are few visible signs of what has gone on in a counselling session and counsellors may find it difficult to give a full explanation of what they do. This is linked with the confusion that arises from understanding the difference between the individual work undertaken by counsellors and the supportive and listening skills that all practitioners in primary care should use in their daily work (see Chapter 1 for a discussion of counselling and counselling skills).

Services can be evaluated by examining the input, throughout, and output of a service (for example information on referral and who is referred, information on the type of work carried out, and information on closure). In addition, any evaluation should also examine outcome—whether the service actually improved the health or well-being of the patient or client. While both types of evaluation are necessary to measure the effectiveness and efficiency of a service, the measurement of outcome is much less frequently carried out in all branches of medicine. For example, surgeons and hospital managers may collect information on waiting lists and the number of operations carried out, but may find it difficult to give figures on how many patients still continued to feel better one year after the operation or even how many had died.

The same is true in terms of researching counselling. It is relatively easy to measure the setting up of a counselling placement, but much more difficult to investigate outcome and prove (or disprove) that counselling 'works'. Unfortunately, both types of evaluation are necessary if we are to answer some of the more important questions, such as whether we are making the best use of the resources available for the treatment of emotional problems and distress.

The researcher into counselling has additional problems. Unlike the evaluation of a drug or a surgical procedure, it is difficult to measure and assess the quality of the counselling. How much better is the qualified counsellor with years of training than a sensitive individual with a few days of training? The type of 'counselling' needed is also likely to vary with the individual. With some distressed individuals, a brief session with a known

GP or health visitor may be more appropriate than a longer period with a counsellor.

This chapter describes some of the methods used to evaluate counselling in general practice, ranging from simple methods that can be used by clinicians to more complex methodologies that would need some input from researchers. It is important to remember, however, that we are at an early stage in refining these methods and the types of instrumentation used. While this can be frustrating, it also means that there is still much work to be done, with clinicians and researchers both having major roles in future development.

EVALUATING COUNSELLING IN GENERAL PRACTICE

Assessing the service

The investigation of what actually happens when a counsellor is employed or attached to a general practice is relatively straightforward as an area of research. Details such as which patient turns up for counselling and which patients were perceived as having been helped will become the basis of making a more objective assessment of the value of the attachment, rather than relying solely on subjective opinions and attitudes. A number of studies of referrals have been reported in the literature which give guidelines on the type of information to collect (Anderson and Hasler 1979; Cohen 1977; Marsh and Barr 1975; Martin and Mitchel 1983; Martin and Martin 1985; Meacher 1977; Waydenfeld and Waydenfeld 1980).

These limited evaluations may be particularly worthwhile as they can aid future decisions regarding the best way to use the counsellor's limited time in the surgery. For example, an evaluation may discover that the consultative role of the counsellor (giving other team members support or advice regarding their patients) is as valuable as the counsellor seeing clients directly. Alternatively, an evaluation can suggest that running a group for clients (for example, a support group for those wishing to withdraw from tranquillizers) is more cost effective than seeing patients individually. Assessments may also yield information on the types of patients who seem to benefit most from seeing a counsellor, as well as those who find it difficult to accept this type of help.

This information can be collected by counsellors filling up forms on daily activity, when patients are referred, and on closure of the case.

Studies can focus on:

1. The roles of the counsellor in general practice—such as individual work with patients, group work, advising, educating, or supporting other team members.

2. The type of patients referred—their characteristics, their health status, and their emotional and social problems. The characteristics of these patients can also be compared with those of patients referred to psychiatrists or psychologists, thus examining the referral process.
3. The number of interviews conducted and the length of time patients are seen. Further details can be obtained on what determines how much work is done with each patient. Is it dependent on the counsellor, GP, or client preference?
4. How acceptable is counselling to those that are referred? How many miss appointments, fail to turn up, or refuse to be referred in the first place? (The latter information would need to be collected by the referral agent.)

Effects on other team members

Ideally, any study should also evaluate the other effects of having a counsellor based in the practice in addition to changes in the actual patients referred. For example, a counsellor may increase the sensitivity of other team members to psychological problems and help them feel more confident in managing some of these problems.

In order to obtain any measures of changes in the attitudes of members of the team towards counselling and counsellors it is important to carry out the initial assessment prior to the start of the attachment. A second assessment can be obtained at a reasonable period after the beginning of the placement. These assessments can be collected by questionnaire, interview, or by group discussion (Ashurst and Ward 1983; Meacher 1977).

Some investigators have also asked random samples of patients their views of the value of having a counsellor in the practice. The results overwhelmingly suggest that patients regard it as beneficial and are generally in favour of self-referral as well as referral from members of the primary care team.

Subjective assessments of outcome

Subjective estimates of the outcome of counselling can be obtained by asking other involved team members (for example, the referral agent) to fill in a short form giving their opinion of any improvement or changes they have perceived in the client either during counselling or in the period afterwards.

Clients seen by the counsellor can be asked to give their views of whether the counselling helped. These views can be assessed by independent researchers interviewing the clients or by sending postal questionnaires. Clients' views can be important and valid sources of feedback and yield tentative information on which clients benefited most from counselling. They may also be helpful in clarifying which therapeutic methods are more acceptable to clients and which types of treatment benefit which problems most. Client feedback may also include other questions to evaluate the service, such as satisfaction with access, hours, waiting lists, reception procedures, concerns over confidentiality, etc. Obtaining clients' views is problematic, however. They are not definitive evidence of outcome, as clients do not know what would have happened if they had not seen a counsellor. In addition, most surveys of client satisfaction in general practice have found consistently high levels. These levels may be more a measure of expectations, in that those with low expectations are likely to be happy with any extra help or time given. By contrast, there may be some clients who will never be satisfied whatever help is received. The majority of patients may also be fearful of displeasing their doctor (or the counsellor) by admitting to any dissatisfaction with the services provided. It is, therefore, crucial that complete confidentiality is assured.

Qualitative research

Many researchers and clinicians consider that the use of clinical trial methodology is inappropriate for the study of counselling. They would argue for the use of qualitative 'in depth' studies. Video or tape recording of the counselling sessions may be undertaken, supplemented by the counsellor making detailed notes after each interview. This could include the client's and the counsellor's perceptions of the problems presented, the plan of action, and whether this was agreed with the client, as well as the client's motivation to be helped. After cessation of counselling, details can be collected on the counsellor's perception of whether the client was helped, details of the therapy, and any arrangements made for future involvement.

Targets can also be set by counsellor and client on appropriate goals, and assessments made during and after counselling on whether these targets are reached. In addition, detailed interviews conducted with the client and important others (for example relatives, carers, the GP, etc.) on their perceptions of improvement (including the targets) and the help received will shed further light on the process from all concerned.

Another similar method of evaluation is by the counsellor performing single case-control studies. In these studies the individual client acts as his/her own control, thus a period before counselling is compared with the period after counselling. These types of studies are commonly conducted by psychologists and behaviour therapists who obtain baseline ratings on symptoms over a period of time and then chart these ratings over the period of contact and again at a follow-up session some weeks or months later. While this is a fairly simple task with some disorders, for example, phobias or anxieties, it is much more difficult with more complex problems including family and interpersonal situations. These types of studies are also more appropriate when a problem solving approach is adopted, with the therapist and client deciding on priority areas which need to be tackled.

Qualitative work or detailed analyses of consultations could also be used to examine whether counselling attachments have altered the behaviour of GPs or other members of the primary care team. Investigations could consider whether their skills of detection and management of psychosocial problems have changed since the counsellor attachment was set up. The techniques used to measures these changes have been developed by Gask and colleagues (1987).

Rates of utilization of medical services and cost-effectiveness

Reductions in medical service utilization and in psychotropic drug prescriptions have also been used to indicate that counselling has been of value in improving the client's health. Thus it is assumed that individuals have improved because they are visiting the doctor less or taking fewer drugs. However, caution does need to be exercised. Doctors may use counselling as an alternative to a psychotropic drug prescription and this may explain the reduction in drug prescription rather than the client getting better. In addition, a reduction in GP attendances may not always be positive. In some clients, ongoing medical contact for physical ailments may be important, and, in some cases, counsellors who are concerned about their client's health may suggest that the client contacts their doctor. It is also likely that there will be fewer visits in the period after a referral than the period before it. Patients are normally referred at a crisis point in their lives when attendances are more likely to be frequent.

Medical service utilization rates are also used to evaluate whether employing a counsellor is cost-effective. One argument in favour of placing a counsellor in the practice is that it may reduce the numbers of times the client visits the doctor or uses other health care services. This off-sets some of the costs of the counsellor. For each client referred to the counsellor, a set time period before counselling is compared to a similar time period during and after cessation of counselling. Thus details of numbers of attendances, prescriptions written, and referrals made to other agencies are collected from the medical notes or by placing special cards in the notes on referral. With the arrival of GP fundholding, it will be easier to determine actual costs in those practices taking part in this initiative.

Many studies have indeed shown a reduction in visits made to the doctor (Marsh and Barr 1975; Waydenfeld and Waydenfeld 1980) after cessation of counselling in contrast with a period before. A similar number of studies have found a reduction in the number of psychotropic and other drugs prescribed (Cohen 1977; Meacher 1977 (unpublished); Waydenfeld and Waydenfeld 1980). Other studies have indicated that there was a reduction in referrals to psychiatrists after a counselling attachment had been instigated (Corney 1992; Illman 1983).

However, proving that counselling is cost-effective is likely to be extremely difficult. Analyses of benefits and costs are extremely difficult to carry out. They should take into account and try to cost the greater sense of well-being of the individuals concerned after counselling and the effects on their families and their physical health. Normally, however, benefits are often only measured in terms of tangible outcomes, such as reduced prescriptions and fewer attendances. These costs may not be very great, particularly as psychotropic drugs are not expensive and most GP attendances are short. There might be only a few cases where the provision of counselling may reduce the use of more expensive treatment, such as referrals for inappropriate medical investigations or out-patient and in-patient treatment.

It is unlikely that by using these limited indices it can be shown that a counsellor is cost-effective in Great Britain, where medical costs in general are low in comparison with other countries such as the United States. In addition, counselling may not reduce time spent by GPs. If an attachment is to be successful, the reduction in GP time spent may only be minimal as doctors need to spend time discussing patients with the counsellor and possibly becoming involved in joint sessions. A counsellor in a practice may also encourage and stimulate others to do some 'counselling' themselves either after the surgery or by arranging a few longer appointment sessions. This will not normally decrease the doctor's workload. Because of these difficulties, practices should collect additional information regarding the quality of the service offered and clients' views in order to justify the value of the attachment rather than solely measuring the costs (see also Chapter 3).

Case-control studies

Some investigators have compared the progress of the counselled clients with a matched group of patients selected from the medical register. These can be useful for direct comparisons between the clients referred and the 'normal' population. However, the controls are usually only matched in terms of age and sex and not in terms of their psychosocial problems. This makes it difficult to compare outcome over time between the counselled groups and the controls.

An example of this type of study was carried out by Martin and Mitchell (1983). They compared the outcome of a group of 87 patients receiving counselling with a matched group of patients drawn from the age—sex register. They found no major differences in outcome between the two groups, although this was only measured in terms of attendance rate and psychotropic drug prescription. The controls were only matched according to their age and sex and not their social/psychological characteristics so it is difficult to draw conclusions from the results.

This group of investigators also studied whether having a counsellor in the practice had altered GP behaviour (Martin and Martin 1985). They tried to investigate this by examining medical notes over a period of time. The notes of 300 patients who had been continuously registered with the practice since 1974 were randomly drawn from the files. The number of psychosocial problems and the number of prescriptions for psychotropic drugs recorded in the years 1975, 1979, and 1982 were noted. They found that the number of patients who had had a psychiatric diagnosis recorded in their notes during one year fell between 1975 and 1982, the number of prescriptions for antidepressant drugs fell, but the prescriptions for tranquillizers and sleeping tablets rose substantially. They hypothesized that the change in psychotropic prescriptions could have been due to the doctor becoming more willing to consider psychogenic problems as being precipitated by stress rather than a biochemical change. The reduction in patients being given a psychiatric diagnosis could be due to early attention to patients' emotional needs preventing later breakdowns. The authors conclude, however, that no major changes were detected over the seven-year-period.

Clinical trials

In medicine, clinical trials are normally undertaken in order to evaluate whether a treatment works or not. In these trials, the outcome of one group of patients receiving the treatment is compared to the outcome of another group who either receive no treatment or treatment of another kind. Ideally, patients entering into clinical trials should be randomly allocated to the experimental group or the control group so that there are no initial differences between the two groups.

The need for a control group is crucial as high proportions of patients with depression and anxiety (those patients most likely to be referred to a counsellor) will get better and resolve their problems themselves without outside help. Patients will normally be referred to a counsellor at a point when their problems are most likely to be at their worst. This means that many patients are likely to show some improvement at a follow-up interview, even without treatment. To show that counselling is effective, we have to obtain even better rates of improvement in those receiving counselling than those receiving routine GP treatment. This makes it extremely difficult to prove statistically that counselling works except by conducting trials with fairly high numbers.

In addition to this major difficulty, the following problems need to be tackled by research workers attempting to conduct a clinical trial:

1. *Deciding on what constitutes improvement*
   Is it better physical or mental health, a reduction in family breakup, a reduction in psychotropic drug prescribing, or a reduction in GP consultations? Deciding on what constitutes improvement may involve a number of value judgements. For example, does effectiveness in marital therapy mean an improvement in the clients' physical and mental health or is it more important to keep clients' marriages together? Marriage guidance counselling may not reduce the number of marriage breakups for example. An effective marriage guidance counsellor may ease the process of a couple splitting up so that a woman trapped in a destructive marriage is given the support to start a new life for herself. Thus a favourable outcome for one client may differ considerably from what is regarded as a favourable outcome for another.

   In practice, most trials should include multiple assessments of health status, personal adjustment (for example self-esteem measures) and social adjustment (for example relationships). This is likely to lead to a fairer trial of counselling than focusing predominantly on health measures.

2. *Deciding when to carry out assessments of change*
   There are no hard and fast rules on this. Some patients may improve rapidly but then relapse; others may take longer but stay well. Some therapists argue that the mental health of clients may need to deteriorate (when first facing their problems) before they can get better. The best solution to this dilemma is to follow-up clients more than once, once shortly after cessation of counselling and again, at least once, at a later time.

3. Inadequate tools of assessment
   Are the tools developed sensitive or subtle enough to measure changes brought about by counselling? Previous studies of counselling have been criticized for using insensitive or inappropriate measures, and it is important that further developmental work is undertaken.

4. *Unlike clinical trials on drugs, no placebos are readily available*
   Patients can not be 'blind' to treatment. Usually the control group receives 'treatment as usual' or is allocated to a waiting list. It may be more appropriate to use a control treatment such as a befriender or an untrained listener spending similar amounts of time with the client.

5. *Motivation of subjects*
   Subjects may participate but lack motivation—this can be linked with the difficulties involved of matching counsellors with subjects. It is perhaps not a fair test of counselling if many of the patients referred to the counsellor are half-hearted about it or perhaps do not want to change their situation.

In addition, there are problems that are common to other types of clinical trials, such as getting the referrer to agree to a clinical trial when they are convinced counselling works, as well as the problems involved in getting an adequate sample (is the sample sufficiently large or representative of those with the particular illness/problem?). The last problem is usually the biggest headache for the researcher, who normally has a limited and set amount of time in which to carry out the study and usually has to be content with a smaller number of subjects than originally proposed.

Quality issues

GPs who wish to employ counsellors may find it difficult to know the standards of experience and training necessary for a counselling placement to succeed. Once the placement is set up, they might be unclear which patient should be referred to the trained (and probably more costly) counsellor and which ones can be referred to a befriender or a listening service (if available). One of the major difficulties for any researcher is the measurement of quality. How do we attempt to measure how good a counsellor is? Is the degree of experience important or the number of years of training, or both? Accreditation of counsellors using specific guidelines is an important step forward (see Chapter 4). However, most practitioners working in this area would also agree that the personal characteristics of a counsellor, which are almost impossible to define or measure, are also important. Some of these are well known, such as empathy, warmth, and genuineness (Traux and Carkhuff 1976), and researchers have developed scales to measure them.

It is perhaps in this area that much research still needs to be conducted. We urgently need to know which clients benefit most from expert help and which ones need less skilful handling. One clinical trial of health visitors who received minimal counselling training indicated that their help was beneficial to women suffering from postnatal depression (Holden *et al.* 1989). It seems likely that a highly trained counsellor not only needs to undertake individual work with clients, but also to work alongside other team members offering them support and help through 'case' discussions.

CONCLUSIONS

Evaluating the outcome of counselling is, therefore, no simple matter and there is a need to work hard at refining the techniques as well as using a variety of qualitative and quantitative methodologies. Collaborative efforts, where the work of practitioners and researchers builds upon that of others, are essential.

REFERENCES

Ashurst, P. M. and Ward, D. F. (1983). *An evaluation of counselling in general practice*. Final report of the Leverhulme Counselling Project. Report available from the Mental Health Foundation, London.

Anderson, S. and Hasler, J. (1979). Counselling in general practice. *Journal of the Royal College of General Practitioners*, **29**, 352–6.

Cohen, J. S. H. (1977). Marital counselling in general practice. *Proceedings of the Royal Society of Medicine*, **70**, 495–6.

Corney, R. (1992). Studies of the effectiveness of counselling in general practice. In *Counselling in general practice*, (ed. R. Corney and R. Jenkins). Routledge, London.

Gask, L., McGrath, G., Goldberg, D., and Miller, T. (1987). Improving the skills of established general practitioners: evaluation of group teaching. *Medical Education*, **21**, 362–8.

Holden, J. M., Sagovsky, R., and Cox, J. L. (1989). Counselling in a general practice setting: controlled study of health visitor intervention in treatment of postnatal depression. *British Medical Journal*, **298**, 223–6.

Illman, J. (1983). Is psychiatric referral good value for money? *British Medical Association*, **9**, 41–2.

Marsh, G. N. and Barr, J. (1975). Marriage guidance counselling in a group practice. *Journal of the Royal College of General Practitioners*, **25**, 73–5.

Martin, E. and Mitchell, H. (1983). A counsellor in general practice: a one-year survey. *Journal of the Royal College of General Practitioners*, **33**, 366–7.

Martin, E. and Martin, P. M. L. (1985). Changes in psychological diagnosis and prescription in a practice employing a counsellor. *Family Practice*, **2**, 241–3.

Meacher, M. (1977). *A pilot counselling scheme with general practitioners: summary report*. Mental Health Foundation, London. (Unpublished.)

Truax, C. B. and Carkhuff, R. R (1976). *Towards effective counselling and psychotherapy training and practice*. Aldine, Chicago.

Waydenfeld, D. and Waydenfeld, S. W. (1980). Counselling in general practice. *Journal of the Royal College of General Practitioners*, **30**, 671–7.

18 Conclusions

Jane Keithley and Geoffrey Marsh

Counselling is now firmly established as one of the range of services which is provided within primary health care, and nearly one-third of general practices have a counsellor. This book has offered a timely review of the major issues in the field. It should help those two-thirds of practices who do not have a counsellor to consider whether they should, as well as encouraging those who do provide this service to reflect on how its contribution to patient care can reach its full potential. This is particularly pertinent in the context of a health service increasingly conscious of the need to deploy resources efficiently, to audit the services provided, and to demonstrate 'value-for money'.

Our conclusions have not been easy to formulate. The philosophy, techniques, and outcomes of counselling are notoriously difficult to evaluate, particularly by means of the 'scientific' model most familiar to GPs. Our contributors have written from their individual perspectives and have not always reached the same conclusions. Indeed, it is unlikely that any one 'blueprint' would fit the variety found among primary health care teams and the different populations they serve.

However, in this final chapter, we aim to draw out and mull over the arguments and evidence presented by our contributors and to reach conclusions of our own regarding counselling in primary health care.

THE NATURE OF COUNSELLING

The growth in counselling and in counselling services is not confined to primary health care. It is symbolized, as Dammers and Wiener point out, by the British Association of Counselling's enrolment of its 10 000th member in May 1993. However, the precise nature of counselling has remained something of a mystery, encouraged by the strict rules of confidentiality surrounding hour-long sessions and the counsellors' own reluctance to be too specific about a 'talking cure' which is often founded on an explicitly non-directive approach.

Many of our contributors have shed light upon this mystery, often by examples of how counselling can help people with particular kinds of health problems. However, it is Tim Bond's chapter on the nature and outcomes of counselling which most directly addresses the question 'what is counselling?'. He clarifies the distinctions between counselling and advice, counselling and psychotherapy (although readers will note that Dammers and Wiener use the terms interchangeably), and counselling and counselling skills. However, he emphasizes that these are *different* ways of offering help and (unlike some proponents of the counselling movement) does not claim that counselling is always the most appropriate or best way of offering help. In particular, he argues that the use of counselling skills can be more skilled than counselling itself and is certainly not a 'lower order activity'. This is of clear relevance to the primary health care team, where a specifically counselling approach should not be seen as replacing, or being in opposition to more 'traditional' ways of responding to patients, such as the giving of advice. Most people approach their GP and other PHCT members seeking advice, and in many cases (probably a good majority) this is the most appropriate response. How far should counselling complement this? To answer this question we need to consider two issues: whether counselling is effective, and whether primary health care is an appropriate setting in which to provide it.

IS COUNSELLING EFFECTIVE AND COST-EFFECTIVE?

Questions of whether counselling works and whether resources should be devoted to counselling rather than other primary health care services must be central to the thinking of GPs. The first (frustrating) response is that it is difficult to tell because, as Corney's chapter makes evident, it is a complex matter to evaluate the outcomes of counselling. Evidence from this book, and from other studies, strongly suggests that counselling does work and we would concur; we have not unearthed irrefutable statistics, but the weight of anecdotal evidence is very considerable. Counsellors and GPs believe it to be a valuable therapeutic tool and a substantial proportion of clients report they have been helped. However, as Rowland and Tolley argue, whether counselling is cost-effective, or leads to measurably better health, or lower expenditure on other health services, is yet to be proved. To provide more evidence on the cost-effectiveness and value of counselling, especially in the new audit-aware environment in general practices, some teams, at least, should try to measure the value of the counsellor who works with them.

The net cost of the service depends on whether it is a substitute for more costly forms of care. There are suggestions that counsellors can save the GP's time; can provide an alternative and more efficacious source of support and help in making decisions for some people with seemingly intractable problems; and can reduce the need for psychotropic drugs. However, the cost of counselling can be quite high (despite counsellors' time being much cheaper than that of GPs) because of the length of each appointment. In addition, research has shown that in the case of the management of depression, psychotropic drugs, combined with brief appointments with a GP, can provide a relatively cheap alternative which seems to produce equally good clinical outcomes.

The impact on the workload of other PHCT members is uncertain. On the one hand, time undoubtedly needs to be devoted to making an attachment work. In addition, the provision of a counselling service could encourage people to seek help from the PHCT for a wider range of problems than before. Set against this, by encouraging people to take more responsibility for their problems and for tackling them and by helping them to clarify the nature of those problems, counselling could encourage patient independence and so lessen the PHCT's workload.

IS COUNSELLING AN APPROPRIATE PART OF PRIMARY HEALTH CARE?

It may well be impossible to demonstrate conclusively that counselling in primary health care saves money. However, this may not be its prime aim, and we are convinced by the enthusiasm and evidence of our contributors that it is a valuable and appropriate addition to primary health services. The chapter on 'The client's perspective' suggests that those who are referred see many advantages and few disadvantages in providing counselling in this setting—even when they personally did not feel counselling helped them.

Studies point to the large proportion of GP consultations which are related to psychological and interpersonal difficulties. An audit by one of us, in which up to four diagnoses could be listed in every consultation, found that 'depression' and 'anxiety state' were the second and third most frequent reasons for consultation, only exceeded by 'upper respiratory tract infection'. Other consultations are for health problems which may well have implications for psychological well-being (for example terminal physical illness). Our contributors also make the case that counselling can be of benefit to individuals with a very wide range of problems which are brought to the primary health care team. Many GPs reading this book—or merely glancing at the chapter titles—will be surprised at the scope and potential of counselling. For example, Street and Soldan's chapter on the need for counselling for those with chronic disease may well be an eye-opener to many GPs and nurses who, year in year out, care for slowly deteriorating patients with chronic respiratory disease, arthritis, neurological disease, and so on. Judicious referrals to a counsellor, particularly of those patients who appear to be most disaffected by their condition, will help more than fine-tuning physical or pharmaceutical treatments. Sharing the emotional burden of the care of patients who patently will never get better will lighten the load of the doctor and nurse. Nor must the needs of their carers go unanswered—'patient home, partner now at risk'.

Referrals to a counsellor are likely to be more appropriate and sensitive if he/she is part of the team. A counselling service which is part of a range of primary health care services, especially if it is provided from the same premises, is generally more acceptable and accessible to practice patients than one at a separate, specialist centre.

Following the pattern of other primary health care services the bulk of counselling care can probably be provided from within the team, especially if that team includes a trained counsellor. However, counselling expertise in the PHCT can also ensure appropriate and sensitive referrals to outside specialist services when necessary, as indicated for example in the chapters by Mason (substance misuse), Bond (HIV), and Jennings (fertility).

The response to the question of whether counselling is an appropriate part of primary health care is thus resoundingly positive. There remain, however, difficult questions to tackle relating to *how much* counselling should be provided in primary health care, what *priority* it should take, and *who* should deliver it. Keeping the lid on this particular Pandora's box requires a hard look at the priority which should be accorded to counselling as compared with other aspects of primary health care. For example, one could argue that, given the training and specific expertise of GPs, their first responsibility should be to diagnose and treat physical and defined psychiatric illness, with attention to psychosocial issues being seen as desirable, but a bonus. Maybe patients should be discouraged from seeing their doctor as a 'secular priest'? While accepting the dangers of creating a role for GPs and for other PHCT members which is all-encompassing, we do not share this view. We would support Campkin's argument that patients expect the PHCT to have a pastoral/listening role as well as a clinical one and that this expectation is justified, not least because of the difficulties and dangers of trying to impose clear distinctions between physical, psychiatric, and psychosocial ill-health.

THE VOLUME PROBLEM: COUNSELLING AS A 'BOTTOMLESS PIT'

It is abundantly clear from the range of contributions to this book that there is a huge potential pool of unmet demand for counselling services in primary health care. To provide a comprehensive service to all who may benefit from it would require a massive redeployment of health care resources. Many would argue that such a redeployment is unnecessary and untenable.

In addition, many of the problems faced by people consulting their GP are part of the life experiences which everyone can expect to face at some time: birth, death, ill-health, and difficult relationships. Most people can and do cope with these without counselling help, especially if they have support from and good communication with relatives, friends, and a familiar and sensitive PHCT (see, for example, the chapters by Thompson and

Poingdestre on bereavement and terminal illness). Assuming that everyone needs to be referred to a counsellor at these times not only has daunting resource implications, but could also be viewed as an unnecessary and undesirable extension of professional intervention into private lives.

Nurses, doctors, and others in primary health care thus have an important task in the filtering of demand, in the selection of individuals for whom counselling is likely to be of most help, and in ensuring appropriate and sensitive referral. Most caring GPs and nurses will determine who needs counselling by first offering the conventional support system of listening, time, patience, empathy, occasional medication and, where appropriate advice, using counselling skills. We would endorse this wholeheartedly. For the great majority of people it is what they are looking for, it works remarkably well and is extremely cost-effective. When it fails, counselling could well be of help.

Once individuals have reached the counsellor, there are resource issues relating to the duration of their counselling. A number of contributors point to the implications of providing long-term counselling even for a few clients, with sessions quickly blocked, waiting-lists lengthening, and access for other potential clients severely curtailed.

However, the ethos of general practice is of continuing care, sometimes involving long-term care. In this context it may be difficult to exclude long-term counselling. Thus Street and Soldan talk, for example, about counselling as being 'regularly about the struggle with chronicity'. At the very least it should be made clear to individuals that they can always return to the counsellor if they feel the need (although the counsellor is not as likely still to be there as the GP!)

WHO SHOULD COUNSEL?

It is useful here to return to the distinction between counselling and counselling skills. There is a consensus among our contributors that all members of the PHCT should acquire and utilize counselling skills to enhance their professional practice, within the confines of the ten minute (or less) consultation. Even in relation to the giving of advice, often seen as the opposite of counselling, Bond suggests that counselling skills can improve the quality of the communication between doctor and patient and thus of the help given. Yet we are extremely doubtful whether more than a tiny percentage of members of the PHCT (and GPs in particular) have had any formal training in counselling skills. The numbers of courses available are growing, but we still see a potential for considerable expansion in this area of teaching. By the same token these skills should be higher on the teaching agenda in schools of medicine and nursing.

It may well be that a team with a high level of counselling skills will seldom need to refer to specialist counsellors. When they do, their referrals are likely to be more appropriate, recognizing that for those whose problems are very complex and/or associated with psychological and interpersonal difficulties, counselling can play a very significant role.

To whom should individuals be referred? Should the role of counsellor be a separate one, involving a new member of the primary health care team, or could one of the existing team, such as a GP or a practice nurse, take this on?

It is evident from our contributors that in some practices, existing PHCT members have the interest and expertise to develop the role. Campkin argues cogently for a wider adoption of a 'counselling attitude' among GPs and describes (as does Freedman) how she has taken on a more formal counselling role in relation to some of her own patients. Forth stresses the significant counselling element in the work of CPNs with individuals suffering from defined mental health problems.

However, as Campkin herself points out, there are some difficulties associated with this counselling role, especially for GPs. Counselling, as many of our contributors emphasize, requires proper training, continuing and regular supervision, and a great deal of time. It is likely that for most GPs, this would be seen as in conflict with their primary role as clinicians and the need to keep their clinical knowledge and skills well honed. There can be no worse scenario than a GP endlessly counselling a lethargic, depressed, overweight patient and failing to diagnose her thyroid deficiency. Furthermore, many may feel a hesitation in embarking on counselling their own patients, given the likelihood of a continuing relationship with them and probably with their families.

We would thus suggest that for most PHCTs, the preferred option would be to have a separate, specialist counsellor in the practice. How can they set about finding the right person for this job?

ENSURING THE QUALITY OF COUNSELLING

Well-established professions such as medicine and nursing have similarly well-established and recognized systems of training and accreditation, which ensure at least a baseline level of competence. This is not so with counselling. The rapid expansion of counselling has been accompanied by the proliferation of counselling courses, but, as Cocksedge and Ball point out, these vary enormously in content, duration, and level. Moreover, anyone can describe themselves as a counsellor without having attended even the briefest of courses.

This lack of regulation of counselling activities seems to reflect a view that anyone can 'counsel' and that counselling cannot do any harm, thus its practitioners do not need the same kind of scrutiny and accreditation as other professionals. We hope that these views have been dispelled by our contributors, who have demonstrated both that the task demands considerable skill and high ethical standards and also that those who receive counselling are often very unhappy and vulnerable individuals, whose interests must be safeguarded.

Cocksedge and Ball outline the current situation relating to training and accreditation and suggest ways forward at a national and local level. There are some sources of guidance for GPs (including, in some parts of the country, the FHSA). In employing a counsellor, GPs should scrutinize the training undertaken, ensure that the counsellor has sufficient, continuing professional support, and make use of the guidelines produced by the Counselling in Primary Care Trust and by the British Association for Counselling, which is developing accreditation for courses and for individual counsellors.

THE INTEGRATION OF COUNSELLORS INTO THE PHCT

Acknowledgement of the significant psychological element in many of the problems brought to the PHCT, of the value of counselling to some patients with these problems, and of the need for careful selection of the counsellor do not constitute in themselves a sufficient basis for setting up a successful service in primary health care. We would refer our readers to a number of chapters, particularly those by Dammers and Wiener, Irving, and Graham for discussion of the issues to be resolved. There must be a clear agreement between the counsellor and the practice about the job description, hours of work, accommodation, and remuneration. Mechanisms for the auditing and simple monitoring of the service must be agreed and in place. All the members of the PHCT, including the counsellor, need to be clear about the nature, meaning, and boundaries of confidentiality; the process of referral; how good communication is to be ensured between the counsellor and other team members; and the scope of the counsellor's role. For example, as well as a role in counselling individual patients, has he/she a part to play in facilitating the staff to work together as a team, or in supporting individual team members who are under stress?

To return to an assertion at the beginning of this chapter, it is unlikely that any one 'blueprint' for a counselling service will fit all practices, with their variety of needs, skills, and circumstances. This book, however, should help practices to work out their own model, by drawing on the expertise and experience of others to highlight opportunities, to avoid some pitfalls, and to ensure counselling plays its part in contributing to patient care.

Index